Essentials of Clinical Geriatrics

Essentials of Clinical Geriatrics

Second Edition

Robert L. Kane, M.D.

Professor and Dean
School of Public Health
University of Minnesota
Minneapolis, Minnesota

Joseph G. Ouslander, M.D.

Medical Director, Jewish Homes for the Aging
of Greater Los Angeles
Multicampus Division of Geriatric Medicine
UCLA School of Medicine
Los Angeles, California

Itamar B. Abrass, M.D.

Professor and Head, Division of Gerontology
and Geriatric Medicine
University of Washington
Seattle, Washington

McGraw-Hill Information Services Company
HEALTH PROFESSIONS DIVISION

New York   St. Louis   San Francisco   Colorado Springs
Auckland   Bogotá   Caracas   Hamburg   Lisbon   London
Madrid   Mexico   Milan   Montreal   New Delhi   Panama   Paris
San Juan   São Paulo   Singapore   Sydney   Tokyo   Toronto

ESSENTIALS OF CLINICAL GERIATRICS
Second Edition

34567890   DOCDOC   943210

ISBN 0-07-051968-4

This book was set in Times Roman by Science Press.
The editors were Avé McCracken and Muza Navrozov;
the production supervisor was Elaine Gardenier;
the cover was designed by Edward R. Schultheis.
R. R. Donnelley & Sons Company was printer and binder.

Library of Congress Cataloging-in-Publication Data

Kane, Robert L., date
  Essentials of clinical geriatrics.

  Includes bibliographies and index.
  1. Geriatrics.   I. Ouslander, Joseph G.
II. Abrass, Itamar B.   III. Title.   [DNLM: 1. Aging.
2. Geriatrics.   WT 100 K16e]
RC952.K36   1989   618.97   88-8334
ISBN 0-07-051968-4

Contents

PART ONE: THE AGING PATIENT AND GERIATRIC ASSESSMENT

PART TWO: DIFFERENTIAL
DIAGNOSIS AND MANAGEMENT

PART THREE: GENERAL MANAGEMENT STRATEGIES

APPENDIX: SUGGESTED GERIATRIC MEDICAL FORMS

List of Tables and Figures

CHAPTER 3

CHAPTER 4

CHAPTER 9

CHAPTER 15

CHAPTER 16

CHAPTER 17

Preface to Second Edition

Essentials of Clinical Geriatrics was intended for a diverse audience of primary care givers. The response to the first edition suggested that we had achieved that goal. We were pleasantly surprised to discover that a number of nonclinical persons interested in the health of older persons also found the book useful. At the same time, we appreciated the comments and suggestions for modifications that many readers generously offered. We have diligently tried to incorporate these into the second edition. This new edition represents a major overhaul of the original edition. Not only have we updated the information, but we have also substantially expanded the supporting material with more figures, tables, and references. We have revised the clinical forms, in addition to the text itself. Two new chapters have been added on topics readers said they wanted information on: the role of the physician in the nursing home and ethical dilemmas.

In the few years since the first edition, geriatrics has grown enormously. Today geriatrics has become more generally recognized as part of the health sciences, with a special certifying examination in several disciplines. Major efforts have been developed to train health care professionals at various levels in the skills needed to improve their care of older patients. There is much more information available, and many more people are interested in using it. We have tried to incorporate this growth in knowledge and to keep constantly in mind the diverse nature of the clinical community caring for older persons.

We continue to view this edition as a book to be used in practice. We have tried to make the information practical, accessible, and useful. It is not designed to replace the more extensive textbook on geriatrics, but rather to be kept as a quick and easy reference and an introduction to stimulate more careful attention to the multiple and complex problems of managing older patients. We believe that much of the battle can be won if the clinician is assisted to organize the large volume of information collected and to approach the multiple problems systematically. We hope that this book, with its focus on problems and problem-solving, will be of some assistance in that important work.

Since the first edition, the authors have each changed jobs. Robert Kane is now Dean of the School of Public Health at the University of Minnesota and Professor of Public Health and Medicine there. Joseph Ouslander is Medical Director of the Jewish Homes for the Aging of Greater Los Angeles and Assistant Professor in the Multicampus Division of Geriatric Medicine in the UCLA School of Medicine. Itamar Abrass is Professor of Medicine and Head, Division of Gerontology and Geriatric Medicine at the University of Washington School of Medicine.

Preface to First Edition

Essentials of Clinical Geriatrics is intended as a practical guide for primary care physicians and other practitioners who provide care to elderly persons. The text presupposes a basic knowledge of medicine. Emphasis is given to those aspects of care that are *different* when treating the elderly. We have deliberately *not* written a handbook of geriatrics. Pathophysiology and basic gerontological research have been held to a minimum in order to emphasize practical information. For those interested in reading more about a subject, we have provided suggested readings at the end of each chapter.

The volume is organized into three parts. The first (Chapters 1 through 3) addresses the medical differences associated with the aging patient and how these are translated into approaches to geriatric assessment. Part 2 (Chapters 4 through 12) uses a problem-based format to discuss the differential diagnosis and management of common problems (and some unique problems) of the elderly. Part 3 (Chapters 13 through 16) deals with general management strategies appropriate to elderly patients.

The Appendix is a set of medical forms to assist practitioners in collecting organized information on geriatric patients. These forms include a basic history and physical assessment, environmental and social assessments, medical records, and specific forms for evaluating dementia, incontinence, and falls.

A number of people have assisted us in preparing *Essentials of Clinical Geriatrics*. Douglas Noffsinger, Alan Robbins, Larry Rubenstein, Richard Weisbart, and Tom Yoshikawa generously shared their materials on relevant areas. Several individuals provided critical reviews of earlier drafts: Chris Foote, Lissy Jarvik, Gabor Jilly, Cindy Layden, Ed Liston, Jim Moore, Jane Murray, Shlomo Raz, Alan Robbins, and Gary Small. We thank everyone who helped, but take full responsibility for the final product.

Dr. Kane is supported by a National Institute on Aging Geriatric Medicine Academic Award; Dr. Ouslander, by a National Institute on Aging Geriatric Academic Award; and Dr. Abrass, by the Geriatric Research, Education and Clinical Center at the Sepulveda Veterans Administration Medical Center.

Part One

The Aging Patient and Geriatric Assessment

Chapter 1

Clinical Implications of the Aging Process

The care of elderly patients differs from that of younger patients for a number of reasons. Some of these can be traced to the changes that occur in the process of aging, some are caused by the plethora of diseases and disruptions that accompany seniority, and still others result from the way old people are treated.

Perhaps one of the most intriguing challenges in medicine is to unravel the process of aging. Although we may be able to see pure aging in a cellular culture, it is very hard to visualize in the intact organism. Discussions about aging seem to imply accumulation of chronic diseases. How then does one separate the changes caused solely by aging from the sequelae of disease? Would a group of disease-free older persons be the appropriate models to help us understand the aging process? The prospect sounds uncomfortably like describing life on the basis of a colony of germ-free mice.

Nonetheless, the distinction between so-called normal aging and pathological changes is critical to the care of elderly people. We wish

3

to avoid both dismissing treatable pathology as simply a concomitant of old age and treating natural aging processes as though they were diseases. The latter is particularly dangerous because the elderly are so vulnerable to iatrogenic effects. A frequently quoted story captures the dilemma: A 102-year-old man complained to his physician about pain in his right knee. The physician dismissed it. "What can you expect at 102?" But the patient retorted, "My left knee is 102 years old, too, and it doesn't hurt" (Butler, 1975, p. 182).

There is growing appreciation that everyone does not age in the same way or at the same rate. The changing composition of today's elderly compared to a generation ago may actually reflect a bimodal shift wherein there are both more disabled people and more healthy older people. Attention has become focused on the variations in aging, with great interest directed toward those described as aging successfully, that is, showing the least decline in function with time (Rowe and Kahn, 1987).

CHANGES ASSOCIATED WITH "NORMAL" AGING

We have already noted the critical and difficult distinction a clinician must make to attribute a finding as either part of the expected course of aging or the result of pathological changes. This distinction perplexes the researcher as well. We currently lack precise knowledge of what constitutes normal aging. Much of our information comes from cross-sectional studies, which compare findings from a group of younger persons with those from a group of older individuals. Such data may reflect differences other than simply the effects of age. The older group grew up in a different environment, perhaps with different diet and activities. They represent a cohort of survivors. We have come to appreciate that what we see in the elderly patient is largely a result of what is brought to old age. For example, the decrease in the frequency of osteoporosis today has been related to the observation that women entering the high-risk period (postmenopause) have stronger bones with thicker cortex.

Many of the changes associated with aging result from gradual loss. These losses may often begin in early adulthood, but, thanks to the redundancy of most organ systems, the decrement does not

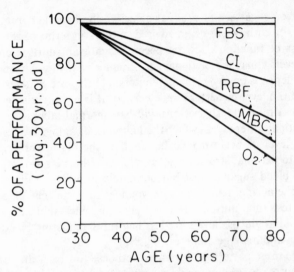

Figure 1-1 Schematic linear projections of physiological function decrements in males. Mean values for 20- to 35-year-old subjects are taken as 100 percent. FBS = fasting blood glucose; CI = resting cardiac index; RBF = renal blood flow; MBC = maximum breathing capacity; O_2 = maximum oxygen uptake. (*After Shock, 1977.*)

become functionally significant until the loss is fairly extensive. Figure 1-1, taken from one of the best-established studies on aging, describes this prevalent pattern. One might generalize to the "1 percent rule." Most organ systems seem to lose function at roughly 1 percent a year beginning around age 30.

These original data were developed from cross-sectional comparisons of groups at different ages (Andres and Tobin, 1977). More recent data (Svanborg, Bergstrom, and Mellstrom, 1982) suggest that the changes in the same people followed longitudinally are much less dramatic and certainly begin well after age 70.

In some organ systems, such as the kidney, a subgroup of persons appear to experience gradually declining function over time, whereas others' function remains constant (Lindeman, Tobin, and Shock, 1985). If these newer findings are substantiated, the earlier theory of gradual loss must be reassessed as reflecting disease rather than aging.

Given a pattern of gradual deterioration, whether from aging, disease, or both, we are best advised to think in terms of thresholds. The loss of function does not become significant until it crosses a given level. Thus the functional performance of an organ in an elderly person depends on two principal factors: (1) the rate of deterioration and (2) the level of performance needed. It is not surprising then to learn that most elderly persons will have normal laboratory values. The critical difference, in fact the hallmark of aging, lies not in the resting level of performance but in how the organ (or organism) adapts to external stress. For example, an older person may show a normal blood sugar at rest but be unable to handle a glucose load within the normal parameters for younger subjects. The glucose tolerance test thus must be reinterpreted for older subjects, and 2-h postprandial glucose levels are less helpful than fasting blood sugars to detect and manage diabetes.

The same pattern of decreased response to stress can be seen in the performance of other endocrine systems or the cardiovascular system. A patient may have a normal resting pulse but be unable to achieve an adequate increase in cardiac output with exercise.

Sometimes the changes of aging work together to produce apparently normal resting values in other ways. For example, although both glomerular filtration and renal blood flow decrease with age, many elderly persons have normal serum creatinine levels because of the concomitant decreases in lean muscle mass and creatinine production. Thus serum creatinine is not as good an indicator of renal function in the elderly as in younger persons. Because knowledge of kidney function is so critical in drug therapy, it is important to get some measure of this parameter. A useful formula for estimating creatinine clearance on the basis of serum creatinine values in the elderly has been developed (Cockcroft and Gault, 1976). (The actual formula is provided in Chapter 14.)

Table 1-1 summarizes some of the pertinent changes that occur with aging. For many items, the changes begin in adulthood and proceed gradually; others may not manifest themselves until well into seniority. Readers interested in more detailed discussion of the changes associated with aging should consult the several excellent reviews on the subject from which this table was derived (Birren and Schaie, 1985; Finch and Schneider, 1985).

Table 1-1   Changes Associated with Aging

Item	Morphology	Function
Overall	Decreased height (stooped posture secondary to increased kyphosis) Decreased weight Increased fat-to-lean-body-mass ratio Decreased total body water	
Skin	Increased wrinkling Atrophy of sweat glands	
Cardiovascular system	Elongation and tortuosity of arteries, including aorta Increased intimal thickening of arteries Increased fibrosis of media of arteries Decreased rate of cardiac hypertrophy Sclerosis of heart valves	Decreased cardiac output Decreased heart rate response to stress Decreased compliance of peripheral blood vessels
Kidney	Increased number of abnormal glomeruli	Decreased creatinine clearance Decreased renal blood flow Decreased maximum urine osmolality
Lung	Decreased elasticity Decreased cilia activity	Decreased vital capacity Decreased maximal oxygen uptake Decreased cough reflex
Gastrointestinal tract	Decreased hydrochloric acid Decreased saliva flow Fewer taste buds	
Skeleton	Osteoarthritis Loss of bone substance	
Eyes	Arcus senilis Decreased pupil size Growth of lens	Decreased accommodation Hyperopia Decreased acuity Decreased color sensitivity Decreased depth perception

Table 1-1   Changes Associated with Aging *(Continued)*

Item	Morphology	Function
Hearing	Degenerative changes of ossicles Increased obstruction of eustachian tube Atrophy of external auditory meatus Atrophy of cochlear hair cells Loss of auditory neurons	Decreased perception in high frequencies Decreased pitch discrimination
Immune system		Decreased T-cell activity
Nervous system	Decreased brain weight Decreased cortical cell count	Increased motor response time Slower psychomotor performance Decreased intellectual performance Decreased complex learning Decreased hours of sleep Decreased hours of REM sleep
Endocrine	Decreased triiodothyronine (T_3) Decreased free (unbound) testosterone Increased insulin Increased norepinephrine Increased parathormone Increased vasopressin	

THEORIES OF AGING

Death from old age generally occurs only in humans and protected animals. Animals in the wild are usually killed or die from environmental causes before they have marked physiological decrements. There is no survival value for species for a life span beyond reproductive maturation. In considering the genetic influence on aging, then, it is not surprising that factors of immortality have not been selected for and that advantages in development may be liabilities for longevity.

More than 20 years ago, Moorhead and Hayflick found that cultured normal human embryonic fibroblasts underwent a finite number (about 50) of population doublings and then died. A finite proliferative capacity has now been demonstrated for a host of other normal cell types and is accepted as a general phenomenon (Hayflick, 1979).

Not only do embryonic cells have a limited number of population doublings, but there is also an inverse relationship between the age of the human donor and the in vitro proliferative capacity. This phenomenon is determined by nuclear factors because nuclear-cytoplasmic fusions between old and young cells demonstrate that the fused cells behave as the cell from which the nucleus has been derived. Limited replication is not confined to in vitro conditions. Serial transplantation of normal somatic tissue to new, young inbred hosts indicates that normal cells do not survive indefinitely.

The possibility that animals age because one or more important cell populations lose their proliferative capacity is unlikely. Other functional losses occur in cells prior to the cessation of mitotic capacity and produce physiological decrements much before their normal cells have reached their maximum proliferative capacity.

Major theories of aging are summarized in Table 1-2. Two major mechanisms are currently proposed as the basis of cellular aging. One concept is based on genetic instability. The second involves damage to the cell from internal or external factors. Both mechanisms probably contribute to the final process of aging.

Genetic instability might include the progressive accumulation of faulty copying in dividing cells or the accumulation of errors in

Table 1-2   Major Theories on Aging

Theory	Mechanisms	Manifestations
Cellular	Genetic instability	Copying errors
	Cellular damage	"Wear and tear"
		Toxins
Autoimmune	Genetic	Cell-mediated immunity
	Environmental	Autoimmune disease
	Endocrine	Malignancy
Neuroendocrine	Neural/endocrine control of gene activity	Multiple end-organ effects

information-containing molecules. The progressive accumulation of errors in the transcription functions could act to initiate secondary changes, which would ultimately be manifest as biological aging.

Damage to the cell from external or internal factors may lead to "wear and tear." Simple effects of use may also potentiate the aging process. Collagen and elastin are relatively inactive metabolically. Continuous extensions and relaxation of these fibers may lead to progressive degeneration.

Cells themselves produce toxins whose cumulative effects over a lifetime may promote the aging process. Free radicals of oxygen arise from a number of reactions within cells. They are highly reactive and can alter most cellular molecules.

An immunologic theory of aging proposes that aging is not primarily a process of passive wearing out of systems but of active self-destruction mediated by the immune system. Whether the immunologic changes are genetically determined (as might be suggested by an association of the major histocompatibility locus with life span), regulated by environmental factors (as suggested by modulation of the immune response by diet), or influenced by endocrine factors (as suggested by thymic hormone replacement) remains to be defined. All three factors probably have a role.

The neuroendocrine theory of aging suggests that neural and endocrine changes may be pacemakers for many cellular and physiological aspects of aging. Changes in gene activity under neural or endocrine control may lead to a spectrum of diseases involving immune function, proliferative changes in arterial walls, malignant growths, and other conditions, which currently set the maximum longevity in mammals.

Despite a host of extrinsic and intrinsic factors that affect life span, the most prominent role in the aging process is that of genetic function. The only way cells can be given immortality is by introduction of a change into the cell genome. Interventions into modifying intrinsic and extrinsic factors will only allow the biological "clock" to run to its full allotted time.

CLINICAL IMPLICATIONS

As we try to understand aging, we appreciate the limitations of available information. As noted earlier, most of the data cited to document changes with age come from cross-sectional studies in which individuals of different ages are compared in terms of group averages. Such an approach generally reveals a gradual decline in organ function with age, beginning in early middle life. A few studies have followed cohorts of people longitudinally as they age. Their conclusions are quite different. In several parameters, performance actually increases with age. For example, cognitive function can improve over time among older persons (Schaie, 1970). Similarly, cardiac function in subjects free of heart disease does not show inevitable decline with age (Gerstenblith, Weisfeldt, and Lakatta, 1985).

The physician must be able to take data derived from group studies and apply them to the individual. It is essential to keep in mind the principle of individual variation. The best predictor of a given patient's performance now is that person's earlier performance rather than an average age-related decline that has been documented in cross-sectional studies. Thus, an 80-year-old runner may well have better cardiovascular function than a 50-year-old sedentary doctor.

Aging is not simply a series of biological changes. That point when we look in the mirror and confront an old person is associated with a variety of alterations in life. Aging is a time of losses: loss of social role (usually through retirement), loss of income, loss of friends and relatives (through death and mobility). It can also be a time of fear: fear for personal safety, fear of financial insecurity, fear of dependency.

In the face of these enormous threats, we should pause to rethink our views about the elderly. Rather than the victims, they are the survivors. Most elderly persons have developed mechanisms to cope with multiple limitations. Most continue to function despite these forces. The physician's role is to enhance this coping ability by identifying and treating remediable problems and by facilitating changes in the environment to maximize function in the face of those problems that remain.

In some instances, the patient's coping skills may make the physician's task more difficult. The elderly patient has often adapted to problems by denying or ignoring them. In such cases, it will be difficult to obtain a good history. Other patients cope with their disabilities by employing adaptive techniques. For example, a person who is hard of hearing may talk a great deal to hide a hearing deficit. A particularly troublesome problem is the skillful compensation for cognitive losses. At least once in every physician's career, he or she will encounter a patient who carries on a perfectly lucid conversation only to discover on closer examination that the patient is completely disoriented to time, place, and person. Because it is easy to miss these cognitive deficits, we recommend that an evaluation of older persons include a formal screening for mental status. A simple method for doing this is described in Chapter 3.

The physician's role is thus a delicate one. The physician must remove barriers erected by coping mechanisms but be equally attentive to restoring and reinforcing those coping skills that enhance functioning.

Coping is not the only factor that complicates getting reliable information from geriatric patients. At the most tangible level, we must first be sure that communication has truly been established. Patients with hearing impairments or severe vision problems may not be receiving the questions and messages we are sending. If they are accustomed to dealing with this deficit by giving ready answers that do not necessarily respond to the questions posed, no useful information is exchanged. It is often helpful to check communication early in the interview by asking the patient to repeat what you have said.

The problems of the geriatric patient may present quite differently from younger patients. Because of the increased prevalence of chronic disease, the presenting problem may not be as distinct as with a younger patient, who is typically well until the onset of a new symptom complex. With an elderly patient, the new problem is generally superimposed on a background of already existing signs and symptoms. The onset may be less clear, the manifestations less precise. In addition, we need to recall that many symptoms and signs are not produced by the disease itself but by the body's response to that insult. One of the hallmarks of aging is the reduced response to stress, including the stress of disease. Thus, the symptom intensity may be dampened by the aged body's decreased responsiveness. The presentation of illness in the geriatric patient can be thought of as a combination of dampened primary sound in the presence of background noise.

When treating the elderly, it is useful to keep in mind that an individual's ability to function depends on a combination of characteristics of the individual (e.g., innate capacity, motivation, pain tolerance) and the setting in which that person is expected to function. The same individual may be functional in one setting and dependent in another. The physician's first responsibility is to treat the patient, to remedy the remediable by searching for and dealing with those conditions that are treatable. Having improved the patient's ability (physiologically and psychologically) as much as possible, the physician's next task is to structure an environment that will facilitate the patient's functioning with maximum autonomy. This latter mandate should not rest exclusively on the doctor's shoulders. A variety of health-related professionals are available in most situations to play major roles in locating and utilizing supportive environments. But the physician must not abrogate this task. To ignore the environment of a disabled individual is tantamount to prescribing drugs and ignoring the patient's compliance with the treatment regimen.

Conversely, the environment can produce dysfunction. At the simplest level, it may produce hazards that lead to falls (see Chapter 7). At a more subtle level, it may require a level of effort that produces decompensation. For example, an elderly person with dyspnea on exertion may get along reasonably well in a ground-floor apartment but become unmanageable in an apartment on the second floor of a building with no elevator. Similarly, patients with compromised pulmonary or cardiac function will show increased morbidity and mortality as air pollution levels increase. Finally, the environment may create disability by fostering dependency. This iatrogenic effect is discussed in Chapter 13.

At a somewhat more subtle level, physicians must be aware of the forces among care givers that foster dependency. Patients may be immobile because of the care they get. One important factor is risk aversion. Nursing personnel may be reluctant to mobilize patients for fear they will fall and sustain injuries. We must provide assurance to staff that they will not be penalized for appropriately activating patients. Nor is risk aversion confined to professionals. Families may be equally protective, insisting on limiting an older relative's activities or moving him or her to a more closely supervised situation. Such fears are often infused with guilt and may manifest as anger. Families can be helped to see the dangers of such restricted activity.

CLASSIFYING GERIATRIC PROBLEMS

Because diagnoses often do not tell the whole story in geriatrics, it is more helpful to think in terms of presenting problems. One aid to recalling some of the common problems of geriatrics uses a series of I's:

- Immobility
- Instability
- Incontinence
- Intellectual impairment
- Infection
- Impairment of vision and hearing
- Irritable colon
- Isolation (depression)
- Inanition (malnutrition)
- Impecunity
- Iatrogenesis
- Insomnia
- Immune deficiency
- Impotence

The list is important for several reasons. Especially with older patients, the expression of the problem may not be a good clue to the etiology. Conversely, a problem may occur for a variety of diverse reasons. For example, an individual may be immobilized by a broken hip, by severe angina, or by arthritis. But the patient may also be immobilized by fear. The elderly patient with a successfully repaired hip fracture may be unwilling to walk again for fear of falling and sustaining another fracture. An elderly person living in a deteriorated neighborhood may be confined to the home, not by physical limitations, but because of a fear of being molested. Such an individual may decide to enter a long-term-care institution to seek a safer environment. In each instance, the physician and co-workers must obtain a sufficient history to understand the true etiology of the problem if they are to develop a successful approach to remedying the condition.

Another factor in generating dependency is cost. It is often much easier and cheaper to do things *for* people with functional limitations than to invest the effort needed to encourage them to do for themselves. Unfortunately such savings are short-ranged; they will increase the level of dependency and ultimately the amount of care needed.

Among the list of I's, we have included iatrogenesis (Chapter 13). The least desirable outcome of medical care is to decrease the patient's health as a result of contact with the care system. In some cases, there is a real risk that untoward consequences of treatment may worsen a patient's health. The risk-benefit calculation as a basis for urging intervention must be performed carefully for each elderly patient in the context of his or her condition. Many risks are within the ordinary bounds of medicine.

We are concerned here with those events that result from indifferent or superficial care. The physician who casually adds another drug to the patient's polypharmacy portfolio is playing with a living chemistry set. The reduced rate of drug metabolism and excretion in many elderly persons exacerbates the problem of drug interactions (Chapter 14). Even more dangerous is the careless, hasty application of clinical labels. The patient who becomes confused and disoriented in the hospital may not be suffering from dementia. The individual who has an occasional urinary accident is not necessarily incontinent. Labeling patients as demented or incontinent is too often the first step toward entering the nursing home, a setting that can make such labels self-fulfilling prophecies. We must exercise great caution in applying such potent labels. They should be reserved for patients who have been carefully evaluated, lest we unnecessarily condemn such persons to a lifetime of institutionalization.

DIAGNOSIS VERSUS FUNCTIONAL STATUS

One of the persistent problems surrounding the growing discussions about the care of the elderly has arisen from the emphasis on functioning. This emphasis on the need to direct clinical attention to the patient's functional status as well as to specific medical conditions has been occasionally misinterpreted. The point is not that functional status is more important or more useful than diagnosis but that both are needed. One is incomplete without the other. Functioning is the result of the innate ability of the patient and the environment that supports those abilities.

Clearly the most desirable management of an elderly patient is to identify a correctable problem and correct it. The first and principal task of the physician is to do precisely that. No amount of rehabilitation, compassionate care, or environmental manipulation will compensate for missing a remediable diagnosis. However, diagnoses alone are usually insufficient. The elderly are the repositories of chronic disease more often cared for than cured.

The process of geriatrics is thus twofold: (1) careful clinical assessment and management to identify remediable problems and (2) equally careful and competent functional assessment to ascertain how the patient autonomy can be maximized by appropriate human and mechanical assistance and environmental manipulations.

Our goal in orienting primary-care providers is to raise their consciousness about the need to consider the whole patient and his or her environment, but never at the cost of neglecting the search for correctable causes for the patient's problems. In that search for causes, the a priori probabilities will often differ substantially from those of younger patients. For this reason, a problem-focused approach, like the I's, may prove useful.

REFERENCES

Andres R, Tobin JD: Endocrine systems, in Finch CE, Hayflick L (eds): *Handbook of the Biology of Aging.* New York, Van Nostrand Reinhold, 1977.

Birren J, Schaie W (eds): *Handbook of the Psychology of Aging* (2d ed). New York, Van Nostrand Reinhold, 1985.

Butler R: *Why Survive? Being Old in America.* New York, Harper & Row, 1975.

Cockcroft DW, Gault MH: Prediction of creatinine clearance from serum creatinine. *Nephron* 16:31–41, 1976.

Finch C, Schneider E (eds): *Handbook of the Biology of Aging* (2nd ed). New York, Van Nostrand Reinhold, 1985.

Gerstenblith G, Weisfeldt ML, Lakatta EG: Disorders of the heart, in Andres R, Bierman EL, Hazzard WR (eds): *Principles of Geriatric Medicine.* New York, McGraw-Hill, 1985.

Hayflick L: Cell biology of aging. *Fed Proc* 38:1847–1850, 1979.

Lindeman RD, Tobin J, Shock NW: Longitudinal studies on the rate of decline in renal function with age. *J Am Geriatr Soc* 33:278–285, 1985.

Rowe JW, Kahn RL: Human aging: Usual and successful. *Science* 237:143–149, 1987.

Schaie KW: A reinterpretation of age-related changes in cognitive structure and functioning, in Goulet LR, Baltes PB (eds): *Life-Span Developmental Psychology: Research and Theory*. New York, Academic Press, 1970.

Shock NW: System integration, in Finch CE, Hayflick L (eds): *Handbook of the Biology of Aging*. New York, Van Nostrand Reinhold, 1977.

Svanborg A, Bergstrom G, Mellstrom D: *Epidemiological Studies on Social and Medical Conditions of the Elderly*. Copenhagen, World Health Organization, 1982.

SUGGESTED READINGS

Binstock RH, Shanas E (eds): *Handbook of Aging and the Social Sciences* (2d ed). New York, Van Nostrand Reinhold, 1985.

Finch CE: The regulation of physiological changes during mammalian aging. *Q Rev Biol* 51:49–83, 1976.

Fries JF, Crapo LM: *Vitality and Aging*. San Francisco, Freeman, 1981.

Haynes SG, Feinleib M: *Second Conference on the Epidemiology of Aging*. U.S. Government Printing Office, 1980.

Portnoi VA: Diagnostic dilemma of the aged. *Arch Intern Med* 141:734–737, 1981.

Rowe JW: Clinical research on aging: Strategies and directions. *N Engl J Med* 297:1332–1336, 1977.

Scoggin GH: The cellular biochemical and genetic basis of aging, in Schrier RW (ed): *Clinical Internal Medicine in the Aged*. Philadelphia, Saunders, 1982.

Shock NW: The physiology of aging. *Sci Am* 206:100–110, 1962.

Shock NW, Greulich RC, Andres R et al: *Normal Human Aging: The Baltimore Longitudinal Study of Aging*. NIH Publ. No. 84-2450. Washington, DC, U.S. Government Printing Office, 1984.

Weindruch RH, Kristie JW, Cheney KE, et al: Influence of controlled dietary restriction on immunologic function and aging. *Fed Proc* 38:2007–2016, 1979.

Williams TF, Hill JG, Fairbank ME, Knox KG: Appropriate placement of the chronically ill and aged: A successful approach by evaluation. *JAMA* 226:1332–1335, 1973.

Chapter 2

The Elderly Patient: Demography and Epidemiology

From the physician's perspective, the demographic curve strongly argues that medical practice in the future will entail a great deal of geriatrics. Persons aged 65 and older currently represent a little over a third of the patients seen by a primary-care physician. In the next century, we can safely predict that at least every other adult patient will be an elderly person.

The concern so often heard about the epidemic of aging stems primarily from two factors: numbers and dollars. We hear a great deal of talk about the incipient demise of Social Security, the bankrupt status of Medicare, the death of the family, and dire predictions of demographic cataclysms. There is indeed cause for concern, but not necessarily for alarm. The message of the numbers is straightforward: We cannot go on as we have; new approaches are needed. The shape of those approaches to meeting the needs of growing numbers of elderly persons in this society will reflect societal values.

GROWTH IN NUMBERS

A few trends will help focus the problem. The numbers of elderly in this country (and in the world) have been growing in both absolute and relative terms, and they are going to continue increasing through the first half of the next century as a result of the post-World War II baby boom. That group of people, born in the late forties and early fifties, will not reach seniority until 2010, at the earliest. Figure 2-1 describes the growth in the age 65+ sector of the population. Not

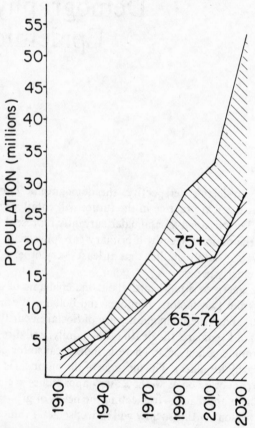

Figure 2-1   Growth in population age 65 and over.

Table 2-1   The Elderly in the United States: Trends

Age	Percent of total population						
	1910	1940	1970	1980	1990	2010	2030
65+	4.3	6.8	9.9	11.3	12.3	12.6	18.3
65–74	3.0	4.8	6.1	6.9	7.3	7.1	10.6
75+	1.3	2.0	3.8	4.4	5.0	5.5	7.7

Note: Future dates assume (1) a fertility level of 2.1 children born per woman and (2) that mortality rates decrease at a rate whereby life expectancy at birth increases by about 0.05 percent per year.
Source: After Kane et al., 1981.

only is this group increasing, but more of the growth is occurring in those over age 75. The impact of this projection can be better appreciated by looking at Table 2-1, which expresses the growth as a percentage of the total population. Although these forecasts can vary with the future birth rate and death rate, they are likely to be reasonably accurate. Thus, since the turn of the century, we have gone from a situation in which 4 percent of the population was 65 or older to a time when 11 percent have reached seniority. By the year 2030, that older population will have almost doubled. Put another way, in 2030 there will be as many people over 75 as there are today over 65.

We recognize that the elderly use more health care services than do younger people. The result is an even greater demand on the health care system and a concomitant rise in total health care costs. Because the elderly use more institutional services (i.e., hospital and nursing home care), their health care costs are higher than those for younger groups. Only 11 percent of the population, those age 65 and over, account for over 30 percent of health expenditures. The per capita cost of health care for the elderly was over $4200 in 1985, compared with about $1700 for the population as a whole.

The increased number of older persons has been accompanied by a number of changes in the way medical care is financed. Although these programs are discussed in more detail in Chapter 16, we note here that the appearance of programs like Medicare and Medicaid, with all their shortcomings, has been associated with a growing expenditure on health care for the elderly and an increasing role in this area for public dollars. It is important to bear in mind that, even in the face of greatly increased public financing, the elderly person

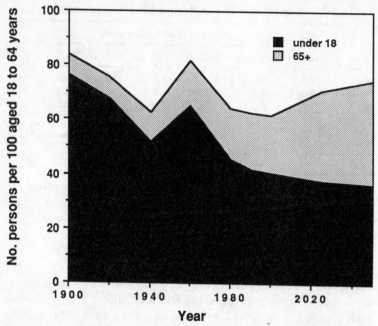

Figure 2-2   Changes in the young and elderly support ratio, 1900–2050. (*From U.S. Senate, 1984.*)

still must bear a considerable share of the financial burden. In fact, in 1986, an elderly person's out-of-pocket costs for health care were about equivalent to those just prior to the passage of Medicare.

The growing numbers of older persons have created great consternation among forecasters. There is a sense of doom, a future in which all resources will go to support the elderly. To counter this ageist misimpression, it is useful to look at the dependency ratio. This index compares the proportion of the population under 18 and over 65 to that between 18 and 64 (the group presumed to be working to support the rest). Figure 2-2 traces the changes in the index and its principal components from 1900 through projections to the year 2050. It is important to note that while the relative contribution of the older population will increase impressively, the total will never be as high as it was in the mid-1960s.

The growth in the number of elderly persons results from improvements in both social living conditions and medical care. Over the course of this century, we have moved from a preponderance of acute diseases (especially infections) to an era of chronic illnesses. Table 2-2 reflects the changes in the common causes of death from 1900 to the present. Many of those common at the turn of the century are no longer even listed. Today the pattern of death among the elderly is generally similar to that of the population as a whole. The leading causes are the same, but there are some differences in the rankings. The leading causes of death are heart disease, cancer, stroke, and influenza/pneumonia. Although the most dramatic re-

Table 2-2   Changes in the Commonest Causes of Death, 1900–1985, All Ages and for Those 65+

| | All ages | | | | 65+ | |
| | 1900 | | 1985 | | 1985 | |
	Rate*	Rank	Rate	Rank	Rate	Rank
Diseases of the heart	13.8	4	32.3	1	217.3	1
Malignant neoplasms	6.4	8	19.3	2	104.7	2
Cerebrovascular disease	10.7	5	6.4	3	46.4	3
Accidents	7.2	7	3.9	4	8.7	6
Influenza and pneumonia	22.9	1	2.8	5	20.6	4
Diabetes mellitus	1.1		1.5	6	9.6	5
Suicide	1.0		1.2	7	2.0	11
Cirrhosis of liver	1.2		1.1	8	3.4	10
Atherosclerosis	NR		1.0	9	8.0	7
Bronchitis, emphysema, asthma	4.5	9	0.9	10	5.7	9
Nephritis and nephrosis	8.9	6	0.9	11	6.1	8
Homicide	0.1		0.8	12	0.4	12
Tuberculosis	19.4	2	0.07		0.4	
Diarrhea and enteritis	14.3	3	NR			
Diphtheria	4.0	11	NR			
Typhoid fever	3.1	12	NR			
Senility	5.0	10	NR			

*Rate per 10,000 population.
Note: NR = not reported.
Sources: For 1900 data: Linder FE, Grove RD: *Vital Statistics Rates in the United States 1900-1940.* Washington DC, U.S. Government Printing Office, 1947. For 1985 data: National Center for Vital Statistics: *Vital Statistics of the United States, 1985,* Vol. II, *Mortality,* Part B. DHHS Publ. No. (PHS) 88-1102, Public Health Service, Washington DC, U.S. Government Printing Office, 1987.

duction of mortality has occurred in infants and mothers, there has been a perceptible increase in survival, even after age 65. This increased survival is plotted in Figure 2-3. Our stereotypes of what to expect from the elderly may therefore need reexamination. The average 65-year-old woman can expect to live another 19 years, and a 65-year-old man, another 15 years. As shown in Figure 2-4, even at age 85, there is an expectation of over 5 years.

However, this gain in survival includes both active and dependent years. Indeed, one of the great controversies of modern gerontologic epidemiology is whether the gain in life expectancy brings with it equivalent gains in years free of dependency. Although the concept of compression of morbidity has been popularized (Fries, 1980), the data available do not support such an optimistic scenario. Katz and his colleagues (1983) have introduced the concept of active life expectancy to distinguish the years spent free of disability. As shown in Figure 2-5, much of the advantage enjoyed by females comes in the form of dependent years. Table 2-3 summarizes some of the research that has examined the changes in disability patterns across birth

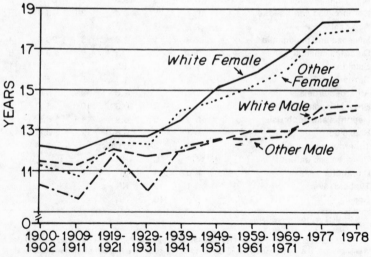

Figure 2-3 Life expectancy at age 65, 1900–1978. (*From Federal Council on Aging, 1981.*)

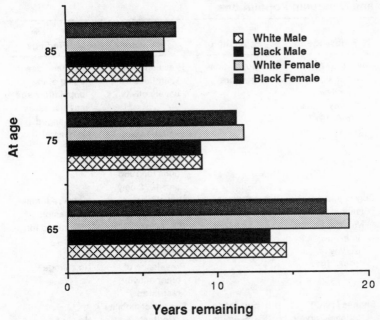

Figure 2-4 Life expectancy of the elderly, 1984. (*From Havlik and Suzman, 1987.*)

cohorts. In general, the weight of present evidence does not show impressive improvements in the age-specific prevalence of disability. If anything, the mean values seem to be getting worse with time.

The observation of worsening morbidity rates with time seems in direct contrast to the clinical observation that older persons seem generally healthier and more robust than even a generation ago. The truth may encompass both sets of findings. If there is a general shift of both survival and disability to older years, we would maintain the same period of disability but delay its onset. In fact, we may be doing more than that. We may be witnessing a bimodal distribution in which part of the population is getting healthier and a part more disabled as a result of increased survivorship from problems that would have been fatal in the past. This bimodality can produce a mean value that seems worse than earlier times, despite a growth in the proportion of those in very good health.

Table 2-3   The Evidence for Compression of Morbidity—Principal Studies of the United States and Canadian Populations

Reference	Population	Disability measure	Findings
Kovar (1977) National Health Interview Survey, 1965–1977	U.S. population 65+ years	Prevalence of limitations in usual activity	Increased due to aging of the population; age specific rates unchanged
		Limitations in mobility due to chronic conditions for 1966 and 1972 only	No change
Colvez and Blanchet (1981) National Health Interview Survey, 1966–1974	U.S. population <45 years 45–64 years 65+ years	Prevalence of main activity	Increase for men impossible
		Prevalence of main activity restricted	Decreased for men
		Prevalence of other activity restricted	No change
Shanas (1982) National Survey of the Aged, 1962 and 1975	U.S. population 65–69 years 70–74 years 75–79 years 80+ years	Degree of mobility	
		Bedfast	No change
		Housebound	No change
		Ambulatory	No change
		Index of incapacity for self-care	
		Goes outdoors	No change
		Walking stairs	Improved
		Walks about house	No change
		Bathes self	No change
		Dresses self	No change
		Cuts toenails	No change
Verbrugge (1984) National Health Interview Survey, 1958–1980	U.S. population 45–64 years 65+ years	Limitation in activity	
		Any limitation	Trend unclear
		Major-activity limitation	Trend unclear
		Secondary-activity limitation	Trend unclear May be a slight increase in major and any-activity limitation after 1970

Table 2-3 The Evidence for Compression of Morbidity—Principal Studies of the United States and Canadian Populations (*Continued*)

Reference	Population	Disability measure	Findings
		Total restricted activity days	For both sexes, declines through 1970 then increases
		Total bed disability days	Steady
Palmore (1986) National Health Interview Survey, 1961–1981	U.S. population 45–64 years 65+ years	Days of restricted activity	No change
		Days of bed disability	Slight decrease
Crimmins (1987) National Health Interview Survey, 1969, 1970, 1971, 1979, 1980, 1981	U.S. population 65 years of age and over Age-specific	Limitation in major activity	Increased for males up to 74 years of age Increased for females up to 72 years of age
		Unable to perform major activity	Increased for males up to 74 years of age No change for females
		Restricted activity days	Increased for both sexes at nearly all ages
		Bed disability days	No change
Wilkins and Adams (1983) Canada Health Survey, 1978–1979	Canadian population 65+ years	Short-term disability Bed days	Unchanged for males Increased for females
		Total days	Unchanged for males Increased for females
Canadian Sickness Survey, 1950–1951		Long-term disability Percent (males)	Unchanged to slight increase
Life expectancy, 1951 and 1978		Percent (females)	Increased

Note: This table was compiled with the assistance of David Radosevich; it draws heavily on the work Guralnik and Schneider (1987).

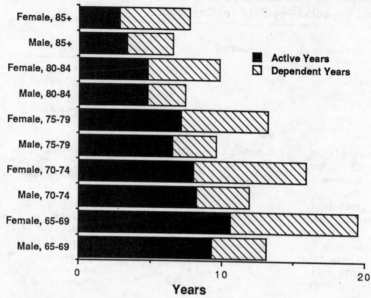

Figure 2-5   Active versus dependent life expectancy, Massachusetts Elderly, 1974. (*From Katz, 1983.*)

DISABILITY

The World Health Organization distinguishes between impairments, disabilities, and handicaps. The distinction is quite useful among the elderly. As shown in Figure 2-6, there is a general pattern of increased impairment in the senses and in orthopedic problems with age. Indeed, not surprisingly, the prevalence of chronic conditions increases with age. However, the nature of survivorship produces the occasional twist. As seen in Figure 2-7, the association between prevalence and age is not absolute. Those afflicted with diabetes and those with chronic lung disease, for example, do not survive as readily to age 85 and above. Despite having more chronic conditions and impairments, the elderly tend to report their health as generally good. This contrast highlights the coping abilities of elderly persons discussed in Chapter 1.

Because physicians tend to see the sick, they may form a distorted picture of the elderly. Most older persons are indeed self-suffi-

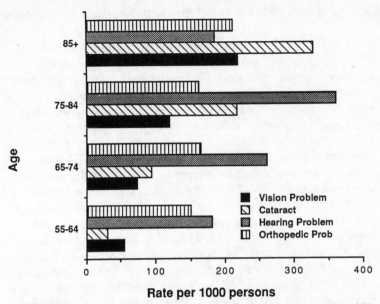

Figure 2-6   Prevalence of impairments among community elderly, 1982-1984. (*From Adams and Collins, 1987.*)

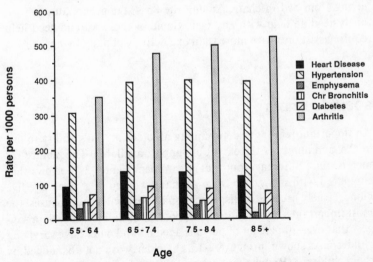

Figure 2-7   Prevalence of chronic conditions among community elderly, 1982-1984. (*From Adams and Collins, 1987.*)

29

cient and able to function on their own or with minimal assistance. Those who need help are likely to be the very old. Functioning can be measured in a variety of ways. Figures 2-8 and 2-9 look at very simple measures: walking and lifting at two levels of performance each. In each case there is a clear age gradient, with decreasing performance with age. Commonly we use the ability to perform specific tasks as a reflection of independence. These are grouped into two classes of measures. Instrumental activities of daily living (IADLs) refer to tasks required to maintain an independent household. They generally demand a combination of both physical and cognitive performances. Figure 2-10 compares the rates of difficulty with common IADLs by age and sex. Even among those at age 85 and above, over half the population living in the community can still perform independently.

The ability to carry out basic self-care activities is reflected in the so-called activities of daily living (ADLs). These dependencies, which tend to occur in a regular fashion beginning with bathing, are less common than IADL losses. As shown in Figure 2-11, even among the oldest groups the prevalence of ADL dependency is quite low. Less than 30 percent of females aged 85 or more living in the community needed assistance with bathing and only 20 percent with transferring from bed to chair. Among the 85+ age group, almost two-thirds need no help with any task. Some of those who do need help require assistance with more than one activity of daily living.

SOCIAL SUPPORT

An important feature in determining an older person's ability to live in the community is the extent of support available. The picture for men is quite different from that for women. Figure 2-12 shows that compared with men, over twice as many women of a given age live alone, largely because of disproportionate survival. After spouses, the most important source of family support is children. Survey data suggest that over 70 percent of persons aged 65 and older have surviving children. As shown in Figure 2-13, the elderly are not abandoned by their children. (Remember that the children of persons age 85 and older may themselves be aged 65 or older.)

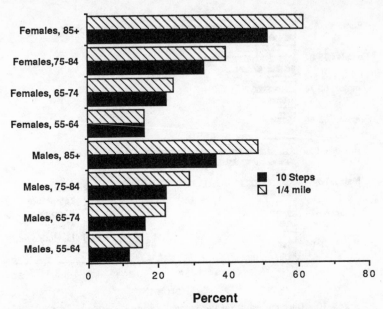

Figure 2-8 Community elderly with difficulty walking, 1984. (*From LaCroix, 1987*.)

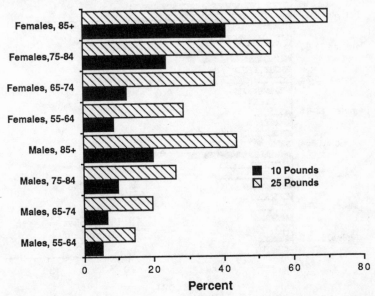

Figure 2-9 Community elderly with difficulty lifting, 1984. (*From LaCroix, 1987*.)

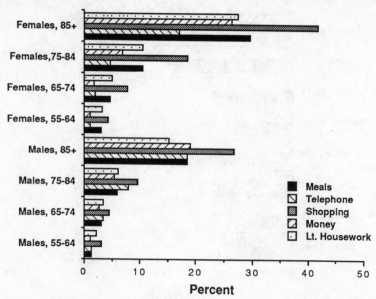

Figure 2-10 Difficulty with IADLs among community elderly, 1984. (*From LaCroix, 1987.*)

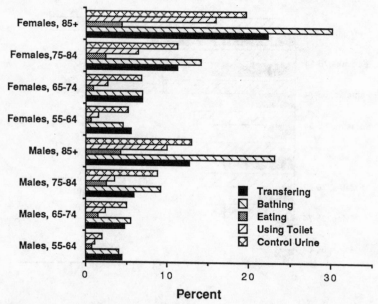

Figure 2-11 Difficulty with ADLs among community elderly, 1984. (*From LaCroix, 1987.*)

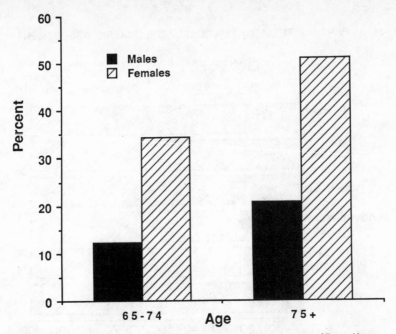

Figure 2-12   Percent of community elderly living alone, 1984. (*From Kovar, 1986.*)

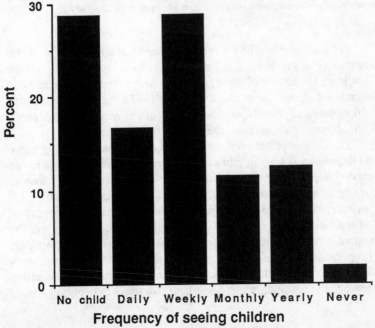

Figure 2-13   Frequency of elderly living alone who saw children, 1984. (*From Kovar, 1986.*)

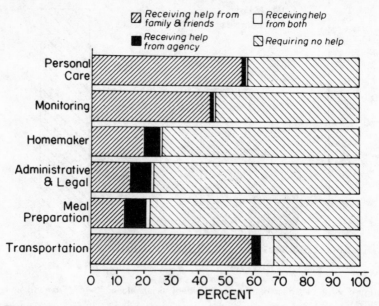

Figure 2-14 Persons 65 and older receiving selected home services provided by family members and agencies, 1975. (*From Allan and Brotman, 1981.*)

In fact, the majority of care provided to elderly persons in the community is given by family members. In a study conducted in Cleveland, the source of assistance for a wide variety of services was ascertained (U.S. Comptroller General, 1977). As shown in Figure 2-14, family and friends provide the bulk of services in each category with, or more often without, the help of formal care givers.

The difference between needing and not needing a nursing home will depend on the availability of such support. The difference in the rates of dependency among community-living elderly and those in nursing homes can seem very dramatic, as shown in Figure 2-15. However, much of this difference is attributable to differences in age and sex ratios. Compare those data to Figure 2-16, which shows the relative rates of dependency for various measures among a single group, namely white females aged 75 to 84, a group that comprises a large share of the nursing home residents. Difficulties in toileting, walking, and continence are only about two times as common among

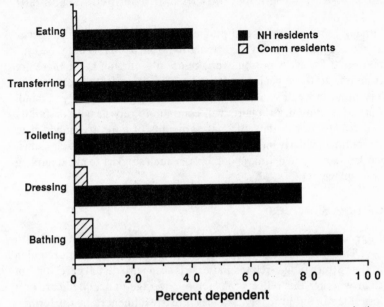

Figure 2-15 Comparative rates of dependency between elderly persons in the community and in nursing homes. (*From Hing, 1987.*)

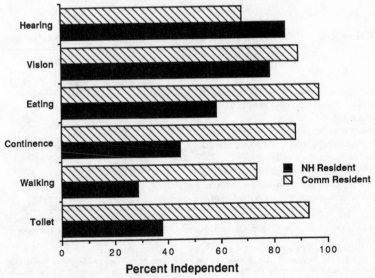

Figure 2-16 White females 75 to 84 years old in nursing home versus in the community. (*From Havlik et al, 1987.*)

nursing home residents, and problems with hearing and vision occur at about equal frequency. Extrapolating from available data, we estimate that for every person over age 65 in a nursing home there are from one to three people equally disabled living in the community. The importance of social support must be kept continuously in mind. Formal community supports will continue to rely heavily on family and friends to see that adequate amounts of care are provided to maintain an elderly individual in the community. The physician must work diligently to maintain and bolster such support to avoid nursing home placement.

USE OF SERVICES

In general, there is an increase in the utilization of health care with age. Table 2-4 summarizes some of these differences. The exception to the pattern of age-related increase is seen with dental care; it is not clear whether this reflects the lack of coverage under Medicare or a loss of teeth, but probably is at least greatly influenced by the former. With the introduction of the new prospective payment system for hospitals under Medicare in 1983, there had been expected some

Table 2-4   Health Services Utilization by Various Age Groups

	Age groups		
	45–64	65–74	75+
Annual hospital discharges / 100	14.2	23.7	33.7
Average length of stay	6.8	8.7	8.3
Short-stay hospital days in past year	9.6	12.5	12.1
Percent of persons with no hospital days	90.3%	84.6%	79.7%
No. of procedures / 100*	19.7	38.7†	
Percent seeing a physician in past year	75.0%	82.2%	87.2%
Average number of physician contacts per year	6.6	8.1	10.6
Percent seeing a dentist in past year	55.9	42.6†	

*Procedures refer to a broader category of activities in short-stay hospitals than just operations; it includes such things as arteriography, angiocardiography, CT scans, diagnostic ultrasound, and endoscopies.

†65 years and over.

Sources: Dawson DA: *Current Estimates from National Health Interview Survey, United States, 1986* Series 10, No. 164, DHHS Publ. No. (PHS)87-1592, Public Health Service, Washington DC, U.S. Government Printing Office, October 1987.

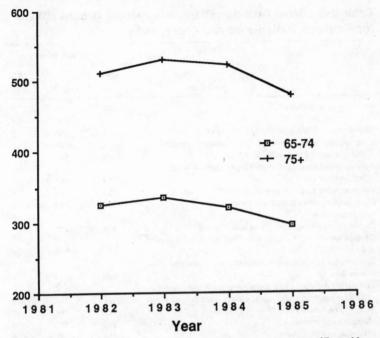

Figure 2-17   Hospital discharges per 1000 persons, 1982–1985. (*From Moss and Moien, 1987.*)

changes in length of stay and admission rates. The use of the Diagnosis-related Group (DRG) as a basis for determining flat rates per admission means that hospitals can vary either the intensity of care per day or the number of days per admission. As expected, length of stay decreased rather sharply, but to the surprise of many, admission rates fell rather than increased. Figures 2-17 and 2-18 trace these falls. Table 2-5 shows the most common DRGs in 1984 and contrasts their rank with that calculated for the situation in 1980, prior to the implementation of DRGs. The top seven have not changed, although their relative order has shifted. Some of the changes seen in the others likely reflect the payment rates accorded the different classifications. It has now become very important to choose the best-paying DRG justified by the clinical findings.

Table 2-5   Most Common Diagnosis-Related Groups (DRGs) for Medicare Patients 65 and Older, 1984

		No. of discharges	
	DRG no.	(1000s)	1980 Rank
Heart failure and shock	127	456	3
Lens procedures	39	394	4
Simple pneumonia & pleurisy age 70 or over &/or CC*	89	350	5
Esophagitis, gastroenteritis, & miscellaneous digestive disease age 70 or over &/or CC	182	345	2
Specific cerebrovascular disorders except transient ischemic attacks	14	339	6
Atherosclerosis age 70 or over &/or CC	132	282	1
Chronic obstructive pulmonary disease	88	272	7
Angina pectoris	140	272	15
Unrelated operating room procedure	468	218	10
Cardiac arrhythmia & conduction disorders age 70 or over &/or CC	138	218	17
Nutritional & miscellaneous metabolic disorders age 70 or over &/or CC	296	203	22
Circulatory disorders with acute myocardial infarction without cardiovascular complications discharged alive	122	191	12
Bronchitis & asthma age 70 or over &/or CC	96	186	16
Medical back problems	243	186	11
Diabetes age 36 or over	294	180	8
Transient ischemic attacks	15	167	14
Kidney & urinary tract infections age 70 or over &/or CC	320	164	18
Transurethral prostatectomy age 70 or over &/or CC	336	158	19
Gastrointestinal hemorrhage age 70 or over &/or CC	174	155	24
Major joint procedures	209	154	25
Respiratory neoplasms	82	148	21
Hip & femur procedures except major joint age 70 or over &/or CC	210	140	20
Hypertension	134	120	13
Red blood cell disorders age 18 or over	395	115	26
Peripheral vascular disorders age 70 or over &/or CC	130	114	23
Major large & small bowel procedures age 70 or over &/or CC	148	112	27
Circulatory disorders with acute myocardial infarction & cardiovascular complications discharged alive	121	102	29

*CC stands for substantial comorbidity and/or complication.

Source: Poktas R: Utilization of short-stay hospitals by diagnosis-related groups, United States, 1980–84. Vital and Health Statistics, Series 13 No. 87 DHHS Pub. No. (PHS)86-1748 Public Health Service, Washington, DC, US Government Printing Office, July 1986.

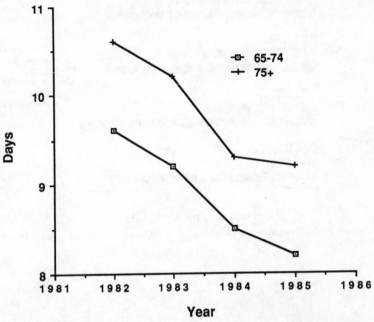

Figure 2-18 Lengths of hospital stay, 1982-1985. (*From Moss and Moien, 1987.*)

Figure 2-19 describes the changes in patterns for ambulatory visits by age. Despite the general principle that bad things are more common with increasing age after 75, not all diagnoses increase with age. The exceptions to the rule reflect a survivorship effect. For several conditions, more persons suffering these problems are likely to die before they reach the older ages. The pattern among the survivors may thus be anomalous.

Nursing Home Use

We are prone to cite a figure of 5 percent for the proportion of elderly in nursing homes at any moment. Such a figure is a potentially misleading generalization. As Figure 2-20 suggests, age is a very important factor. Among those 65 to 74 years old, the rate is less than 2 percent. It rises to about 7 percent for those age 75 to 84, and then jumps to 20 percent for those 85 and older. It is also helpful to distinguish between these prevalence rates and the lifetime probability of

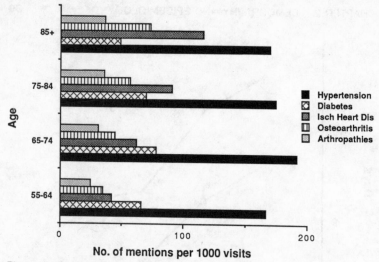

Figure 2-19 Frequency of diagnoses in ambulatory visits, 1980–1981. (*From Koch and Havlik, 1987.*)

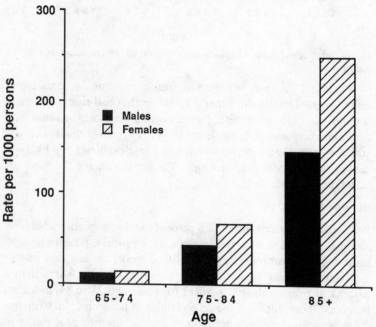

Figure 2-20 Nursing home use by the elderly, 1985. (*From Hing, 1987.*)

entering a nursing home. Longitudinal studies suggest that persons age 65 have between a 25 and 40 percent chance of spending some time in a nursing home before they die (Vicente, Wiley, and Carrington, 1979).

The need for nursing homes is not simply because of the presence of diseases or even functional disabilities. It is also a result of a lack of social support. Often the family becomes exhausted after caring for an elderly patient for a long period. Family fatigue is especially a problem when the patient has symptoms that are very disruptive. Among the most disturbing are incontinence and behavior problems that involve wandering or disruptive behavior. Table 2-6 summarizes the factors associated with increased likelihood of nursing home placement.

About three-fourths of nursing home admissions come from hospitals. A 3-day hospital stay is a prerequisite for even the limited nursing home coverage available under Medicare. Often the hospitalization represents the last step in a series of steps involving the deterioration of the patient and the patient's social supports. For others, the hospitalization results from an acute event, e.g., a broken hip or a stroke, which then requires long-term care.

Less than 10 percent of hospital patients age 65 and older is discharged to nursing homes. As with those from the community, the rate of nursing home placement increases with age and is greater for females than for males. Table 2-7 summarizes some of the factors that can identify those elderly patients in hospitals at risk of nursing home placement. In addition to age and sex, medical patients are more likely to be placed in nursing homes than are surgical patients, and those with mental diagnoses (especially in addition to physical diagnoses) are at higher risk.

Talk about nursing home patients must carefully distinguish between data based on a study of those resident in a facility at a given time and those entering or leaving the facility. The conclusions reached about nursing home patients may be quite different depending on which groups are examined. Researchers have identified two streams of patients entering the nursing home—one group will leave fairly quickly (within 3 to 6 months); the other will stay several years (Keeler, Kane, and Solomon, 1981). These two groups have distinct characteristics. The short-term patients tend to be younger, have

Table 2-6　Factors Affecting the Need for Nursing Home Admission

Characteristics of the individual:
　Age, sex, race
　Marital status
　Living arrangements
　Degree of mobility
　Activities of daily living
　Instrumental activities of daily living
　Urinary continence
　Behavior problems
　Mental status
　Memory impairment
　Mood disturbance
　Vertigo and falls
　Ability to manage medication
　Clinical prognosis
　Income
　Payment eligibility
　Need for special services
Characteristics of the support system:
　Family capability
　　For married respondents, age of spouse
　　Presence of responsible relative (usually adult child)
　　Family structure of responsible relative
　　Employment status of responsible relative
　Physician availability
　Amount of care currently received from family and others
Community resources:
　Formal community resources
　Informal support systems
　Presence of long-term care institutions
　Characteristics of long-term care institutions

more physical problems, and enter from the hospital. The long-term patients are more likely to be older, confused, and incontinent. At admission, the patients are about equally distributed between short-term and long-term patients, but a study of residents will find about nine times as many long-term patients.

Nursing home data can be very confusing. Not only must one distinguish between admissions and residents; one must also look at

**Table 2-7   Percentage of
Hospital Patients 65 and
Over Discharged to a
Nursing Home**

Characteristic	Percent
Sex:	
Male	6.0
Female	11.1
Age:	
65–69	2.8
70–74	5.1
75–79	8.3
80–84	14.3
85+	22.7
Surgical procedure:	
Yes	7.3
No	11.4
Diagnoses:	
Physical	9.1
Mental	16.9
Mixed	27.2

Source: Kane, Matthias, and Sampson (1983).

the time course of former residents to appreciate the true nature of such long-term care. On the one hand, the picture is much more dynamic than is usually suspected. Over half the persons admitted to a nursing home are discharged within 3 months. On the other hand, many of these people die in the nursing home, and many of the discharges are really transfers to hospitals. From there a majority of patients either return to the nursing home or die in hospital. About a third of nursing home discharges do go back to the community, but even then many return to a nursing home in time. Figure 2-21 offers a simplified portrayal of the true dynamics of nursing home discharges and the transitions involved. It is more accurate to talk about long-term care "careers" than to think in terms of discrete episodes.

As we enter an era of more aged persons with chronic disease, physicians will find themselves working increasingly in institutions such as nursing homes. They will be challenged to provide leadership in upgrading the care available in such settings. They will need to be

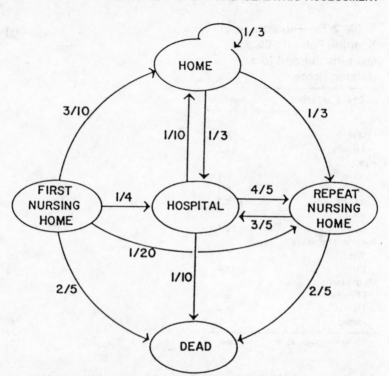

Figure 2-21 Natural history of patients discharged from nursing homes. Transfer patterns of nursing home patients. The fractions indicate the approximate proportion of patients moving from one status to another. For example, about three-tenths of first admissions went home on discharge, a fourth went to the hospital, a twentieth went to another nursing home, and two-fifths died. Of those going home, a third stayed at home, a third went to the hospital and a third went back to a nursing home. (*From Lewis, 1985.*)

familiar with the array of resources available to meet the needs of their patients and the factors determining access to these resources. A guide to long-term-care resources is presented in Chapter 16.

REFERENCES

Adams PF, Collins G: Measures of health among older persons living in the community, in Havlik RJ, Liu MG, Kovar MG, et al (eds): *Health Statistics on Older Persons, United States, 1986. Vital and Health Statistics,* Series 3, No. 25. DHHS Publ. No. (PHS)87-1409. Public Health

Service, Washington, DC, U.S. Government Printing Office, June 1987.

Allan CA, Brotman H (compilers): *Chartbook on Aging in America*. The 1981 White House Conference on Aging, 1981.

Colvez A, Blanchet M: Disability trends in the United States population 1966–76: analysis of reported causes. *Am J Public Health* 71:464–471, May 1981.

Crimmins EM: Evidence on the compression of morbidity. *Gerontologica Perspecta* 1:45–49, 1987.

Federal Council on the Aging: *The Need for Long-Term Care: A Chartbook of the Federal Council on the Aging*. OHDS 81-20704. U.S. Government Printing Office, 1981.

Fries JF: Aging, natural death, and the compression of morbidity. *N Engl J Med* 303:130–136, 1980.

Guralnik JM, Schneider EL: The compression of morbidity: a dream which may come true someday! *Gerontologica Perspecta* 1:8–14, 1987.

Havlik RJ, Liu MG, Kovar MG, et al (eds): *Health Statistics on Older Persons, United States, 1986. Vital and Health Statistics*, Series 3, No. 25. DHHS Publ. No. (PHS)87-1409. Public Health Service, Washington, DC, U.S. Government Printing Office, June 1987.

Havlik RJ, Suzman R: Health status—mortality, in Havlik RJ, Liu MG, Kovar MG, et al (eds): *Health Statistics on Older Persons, United States, 1986. Vital and Health Statistics*, Series 3, No. 25. DHHS Publ. No. (PHS)87-1409. Public Health Service, Washington, DC, U.S. Government Printing Office, June 1987.

Hing E: Use of nursing homes by the elderly: Preliminary data from the 1985 National Nursing Home Survey, in *Advance Data from Vital and Health Statistics*, No. 135. DHHS Publ. No. (PHS)87-1250. Hyattsville, MD, Public Health Service, May 14, 1987.

Kane RL, Solomon DH, Beck JC, et al: *Geriatrics in the United States: Manpower Projections and Training Considerations*. Lexington, MA, Heath, 1981.

Kane RL, Matthias R, Sampson S: The risk of nursing-home placement after acute hospitalization. *Med Care* 21:1055–1061, 1983.

Katz S, Branch LG, Branson MH, et al: Active life expectancy. *N Engl J Med* 309:1218–1224, 1983.

Keeler EB, Kane RL, Solomon DH: Short- and long-term residents of nursing homes. *Med Care* 19:363–369, 1981.

Koch H, Havlik RJ: Use of health care—ambulatory medical care, in Havlik RJ, Liu MG, Kovar MG, et al (eds): *Health Statistics on Older Persons, United States, 1986. Vital and Health Statistics*, Series 3, No. 25.

DHHS Publ. No. (PHS)87-1409. Public Health Service, Washington, DC, U.S. Government Printing Office, June 1987.

Kovar MG: Elderly people: the population 65 years and over. Health—United States—1976–1977. DHEW Publ. No. (HRA)77-1232. Washington, DC: U.S. Department of Health, Education, and Welfare, 1977.

Kovar MG: Aging in the eighties, age 65 and over and living alone, contacts with family, friends, and neighbors. Preliminary data from the Supplement on Aging to the National Health Interview Survey: United States, January–June, 1984, in *Advance Data from Vital and Health Statistics*, No. 116. DHHS Publ. No. (PHS)86-1250. Hyattsville, MD, Public Health Service, May 9, 1986.

LaCroix AZ: Determinants of health—exercise and activites of daily living, in Havlik RJ, Liu MG, Kovar MG, et al (eds): *Health Statistics on Older Persons, United States, 1986. Vital and Health Statistics*, Series 3, No. 25. DHHS Publ. No. (PHS)87-1409. Public Health Service, Washington, DC, U.S. Government Printing Office, June 1987.

Lewis MA, Cretin S, Kane RL: The natural history of nursing home patients. *Gerontologist* 25:382–388, 1985.

Moss AJ, Moien MA: Recent declines in hospitalization: United States, 1982–86, in *Advance Data from Vital and Health Statistics*, No. 140. DHHS Publ. No. (PHS)87-1250. Hyattsville, MD, Public Health Service, September 24, 1987.

Palmore EB: Trends in the health of the aged. *Gerontologist* 26:298–302, 1986.

Shanas E: National survey of the aged. DHHS Publ. No. (OHDS)83-20425. Washington, DC: U.S. Department of Health and Human Services, 1982.

U.S. Comptroller General: *The Well-Being of Older People in Cleveland, Ohio.* HRD 77-70. General Accounting Office, 1977.

U.S. Senate Special Committee on Aging: Aging America: trends and projections. Washington DC, 1984.

Vaupel JW, Yashin AI: Heterogeneity's ruses: some surprising effects of selection on population dynamics. *Am Statistician*, 39:176–185, 1985.

Verbrugge LM: Longer life but worsening health? Trends in health and mortality of middle-aged and older persons. *Milbank Memorial Fund Quarterly/Health and Society* 62:475–519, 1984.

Vicente L, Wiley JA, Carrington RA: The risk of institutionalization before death. *Gerontologist* 19:361–366, 1979.

Wilkins R, Adams OB: Changes in the healthfulness of life of the elderly population: an empirical approach. *Rev Epidemiol Sante Publique* 35:225–235, 1987.

Chapter 3

Evaluating the Elderly Patient

Comprehensive evaluation of an elderly individual's health status is one of the most challenging aspects of clinical geriatrics. It requires a sensitivity to the concerns of elderly people, an awareness of the many unique aspects of their medical problems, an ability to interact effectively with a variety of health professionals, and often a great deal of patience. Most importantly, it requires a perspective different from that used in the evaluation of younger individuals. Not only are the a priori probabilities of diagnoses different; one must be attuned to more subtle findings. Progress may be measured on a finer scale. Special tools are needed to ascertain relatively small improvements in chronic conditions and overall function, compared with the more dramatic cures of acute illnesses often possible in younger patients.

The purposes of the evaluation and the setting in which it takes place will determine its focus and extent. Considerations important in admitting an elderly woman with a fractured hip and pneumonia to an acute care hospital during the middle of the night are obviously different from those in the evaluation of an elderly demented patient exhibiting disruptive behavior in a nursing home. Elements included in screening for treatable conditions in an ambulatory clinic are different from those in assessment of elderly individuals in their own homes.

Despite the differences dictated by the purpose and setting of the evaluation, several essential aspects of evaluating elderly patients are common to all purposes and settings. Figure 3-1 depicts these aspects; they can be summarized as follows:

1 Physical, psychological, and socioeconomic factors interact in complex ways to influence the health and functional status of the elderly.

2 Comprehensive evaluation of an elderly individual's health status will require an assessment of each of these domains. The coordinated efforts of several different health care professionals will therefore be needed.

3 Functional abilities should be a central focus of the comprehensive evaluation of an elderly individual. Other more traditional measures of health status (such as diagnoses and physical and laboratory findings) are useful in dealing with underlying etiologies and

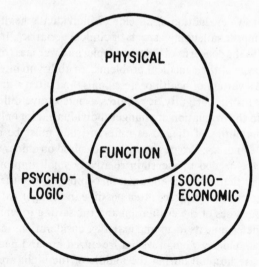

Figure 3-1 Components of assessment of the elderly.

detecting treatable conditions, but, in the elderly, measures of function are often essential in determining overall health, well-being, and the need for health and social services.

Just as function is the common language of geriatrics, assessment lies at the heart of its practice. Special techniques that utilize comprehensive examinations of the multiple problems and their functional consequences offer a way to structure the approach to these often complicated dilemmas. Geriatric assessment has been tested in a variety of forms. The findings from a number of randomized controlled trials of different approaches to geriatric assessment are summarized in Table 3-1 and reviewed in detail elsewhere (Rubenstein, 1987). Despite the dramatic variation in approach to targeting, personnel used, and measures employed, a clear pattern of effectiveness has emerged. Taken together, these results are both heartening and cautioning. Systematic approaches to patient care are obviously desirable. The issue is more how formalized these services should be. Is there a generic model to fit all circumstances, or is it simply a question of doing something? The results of the studies published until now suggest that the specifics of the assessment process seem to be less important than the very act of systematically approaching elderly people with the belief that improvement is possible. More work needs to be done on defining the most appropriate assessment strategies for different patient groups and for different clinical settings.

Because of the multidimensional nature of many elderly patients' problems and the frequent presence of multiple interacting medical conditions, comprehensive evaluation of the geriatric patient can be time-consuming and thus costly. The development of a close-knit multidisciplinary team with minimal redundancy in the assessments performed, the use of carefully designed questionnaires which reliable patients and/or care givers can complete before an appointment, and the effective use of assessment forms (including the incorporation of these forms into computer data bases) are examples of strategies that can make the evaluation process more efficient.

As geriatric assessment becomes more prevalent, there will be conspicuous overlap with the emerging practice of case management. In the best of all possible worlds, these are complementary, not competing, activities. The value of assessment lies in its consequent actions. Case management represents a similarly systematic ap-

Table 3-1 Randomized Controlled Trials of Geriatric Assessment

Reference	Target group	Intervention	Major findings
Rubenstein et al. (1984)	VA patients from acute care hospital felt to need nursing home	Multidisciplinary geriatric assessment team; rehabilitation; outpatient follow-up	Reduced mortality; improved function; reduced hospital and nursing home use
Hendriksen et al. (1984)	Urban community residents aged 75+	Social worker's social assessment and referral to general practitioner	Reduced mortality; reduced hospital use
Vetter et al. (1979)	Urban and community residents aged 70+	Health visitor's nursing assessment and referral to general practitioner	Reduced mortality (urban only); no difference in function or anxiety
Williams (1987)	Applicants to long-term care program	Multidisciplinary outpatient assessment	Reduced hospital use; no difference in function or mortality
Allen et al. (1986), Becker et al. (1987), Saltz et al. (1988)	VA hospital patients aged 75+	Geriatric consultation team; 71% compliance with recommendations	No difference in hospital complication rates, likelihood of being discharged back home, or 6 months rehospitalization or reinstitutionalization rates
Hogan et al. (1987)	Medicine hospital patients aged 75+	Geriatric consultation team; no compliance rate reported	Improved mental status; fewer oral medications; more referrals for community services; reduced posthospital mortality

proach to coordinating a care plan. Although most case managers are not physicians, they rely on physician input as an important building block for the care plans. Conversely, many geriatric assessment programs may offer ongoing case management services, although this will often lead to a confusion between assessment and primary care. (See also the discussion of case management in Chapter 16.)

This chapter will focus on the more general aspects of assessing the geriatric patient. Sections on geriatric consultation, preoperative evaluation, and environmental assessments are included at the end of the chapter. Chapter 17 is devoted to the assessment and management of geriatric patients in the nursing home setting.

THE HISTORY

Sir William Osler's aphorism "Listen to the patient, he'll give you the diagnosis" is as true in the elderly as it is in the young. In the elderly, however, several factors make taking histories more challenging, difficult, and time-consuming.

Table 3-2 lists difficulties commonly encountered in taking histories of the elderly, the factors involved, and some suggestions for overcoming these difficulties. Impaired hearing and vision (despite corrective devices) are common and can interfere with effective communication. Techniques such as eliminating extraneous noises, speaking slowly and in deep tones while facing the patient, and providing adequate lighting can be helpful. The use of simple, inexpensive amplification devices with "walkman"-style earphones can be especially effective, even among the severely hearing impaired. Patience is truly a virtue in obtaining a history; because thought and verbal processes are often slower in elderly than in younger individuals, patients should be allowed adequate time to answer in order not to miss potentially important information.

Many elderly individuals underreport potentially important symptoms because of their cultural and educational backgrounds, as well as their expectations of illness as a normal concomitant of aging. Fear of illness and disability or depression accompanied by a lack of self-concern may also render the reporting of symptoms less frequent. Altered physical and physiological responses to disease processes (see Chapter 1) can result in the absence of symptoms (such as painless

Table 3-2 Potential Difficulties in Taking Histories from the Elderly

Difficulty	Factors involved	Suggestions
Communication	Diminished vision Diminished hearing	Use well-lit room Eliminate extraneous noise Speak slowly in a deep tone Face patient, allowing patient to see your lips Use simple amplification device for severely hearing impaired If necessary, write questions in large print
	Slowed psychomotor performance	Leave enough time for the patient to answer
Underreporting of symptoms	Health beliefs Fear Depression Altered physical and physiological responses to disease process Cognitive impairment	Ask specific questions about potentially important symptoms (see Table 3-3) Use other sources of information (relatives, friends, other care givers) to complete the history
Vague or nonspecific symptoms	Altered physical and physiological responses to disease process Altered presentation of specific diseases Cognitive impairment	Rule out treatable diseases, even if the symptoms (or signs) are not typical or specific Use other sources of information to complete history
Multiple complaints	Prevalance of multiple coexisting diseases Somatization of emotions—"masked depression" (see Chapter 5)	Attend to all somatic symptoms, ruling out treatable conditions Get to know the patient's complaints; pay special attention to new or changing symptoms Interview the patient on several occasions to complete the history

myocardial infarction or ulcer and pneumonia without cough). Symptoms of many diseases can be vague and nonspecific because of these age-related changes. Impairments of memory and other cognitive functions can result in an imprecise or inadequate history and compound these difficulties. Asking specifically about potentially important symptoms (such as those listed in Table 3-3) and using other sources of information (such as relatives, friends, and other care givers) can be very helpful in collecting more precise and useful information in these situations.

At the other end of the spectrum, elderly patients with multiple complaints can frustrate the health care professional who is trying to sort them all out. The multiplicity of complaints can relate to the prevalence of coexisting chronic and acute conditions in many elderly patients. These complaints may, however, be deceiving. Somatic symptoms are commonly manifestations of underlying emotional distress in the elderly rather than symptoms of a physical illness, and symptoms of physical conditions may be exaggerated by emotional distress (see Chapter 5). Getting to know patients and their com-

Table 3-3   Important Aspects of the History in the Elderly

Social history

Living arrangements
Relationships with family and friends
Economic status
Abilities to perform activities of daily living (Table 3-8)
Social activities and hobbies
Mode of transportation

Past medical history

Previous surgical procedures
Major illnesses and hospitalizations
Immunization status
    Influenza, pneumococcal, tetanus
Tuberculosis history and testing
Medications (use the "brown bag" technique; see text)
    Previous allergies
    Knowledge of current medication regimen
    Compliance
Perceived beneficial or adverse drug effects

Table 3-3   Important Aspects of the History in the Elderly (Continued)

Systems review
Ask questions about general symptoms that may indicate treatable underlying disease such as fatigue, anorexia, weight loss, and insomnia. Attempt to elicit key symptoms in each organ system, including:

System	Key symptoms
Respiratory	Increasing dyspnea
	Persistent cough
Cardiovascular	Orthopnea
	Edema
	Angina
	Claudication
	Palpitations
	Dizziness
	Syncope
Gastrointestinal	Difficulty chewing
	Dysphagia
	Abdominal pain
	Change in bowel habit
Genitourinary	Frequency
	Urgency
	Nocturia
	Hesitancy, intermittent stream, straining to void
	Incontinence
	Hematuria
	Vaginal bleeding
Musculoskeletal	Focal or diffuse pain
	Focal or diffuse weakness
Neurological	Visual disturbances (transient or progressive)
	Progressive hearing loss
	Unsteadiness and / or falls
	Transient focal symptoms
Psychological	Depression
	Anxiety and / or agitation
	Paranoia
	Forgetfulness and / or confusion

plaints and paying particular attention to new or changing symptoms are helpful in detecting potentially treatable conditions.

Table 3-3 lists aspects of the history that are especially important in the elderly. It is often not feasible to gather all information in one session; shorter interviews in a few separate sessions may prove more effective in gathering these data from many elderly patients. Often shortchanged in medical evaluations, the social history is a critical component. Understanding the patient's socioeconomic environment and ability to function within it is crucial in determining the potential impact of an illness on an individual's overall health and need for health services. Unlike younger patients, elderly patients have often had multiple prior illnesses. The past medical history is, therefore, important in putting the patient's current problems in perspective; this can also be diagnostically important. For example, vomiting in an elderly patient who has had previous intraabdominal surgery should raise the suspicion of intestinal obstruction from adhesions; nonspecific constitutional symptoms (such as fatigue, anorexia, and weight loss) in a patient with a history of depression should prompt consideration of a relapse. Because elderly individuals are often treated with multiple medications, they are at increased risk of noncompliance and adverse effects (see Chapter 14). A detailed medication history (including both prescribed and over-the-counter drugs) is essential. The "brown bag" technique is very helpful in this regard; have the patient or care giver empty the patient's medicine cabinet into a brown paper bag and bring it at each visit. More often than not, one or more of these medications can, at least in theory, contribute to geriatric patients' symptoms.

A complete systems review, focusing on potentially important and prevalent symptoms in the elderly, can help overcome many of the difficulties described above. Although not intended to be all-inclusive, Table 3-3 lists several of these symptoms. The complexities of interpreting these symptoms in elderly patients should be emphasized. The overlap between symptoms of physical illness and emotional disorders has been mentioned and is further discussed in Chapter 5.

General symptoms can be especially difficult to interpret. Fatigue can result from a number of common conditions such as depression, congestive heart failure, anemia, and hypothyroidism. Anorexia and weight loss can be symptoms of an underlying malignancy, depression, or poorly fitting dentures and diminished taste sensation. Age-related changes in sleep patterns, anxiety, congestive heart failure with orthopnea, or urinary frequency and nocturia can underlie complaints of insomnia. Even relatively specific symptoms can have multiple causes in the elderly. For example, back pain can result from degenerative arthritis, osteoporosis and vertebral compression fractures, metastatic cancer, abdominal aortic aneurysm, retroperitoneal masses, or several other processes. Urinary frequency and nocturia can be caused by heart failure, on the one hand, or by mobilization of lower extremity edema secondary to venous insufficiency, on the other.

THE PHYSICAL EXAMINATION

The common occurrence of multiple pathological physical findings superimposed on age-related physical changes complicates interpretation of the physical examination. Table 3-4 lists common physical

Table 3-4   Common Physical Findings and Their Potential Significance in the Elderly

Physical findings	Potential significance
Vital signs	
Elevated blood pressure	Increased risk for cardiovascular morbidity (see Chapter 9)
	Therapy should be considered if repeated measurements are high, especially with a history of congestive heart failure, stroke, TIA, or dementia
Postural changes in blood pressure	May be asymptomatic and occur in the absence of dehydration
	Aging changes, deconditioning, and drugs may play a role
	Can be exaggerated after meals
	Can be worsened and become symptomatic with antihypertensive, vasodilator, and tricyclic antidepressant therapy
Irregular pulse	Arrhythmias are relatively common in otherwise asymptomatic elderly; seldom need specific evaluation or treatment (see Chapter 9)

Table 3-4   Common Physical Findings and Their Potential Significance in the Elderly (*Continued*)

Physical findings	Potential significance
Tachypnea	Baseline rate should be accurately recorded to help assess future complaints (such as dyspnea) or conditions (such as pneumonia or heart failure)
Weight changes	Weight gain should prompt search for edema or ascites
	Gradual loss of small amounts of weight common; losses in excess of 10% of usual body weight over 3 months or less should prompt search for underlying disease

General appearance and behavior	
Poor personal grooming and hygiene (e.g., poorly shaven, unkempt hair, soiled clothing)	Can be signs of poor overall function and/or depression; often indicates a need for intervention
Slow thought processes and speech	Usually represents an aging change; Parkinson's disease and depression can also cause these signs
Ulcerations	Lower extremity vascular and neuropathic ulcers common; careful evaluation needed
	Pressure ulcers common and easily overlooked in immobile patients
Diminished turgor	Often results from atrophy of subcutaneous tissues rather than volume depletion; when dehydration suspected, skin turgor over chest and abdomen most reliable

Ears (see Chapter 11)	
Diminished hearing	High-frequency hearing loss common; patients with difficulty hearing normal conversation should be evaluated further
	Usual 512-frequency tuning fork is too low for screening

Eyes (see Chapter 11)	
Decreased visual acuity (often despite corrective lenses)	May have multiple causes; all patients should have thorough ophthalmologic examination
	Hemianopsia is easily overlooked and can usually be ruled out by simple confrontation testing

Table 3-4   Common Physical Findings and Their Potential Significance in the Elderly (*Continued*)

Physical findings	Potential significance
Cataracts and other abnormalities of the pupil and lens	Fundoscopic examination often difficult and limited; if retinal pathology suspected, thorough ophthalmologic examination necessary
Mouth	
Missing teeth	Dentures often present; they should be removed to check for evidence of poor fit and other pathology in oral cavity Area under the tongue is a common site for early malignancies
Skin	
Multiple lesions	Actinic keratoses and basal cell carcinomas common; most other lesions benign
Chest	
Abnormal configuration	Kyphosis very common, especially in women with vertebral compression fractures; evidence of new or active fractures (focal vertebral tenderness) should be sought
Abnormal lung sounds	Rales can be heard in the absence of pulmonary disease and heart failure; often indicate atelectasis or age-related fibrotic changes in lung
Cardiovascular (see Chapter 9)	
Irregular rhythms	See Vital Signs, above
Systolic murmurs	Very common and most often benign; clinical history and bedside maneuvers can help to differentiate those needing further evaluation
Extra heart sounds	S_4 common and usually related to hypertension; S_3 has important prognostic and therapeutic implications
Vascular bruits	Carotid bruits may need further evaluation Femoral bruits often present in patients with symptomatic peripheral vascular disease
Diminished distal pulses	Presence or absence should be recorded; this information may be diagnostically useful at a later time (e.g., if symptoms of claudication or an embolism develop)

Table 3-4 Common Physical Findings and Their Potential Significance in the Elderly (*Continued*)

Physical findings	Potential significance
Abdomen	
Prominent aortic pulsation	Abdominal aneurysms close to 5 cm in width should be evaluated and followed by ultrasound
Genitourinary	
Atrophy	Testicular atrophy normal; atrophic vaginal tissue may cause symptoms (such as dyspareunia and dysuria) and treatment may be beneficial
Pelvic prolapse (cystocele, rectocele)	Common and may be unrelated to symptoms; gynecologic evaluation helpful if patient has bothersome, potentially related symptoms
Extremities	
Periarticular pain	Can result from a variety of causes and is not always the result of degenerative joint disease
	Each area of pain should be carefully evaluated and treated (see Chapter 8)
Limited range of motion	Often caused by pain resulting from active inflammation, scarring from old injury, or neurological disease; if limitations impair function, a rehabilitation therapist could be consulted
Edema	Can result from venous insufficiency and/or heart failure; mild edema often a cosmetic problem; treatment necessary if impairing ambulation, predisposing to skin breakdown, or causing discomfort
	Unilateral edema should prompt search for a proximal obstructive process
Neurological	
Abnormal mental status (i.e., confusion, depressed affect)	See Chapters 4, 5, 11
Weakness	Arm drift may be the only sign of residual weakness from a stroke; proximal muscle weakness (e.g., inability to get out of chair) should be further evaluated (see Chapter 8)

Table 3-4   Common Physical Findings and Their Potential Significance in the Elderly (*Continued*)

Physical findings	Potential significance
Sensory abnormalities	Diminished vibratory sensation in toes common without other pathology; peripheral neuropathies may be subtle and difficult to elicit
Abnormal reflexes	Decreased or absent ankle jerks common without other pathology; pathological reflexes (such as grasp, palmomental, and glabellar reflexes) can also occur without other clinical evidence of CNS disease
Abnormal posture and gait	Stooped, short-stepped, wide-based gaits common and do not necessarily indicate Parkinson's disease
	Standardized gait assessment is helpful (see Chapter 7)
	Unsteadiness should be evaluated further (see Chapter 7)

findings and their potential significance in the elderly. An awareness of age-related physical changes is important to the interpretation of many physical findings and therefore subsequent decision making. For example, age-related changes in the skin and postural reflexes can influence the evaluation of hydration; age-related changes in the lung and lower extremity edema secondary to venous insufficiency can complicate the evaluation of symptoms of heart failure. Certain aspects of the physical examination are of particular importance in the elderly. Detection and further evaluation of impairments of vision and hearing can lead to improvements in quality of life for many elderly. Evaluation of gait may uncover correctable causes of unsteadiness and thereby prevent potentially devastating falls (see Chapter 7). Careful palpation of the abdomen may reveal an aortic aneurysm, which, if large enough, might warrant consideration of surgical removal. The mental status examination is especially important in the elderly; this aspect of the physical examination is discussed further below and in detail in Chapters 4 and 5.

LABORATORY ASSESSMENT

Abnormal laboratory findings are often attributed to "old age." While it is true that abnormal findings are common in the elderly, few are true aging changes. Misinterpretation of an abnormal laboratory value as an aging change can lead to underdiagnosis and undertreatment in some instances (such as anemia); failure to appreciate age-related changes can lead to overdiagnosis and overtreatment in others (such as hyperglycemia).

Table 3-5 lists those laboratory parameters unchanged in the elderly and those commonly abnormal. Abnormalities in the former group should prompt further evaluation; abnormalities in the latter group should be interpreted carefully. Important considerations in interpreting commonly abnormal laboratory values are also noted in Table 3-5.

FUNCTIONAL ASSESSMENT

Ability to function should be a central focus of the evaluation of elderly patients (Figure 3-1). Medical history, physical examination, and laboratory findings are all of obvious importance in diagnosing and managing acute and chronic medical conditions in the elderly, as they are in all age groups. But once the dust settles, functional abilities are just as, if not more, important to the overall health, well-being, and potential need for services of the elderly individual. For example, in an elderly patient with hemiparesis, the nature, location, and extent of the lesion may be important in the management, but whether the patient is continent and can climb the steps to an apartment will make the difference between going home to live or going to a nursing home.

The concern about function as a core component of geriatrics deserves special comment. Functioning is the end result of the various efforts of the geriatric approach. Achieving it requires integrating efforts on several fronts. It may be helpful to think of functioning as an equation:

$$\text{Function} = \frac{\text{physical capabilities} \times \text{medical management} \times \text{motivation}}{\text{social and physical environment}}$$

This admitted oversimplification is meant as a reminder that function can be influenced on at least three levels. The first step is to remediate the remediable. Careful medical diagnosis and appropriate treatment are essential in good geriatric care. There is no virtue in the most

Table 3-5 Laboratory Assessment of the Elderly

Laboratory parameters unchanged*

Hemoglobin and hematocrit
White blood cell count
Platelet count
Electrolytes (sodium, potassium, chloride, bicarbonate)
Blood urea nitrogen
Liver function tests (transaminases, bilirubin, prothrombin time)
Free thyroxine index
Thyroid-stimulating hormone
Calcium
Phosphorus

Common abnormal laboratory parameters†

Parameter	Clinical significance
Sedimentation rate	Mild elevations (10–20 mm) may be an age-related change
Glucose	Glucose tolerance decreases (see Chapter 10)
Creatinine	Because lean body mass and daily endogenous creatinine production decline, high-normal and minimally elevated values may indicate substantially reduced renal function
Albumin	Average values decline (<0.5 g/ml) with age, especially in hospitalized elderly, but generally indicate undernutrition
Alkaline phosphatase	Mild elevations common in asymptomatic elderly; liver and Paget's disease should be considered if moderately elevated
Serum iron and iron-binding capacity	Decreased values are not an aging change and usually indicate undernutrition and/or gastrointestinal blood loss
Urinalysis	Asymptomatic pyuria and bacteriuria are common and rarely warrant treatment; hematuria is abnormal and needs further evaluation (see Chapters 6 and 10)
Chest radiographs	Interstitial changes are a common age-related finding; diffusely diminished bone density should generally indicate advanced osteoporosis (see Chapter 10)
Electrocardiogram	ST-segment and T-wave changes, atrial and ventricular arrhythmias, and various blocks are common in asymptomatic elderly and may not need specific evaluation or treatment (see Chapter 9)

*Aging changes do not occur in these parameters; abnormal values should prompt further evaluation.
†Includes normal aging and other age-related changes.

compassionate management of a condition that could have been eliminated by proper treatment.

Adequate medical management, then, is necessary but not sufficient. Once those conditions amenable to treatment have been addressed, the next step is to develop the environment that will best support the patient's autonomous function. Environmental barriers can be both physical and psychological. It is easier to recognize the former: stairs for the person with dyspnea, inaccessible cabinets for the wheelchair-bound, and so on. Psychological barriers refer especially to the dangers of risk aversion. Those most concerned about the patient may restrict activity in the name of protecting the patient or the institution. Hospitals are notoriously averse to risk; they will wheel patients rather than risk them falling when walking.

Risk aversion may be compounded by concerns about efficiency. Personal care is personnel-intensive. Rehabilitation is more time-consuming than providing the service. It takes much more time and patience to work with patients to encourage them to do things for themselves than to step in and do the task. But that pseudoefficiency breeds dependence.

Closely akin to this concept is the importance of motivation. The care of the elderly can be a story of negative spirals. If the care providers believe that the patient cannot improve, they will likely induce despair and discouragement in their charges. The effort becomes a self-fulfilling prophecy. Indeed, the opposite belief—that improvement is quite likely with work—may be the critical element in the success of geriatric evaluation units (Kane, 1988). Belief in the possibility of improvement can play another critical role in the care of the elderly. Psychologists have developed a useful paradigm referred to as "the innocent victim" (Lerner and Simmons, 1966; Lerner and Lichtman, 1968). The basic concept is that care givers respond in a hostile manner to those they feel impotent to help. If given a sense of empowerment, perhaps by using assessment tools such as the ones provided in this book, to gain a sense of a method for approaching the complex problems of the older persons, the care providers are likely to feel more positive toward those individuals and be more willing to work with them rather than avoid them. The more an information system can provide feedback on accomplishments and progress toward improved function, the more the provider will feel a positive sense about the older patient.

Several other important concepts about comprehensive functional assessment in the geriatric population were identified in a Consensus Development Conference at the National Institutes of Health in late 1987 (NIH, 1988) and are summarized in Table 3-6. To a large extent the nature of the assessment process is dictated by the purpose, setting, and timing of the assessment. Table 3-7 lists the different purposes and objectives of functional status measures. Generally functional assessment begins with a case-finding or screening approach in order to identify individuals for whom more in-depth and multidisciplinary assessment might be of benefit. Assessment is often carried out at points of transition, such as a threatened or actual

Table 3-6   Important Concepts for Geriatric Functional Assessment

The nature of the assessment should be dictated by its purpose, setting, and timing (see Table 3-7)

Input from multiple disciplines is often helpful, but routine multidisciplinary assessment is seldom cost-effective

Assessments should be targeted:
Initial screening to identify disciplines needed
Times of threatened or actual decline in status, impending change in living situation, and other stressful situations may yield greatest benefits

Standard instruments are useful, but there are numerous potential pitfalls:
Instruments should be reliable, sensitive, and valid for the purposes and setting of the assessment
How questions are asked can be critically important (e.g., performance vs. capability)
Discrepancies can arise between different informants (e.g., self-report vs. care giver's report)
Most standard instruments have not been tested for reliability and sensitivity to changes over time
Open-ended questions are helpful in complementing information from standardized instruments

The family's capabilities and willingness to provide care must be explored

The patient's preferences should be elicited and considered paramount in planning services

A strong link must exist between the assessment process and follow-up in the provision of services

Table 3-7 Purposes and Objectives of Functional Status Measures

Purpose	Objectives
Description	Develop normative data
	Depict elderly population along selected parameters
	Assess needs
	Describe outcomes associated with various interventions
Screening	Identify from among population at risk those individuals who should receive further assessment
Assessment	Make diagnosis
	Assign treatment
Monitoring	Observe changes in untreated conditions
	Review progress of those receiving treatment
Prediction	Permit scientifically based clinical interventions
	Make prognostic statements of expected outcomes on the basis of given conditions

decline in health status, or impending change in living situation. Without this type of targeting, the assessment of elderly people may be time-consuming and not cost-effective. Numerous standardized instruments are available to assist in the assessment process. Several examples of these instruments are presented in this chapter. Open-ended questioning can complement the information obtained using standard instruments in developing a more global assessment of the individual. For the most part, no one instrument has been shown to be better than others which assess the same domain, and there are numerous potential pitfalls in the use of standardized assessment instruments, which are discussed in detail elsewhere (Kane and Kane, 1981). The critical concept in using standardized instruments is that they should fit the purposes and setting for which they are intended, and there must be a solid link between the assessment process and the follow-up in providing services.

In this chapter, we will focus on the assessment of physical and mental function. The latter is discussed in greater detail in Chapter 4. Examples of measures of physical functioning are shown in Table 3-8. Physical functioning is measured along a spectrum. For disabled persons, one may focus on the ability to perform basic self-care tasks, often referred to as *activities of daily living* (ADL). The patient is

Table 3-8   Examples of Measures of Physical Functioning

Basic activities of daily living (ADL):
  Feeding
  Dressing
  Ambulation
  Toileting
  Bathing
  Transfer (from bed and toilet)
  Continence
  Grooming
  Communication
Instrumental activities of daily living (IADL):
  Writing
  Reading
  Cooking
  Cleaning
  Shopping
  Doing laundry
  Climbing stairs
  Using telephone
  Managing medication
  Managing money
  Ability to perform paid employment duties or outside work (e.g., gardening)
  Ability to travel (use public transportation, go out of town)

assessed on ability to conduct each of a series of basic activities. Data usually come from the patient or from a care giver (e.g., a nurse or family member) who has had a sufficient opportunity to observe the patient. In some cases, it may be more useful to have the patient actually demonstrate the ability to perform key tasks. Grading of performance is usually divided into three levels of dependency: (1) ability to perform the task without human assistance (one may wish to distinguish those persons who need mechanical aids like a walker but are still independent), (2) ability to perform task with some assistance, and (3) inability to perform, even with assistance. Sometimes the latter two classes can be collapsed to form a single category—dependent—which would be contrasted with independent functioning (with or without mechanical assistance).

One commonly used measure of functional status is the index of activities of daily living (ADL), developed by Katz and colleagues (Katz et al., 1963). Others, such as the Barthel Index, can be found elsewhere (Kane and Kane, 1981). The Katz ADL scale, shown in Table 3-9, provides a simple means of summarizing a person's ability to carry out basic tasks needed for self-care. Experience with it suggests that these functional abilities tend to be lost in a generally constant order from bathing to feeding. The ADL score provides an easy means of monitoring change in the basic functioning of an elderly patient and correlating the effects of intervention with that change. A few caveats should be noted:

1   A functional assessment of a patient in an acute state is likely to be invalid (e.g., a patient transferred from a natural environment to the alien world of the hospital, particularly at a time of stress).

2   With the ADL scale, the patient's motivation and the environmental structure are important determinants of performance.

3   It is critical to distinguish what a patient can do under proper circumstances and what is actually done during the patient's daily life. For example, it is not realistic to expect a nursing home patient to show self-care in bathing if the nursing home's policy forbids unattended bathing, or independence in dressing if the staff insists on dressing them as a matter of expectancy.

4   The ADL scale looks at only the lower bound of functioning. For persons able to perform ADL, we are concerned about their ability to do slightly more complex tasks necessary to function in our society. These tasks have been referred to as instrumental activities of daily living (IADL). Such tasks require a combination of physical and cognitive ability. They can be assessed in the same manner as ADL, both by report and by direct observation. Examples of IADL are shown in Table 3-8.

Assessing physical functioning is more complex than just asking if the patient wets the bed, can take a shower, or can do the laundry. Depending on the purposes and objectives of the assessment and the setting in which the assessment takes place, different techniques are useful. For example, ability to perform instrumental activities of daily living is critical in planning the hospital discharge of an elderly widower to his own home, whereas many IADL are less relevant if the

Table 3-9 Katz Index of Independence in Activities of Daily Living (ADL)

The index of independence in activities of daily living is based on an evaluation of the functional independence or dependence of patients in bathing, dressing, going to the toilet, transferring, continence, and feeding. Specific definitions of functional independence and dependence appear below the index.

A. Independent in feeding, continence, transferring, toileting, dressing, and bathing

B. Independent in all but one of these functions

C. Independent in all but bathing and one additional function

D. Independent in all but bathing, dressing, and one additional function

E. Independent in all but bathing, dressing, toileting, and one additional function

F. Independent in all but bathing, dressing, toileting, transferring, and one additional function

G. Dependent in all six functions

Other Dependent in at least two functions, but not classifiable as C, D, E, or F.

Independence means without supervision, direction, or active personal assistance, except as specifically noted below. This is based on actual status and not on ability. Patients who refuse to perform a function are considered as not performing the function, even though they are deemed able.

Bathing (sponge, shower, or tub)

Independent: needs assistance only in bathing a single part (as back or disabled extremity) or bathes self completely

Dependent: needs assistance in bathing more than one part of body and in getting in or out of tub or does not bathe self

Dressing

Independent: gets clothes from closets and drawers; puts on clothes, outer garments, braces; manages fasteners; act of tying shoes is excluded

Dependent: does not dress self or remains partly undressed

Toileting

Independent: gets to toilet; gets on and off toilet; arranges clothes, cleans organs of excretion (may manage own bedpan used at night only and may not be using mechanical supports)

Dependent: uses bedpan or commode or receives assistance in getting to and using toilet

Transfer

Independent: moves in and out of bed independently and moves in and out of chair independently (may or may not be using mechanical supports)

Dependent: assistance in moving in or out of bed and/or chair; does not perform one or more transfers

Continence

Independent: urination and defecation entirely self-controlled

Dependent: partial or total incontinence in urination or defecation, partial or total control by enemas, catheters, or regulated use of urinals and/or bedpans

Feeding

Independent: gets food from plate or its equivalent into mouth (precutting of meat and preparation of food, as buttering bread, are excluded from evaluation)

Dependent: assistance in act of feeding (see above); does not eat at all or parenteral feeding patient lives in an institution. Conflicting information may be obtained, depending on who provides it—the patient, a relative, or other care giver—but the discrepancy provides important insights. To add to these complexities, the interaction of physical function with psychological and socioeconomic functions must be considered.

Because many critical parameters of aging involve changes in cortical function, the clinician cannot ignore the intellectual performance of elderly patients. In Chapter 1 we noted how the elderly person's ability to cope may mask deficits. Perhaps nowhere is this capacity more pertinent than in assessing cognition. At some time in your career, you will encounter an older patient who appears perfectly lucid and able to conduct an informed conversation. Another clinician (too likely a supervisor) performing a more structured evaluation of mental status will uncover marked deficits in this presumably normal patient. A structured assessment of cognitive function should therefore be part of every complete geriatric assessment; at a minimum, it should test for orientation and memory. Two standardized mental status tests commonly used in the elderly are shown in Table 3-10 and Figure 3-2 (Folstein et al., 1975). Although these tests do not probe the variety of intellectual functions appropriate for a more detailed assessment, they are quick, easy, scorable, and reliable. More detailed assessment of cognitive function is discussed in Chapter 4.

The complexities of functional assessment should not overshadow the importance of this process to the evaluation of the elderly patient. It is beyond the scope of this text to review all the intricacies of functional assessment. Examples of commonly used standard assessments of the different functional domains and further details about the assessment process are available elsewhere (Kane and Kane, 1981; McDowell and Newell, 1987).

ENVIRONMENTAL ASSESSMENT

In Chapter 1 and earlier in this chapter we noted that patient function is the result of innate ability and environment. The geriatrician must thus be particularly concerned with the patient's environment. For many patients, an assessment should include an evaluation of the available and potential resources to maintain functioning.

Table 3-10   Short Portable Mental Status Questionnaire (SPMSQ)

Pertinent questions	Scoring
1. What is the date today (month/day/year)?	0–2 errors = intact
2. What day of the week is it?	3–4 errors = mild intellectual impairment
3. What is the name of this place?	5–7 errors = moderate intellectual impairment
4. What is your telephone number? (If no telephone, what is your street address?)	8–10 errors = severe intellectual impairment
5. How old are you?	
6. When were you born (month/day/year)?	Allow one more error if subject had no grade-school education
7. Who is the current president of the United States?	Allow one fewer error if subject has had education beyond high school
8. Who was the president just before him?	
9. What was your mother's maiden name?	
10. Subtract 3 from 20 and keep subtracting 3 from each new number all the way down.	

We are accustomed to the basic paradigm of assessment as a basis for medical treatment. It is considered poor practice to prescribe a drug in the absence of at least a working hypothesis about the derangement it is intended to correct. In a larger sense, these derangements represent disequilibria for which we offer chemical interventions. In older patients, the disequilibrium may be such that chemical responses are less appropriate to the problem. Just as physicians comfortably prescribe drugs, they should also be prepared to prescribe environmental interventions when necessary.

To continue the metaphor, the physician is no longer expected to compound or dispense drugs, nor to develop or obtain the social and environmental resources. The counterparts to the pharmacist are thus the social worker, the public health nurse, and the rehabilitation ther-

---

Figure 3-2   Example of a standardized mental status test (mini-mental state). ▶

I. ORIENTATION (Maximum score 10)

Ask "What is today's date?" Then ask specifically
for parts omitted; eg, "Can you also tell me
what season it is?"

Ask "Can you tell me the name of this hospital?"
"What floor are we on?"
"What town (or city) are we in?"
"What county are we in?"
"What state are we in?"

Date (eg, Jan.21) ____
Year .... —
Month.............. —
Day (eg, Monday)____
Season............ —
Hospital............ —
Floor............... —
Town/City......... —
County......... —
State .... —

II. REGISTRATION (Maximum score 3)

Ask the subject if you may test his/her memory, then say "ball", "flag", "tree"
clearly and slowly, about one second for each. After you have said all 3 words,
ask subject to repeat them. This first repetition determines the score (0–3) but
keep saying them (up to 6 trials) until the subject can repeat all 3 words. If
(s)he does not eventually learn all three, recall cannot be meaningfully tested

"ball"............... —
"flag"............... —
"tree"............... —

III. ATTENTION & CALCULATION (Maximum score 5)

Ask the subject to begin at 100 and count backward by 7. Stop after
5 subtractions (93, 86, 79, 72, 65). Score one point for each
correct number.

"93"................. —
"86"................. —
"79"................. —
"72"................. —
"65"................. —
or

If the subject cannot or will not perform this task, ask him/her to
spell the word "world" backwards (D,L,R,O,W). The score is one point
for each correctly placed letter, eg, DLROW=5, DLORW=3. Record how
the subject spelled "world" backwards: _____
DLROW

\# of correctly–
placed letters.... —

IV. RECALL (Maximum score 3)

Ask the subject to recall the three words you previously asked him/her
to remember (learned in Registration)

"ball"............... —
"flag"............... —
"tree"............... —

V. LANGUAGE (Maximum score 9)

Naming: Show the subject a wrist watch and ask "What is this?"
Repeat for pencil. Score one point for each item named correctly

Watch............. —
Pencil............. —

Repetition: Ask the subject to repeat, "No ifs, ands, or buts."
Score one point for correct repetition

Repetition........... —

3–Stage Command: Give the subject a piece of blank paper and say,
"Take the paper in your right hand, fold it in half and put it
on the floor," Score one point for each action performed correctly

Takes in rt. hand____
Folds in half........ —
Puts on floor...... —

Reading: On a blank piece of paper, print the sentence "Close your eyes."
in letters large enough for the subject to see clearly. Ask subject
to read it and do what it says. Score correct only if (s)he
actually closes his/her eyes

Closes eyes....... —

Writing: Give the subject a blank piece of paper and ask him/her
to write a sentence. It is to be written spontaneously. It must
contain a subject and verb and make sense. Correct grammer and
punctuation are not necessary

Writes sentence.____

Copying: On a clean piece of paper, draw intersecting pentagons,
each side about 1 inch, and ask subject to copy it exactly as
it is. All 10 angles must be present and two must intersect
to score 1 point. Tremor and rotation are ignored
Eg,

Draws pentagons ____

TOTAL SCORE _____

apist. The physician must know both the patient's problem and the appropriate drug therapy, as well as have the understanding to write an appropriate environmental prescription. Such an environmental prescription may include alterations in the physical environment (e.g., ramps, ground-floor apartment, grab bars, and elevated toilet seats for the bathroom), special services (e.g., meals on wheels, home-making, home nursing), increased social contact (e.g., friendly visiting, telephone reassurance, participation in recreational activities), or provision of critical elements (e.g., food or money).

The assessment of environment hinges on a previous assessment of functioning. The patient who is functioning well will likely require few environmental supports unless one expects an imminent change in functioning. However, the patient with decreased function deserves a careful assessment of the resources needed to enhance that functioning. In many instances, the resource assessment is geared to the functional problem. For example, does one with dyspnea on exertion have to climb stairs to get to one's apartment? Is someone available at critical times to assist a patient who is unable to transfer to get out of bed in the morning and back in at night? Is there someone to check on a patient from time to time, or is there someone to supervise medications? Is the environment safe, especially from factors that might contribute to falls? (See Chapter 7 and the Appendix for a Fall Hazard Checklist.)

The ability to identify the supports needed to maintain activity in the community may be the essential difference between enabling an older person to remain at home and transferring that person to an institution. Although identifying the need is not tantamount to providing the resource, it is an important first step. Sending a patient to a social worker with an unspecified request for help is equivalent to sending the patient to the pharmacist with a request for "drugs." We would hope that both professionals, the social worker and the pharmacist, will take pains to review the request critically and suggest more effective or less expensive treatments when appropriate. The prescription, whether for drugs or environmental modifications, is not ironclad, but it is an important document for conveying information. It is also important, and an unfortunate fact, that physicians and social workers should be especially alert to the possibility of elder abuse and search for clues suggestive of physical or emotional effects of such circumstances.

PREOPERATIVE EVALUATION

Internists and geriatricians are often called upon by surgeons and anesthesiologists to assess elderly patients before surgical procedures. Many excellent articles and texts are available which provide comprehensive reviews of the literature on perioperative care of the elderly patient and detailed recommendations (Gross and Kammerer, 1981; Goldman et al., 1982; Goldman, 1983; Kroenke, 1987; Cygan and Waitzkin, 1987). Table 3-11 lists several of the key factors involved in the preoperative evaluation of geriatric patients. Although numerous studies have examined the relative risk of various surgical procedures in elderly compared with younger populations, none have shown convincingly that age alone increases risk of surgical morbidity and mortality (Djokovik and Hedley-Whyte, 1979; Linn et al., 1982). Morbidity and mortality, however, are influenced by the presence and severity of systemic illnesses and whether the procedure is elective versus emergent. Thus, evaluating an elderly patient's preoperative status and risk for surgery requires a thorough assessment of cardiopulmonary and renal function, as well as nutritional and hydration status. Patients with a recent history of myocardial infarction, active angina, pulmonary edema, and severe aortic stenosis are at especially high risk (Goldman, 1983; Kroenke, 1987). Because physiological reserve declines with age, especially in the cardiovascular, pulmonary, and renal systems, routine preoperative measurement of physiological capacity is helpful in certain situations. A baseline arterial blood gas, assessment of pulmonary function, measurement of creatinine clearance, and in some patients modified exercise testing and/or dipyridamole thallium scanning may be indicated if specific indications exist (see Table 3-11). Underlying conditions that are prevalent in the elderly, such as hypertension, congestive heart failure, chronic obstructive lung disease, anemia, and undernutrition, need particularly careful management in the preoperative period. Medication regimens should be scrutinized in order to determine whether specific drugs should be continued or withheld (Cygan and Waitzkin, 1987). Careful consideration should also be given to perioperative prophylactic measures for the prevention of thromboembolism and infection, many of which have documented efficacy in specific situations (NIH, 1986; Oster et al., 1987; Yoshikowa and Norman, 1987).

Table 3-11   Key Factors in the Preoperative Evaluation of the Geriatric Patient

Age >70 is associated with an increased risk of complications and death
  Risk varies with the type of procedure and local complication rates
  Emergency procedures are associated with much higher risk
  Comorbid conditions, especially cardiovascular, are more important risk factors than age per se
The appropriateness and risk-benefit ratio of the proposed surgery must be carefully considered
Underlying conditions must be evaluated and optimally managed before nonemergent surgery:
  Cardiovascular disease, especially heart failure
  Pulmonary status
  Renal function
  Diabetes mellitus
  Thyroid disease (which is often occult)
  Anemia
  Nutrition
  Hydration, especially in patients on diuretics
Medication regimens should be carefully planned; some drugs should be continued, others should be withheld, and some require dosage adjustments*
Several cardiovascular conditions substantially increase risk:
  Myocardial infarction within 6 months
  Pulmonary edema
  Angina (especially if unstable)
  Severe aortic stenosis
Specific laboratory evaluations may be helpful in some situations, e.g.:
  Pulmonary function tests and arterial blood gas with respiratory symptoms, obesity, chest deformity (e.g., kyphoscoliosis), abnormal chest radiographs, planned thoracic or upper abdominal procedure
  Exercise test or dipyridamole-thallium scanning with uncertain or borderline cardiovascular status
  Creatinine clearance with unstable or borderline renal function, or the use of nephrotoxic or renally excreted drugs
The documented effectiveness, risks, and benefits of perioperative prophylactic measures should be considered†
  Antithrombotic prophylaxis
  Antimicrobial prophylaxis

---

*See Kroenke (1987).
†See NIH (1986), Oster et al. (1987), and Yoshikowa and Norman (1987).

Although many surgeons and anesthesiologists tend to favor regional over general anesthesia for the elderly, there are little, if any, data to support this bias. Comparisons of mortality rates after different types of anesthesia for hip fracture repair do not show differences in mortality (Wickstrom et al., 1982; Davis et al., 1987). Local and regional anesthesia (e.g., epidural), in fact, have several potential disadvantages. Many elderly patients in whom these techniques are used require added intravenous sedation and/or analgesia, thus increasing the risks of perioperative cardiovascular and mental status changes. Significant cardiovascular changes can, in fact, occur during regional anesthesia; thus invasive monitoring may be required in some patients. Neither the incidence of deep vein thrombosis nor the amount of blood loss seems to be substantially decreased compared to general anesthesia. Finally, many patients fail attempts at regional anesthesia and preoperative preparation for general anesthesia must be done anyway. Thus, decisions about the type of anesthesia should be carefully individualized on the basis of patient factors, the nature of the procedure, and the preferences of the surgical team.

Finally, part of the role of the geriatrician in the preoperative assessment is to provide input on the appropriateness of the procedure. Recent publications have suggested that a substantial proportion of major procedures may be performed for inappropriate indications, on the basis of expert panel consensus (Chassin et al., 1987; Winslow et al., 1988). Geriatricians will need to become familiar with these types of studies and apply the data to the many other individual factors that determine the appropriateness and timing of surgical procedures in the elderly.

The Appendix offers a set of suggested medical forms for recording history and physical examination information particularly germane to the management of elderly patients. In addition to these forms, forms for social and environmental assessment are also provided.

REFERENCES

Allen CM, Becker PM, McVey LJ, et al: A randomized controlled clinical trial of a geriatric consultation team: Compliance with recommendations. *JAMA* 255:2617–2621, 1986.

Becker PM, McVey LJ, Slatz CC, et al: Hospital-acquired complications in a randomized controlled clinical trial of a geriatric consultation team. *JAMA* 257:2313–2317, 1987.

Chassin MR, Kosecoff J, Park RE, et al: Does inappropriate use explain geographic variations in the use of health care services. *JAMA* 256:2533–2537, 1986.

Cygan R, Waitzkin H: Stopping and restarting medications in the perioperative period. *J Gen Intern Med* 2:270–283, 1987.

Davis FM, Woolner DF, Frampton C, et al: Prospective multicenter trial of mortality following general or spinal anaesthesia for hip fracture surgery in the elderly. *Br J Anaesth* 59; 1080–1088, 1987.

Djokovik JL, Hedley-Whyte J: Prediction of outcome of surgery and anesthesia in patients over 80. *JAMA* 242:2301–2306, 1979.

Folstein MF, Folstein S, McHuth PR: Mini-mental state: A practical method for grading the cognitive state of patients for the clinician. *J Psychiatr Res* 12:189–198, 1975.

Goldman DR, Grown FH, Levy WK, et al (eds): *Medical Care of the Surgical Patient—A Problem-Oriented Approach to Management.* Philadelphia, Lippincott, 1982.

Goldman L: Cardiac risks and complications of noncardiac surgery. *Ann Intern Med* 98:504–513, 1983.

Gross R, Kammerer W: Medical consultation on surgical services: An annotated bibliography. *Ann Intern Med* 95:523–529, 1981.

Hendriksen C, Lund E, Stromgard E: Consequences of assessment and intervention among elderly people: Three year randomized controlled trial. *Br Med J* 289:1522–1524, 1984.

Hogan DB, Fox RA, Bradley BWD, et al: Effect of a geriatric consultation service on management of patients in an acute care hospital. *Can Med Assoc J* 136:713–717, 1987.

Kane RL, Kane RA: *Assessing the Elderly: A Practical Guide to Measurement.* Lexington, MA, Heath, 1981.

Kane RL, Beyond caring: The challenge to geriatrics. *J Am Geriatr Soc* 36:467–472, 1988.

Katz S, Ford A, Moskowitz R, et al: The index of ADL: A standardized measure of biological and psychosocial function. *JAMA* 185:914–919, 1963.

Kroenke MK: Preoperative evaluation: The assessment and management of surgical risk. *J Gen Intern Med* 2:257–269, 1987.

Lerner MJ, Simmons CH: Observer's reaction to the "innocent victim": Compassion or rejection? *J Pers Soc Psychol* 4:203–210, 1966.

Lerner MJ, Lichtman PR: Effects of perceived norms on attitudes and altruistic behavior toward a dependent other. *J Pers Soc Psychol* 9:226–232, 1968.

Linn BS, Linn MW, Warren N: Evaluation of results of surgical procedures in the elderly. *Ann Surg* 195:90–96, 1982.

McDowell I, Newell C: *Measuring Health: A Guide to Rating Scales and Questionnaires.* New York, Oxford University Press, 1987.

NIH Consensus Conference: Prevention of venous thrombosis and pulmonary embolism. *JAMA* 256:744–749, 1986.

NIH Consensus Development Conference Statement: Geriatric assessment methods for clinical decision-making. *J Am Geriatr Soc* 36:342–347, 1988.

Oster G, Tuden RL, Colditz GA: A cost-effectiveness analysis of prophylaxis against deep-vein thrombosis in major orthopedic surgery. *JAMA* 257:203, 1987.

Rubenstein LZ: Geriatric assessment: An overview of its impacts. *Clin Geriatr Med* 3:1–27, 1987.

Rubenstein LZ, Josephson KR, Wieland GD, et al: Effectiveness of a geriatric evaluation unit: A randomized clinical trial. *N Engl J Med* 311:1664–1670, 1984.

Saltz CC, McVey LJ, Becker PM, et al: Impact of a geriatric consultation team on discharge placement and repeat hospitalization. *Gerontologist* 28:344–350, 1988.

Vetter NJ, Jones DA, Victor CR: Effects of health visitors working with elderly patients in general practice. *J Roy Coll Gen Pract* 29:733–742, 1979.

Wickstrom I, Holmberg I, Steffanson T: Survival of female patients after hip fracture surgery: A comparison of five anesthetic methods. *Acta Anaesth Scand* 26:602–614, 1982.

Williams M: Outpatient geriatric evaluation. *Clin Geriatr Med* 3:175–184, 1987.

Winslow CM, Solomon DH, Chassin MR, et al: The appropriateness of carotid endarterectomy. *N Engl J Med* 318:721–727, 1988.

Yoshikowa TT, Norman DC: *Aging and Clinical Practice: Infectious Diseases.* New York, Igaku-Shoin, 1987.

SUGGESTED READINGS

Applegate WB: Use of assessment instruments in clinical settings. *J Am Geriatr Soc* 35:45–50, 1987.

Besdine RW: The educational utility of comprehensive functional assessment in the elderly. *J Am Geriatr Soc* 31:651–656, 1983.

Deyo RA, Inui TS: Toward clinical applications of health status measures: Sensitivity of scales to clinically important changes. *Health Serv Res* 19:275–289, 1984.

Duke University Center for the Study of Aging and Human Development: *Multidimensional Functional Assessment: The OARS Methodology* (2d ed). Durham, NC, 1978.

Falcone AR: Comprehensive functional assessment as an administrative tool. *J Am Geriatr Soc* 31(11):642–650, 1983.

Feinstein AR, Josephy BR, Wells CK: Scientific and clinical problems in indexes of functional disability. *Ann Intern Med* 105:413–420, 1986.

Fillenbaum GG: Screening the elderly: A brief instrumental activities of daily living measure. *J Am Geriatr Soc* 33:698–706, 1985.

Katz S, Branch LG, Branson MH, et al: Active life expectancy. *N Engl J Med* 309:1218–1224, 1983.

Libow LS, Sherman FT: Interviewing and history taking, in Libow LS, Sherman FT (eds): *The Core of Geriatric Medicine*. St Louis, Mosby, 1981.

Rubenstein LZ, Campbell LJ, Kane RL (eds): Geriatric assessment. *Clin Geriatr Med* 3:1–230, 1987.

Part Two

Differential Diagnosis and Management

Chapter 4

Confusion

Few topics in geriatric medicine are as confusing as confusion. Nor is any topic of greater importance. The appropriate diagnosis and management of elderly patients exhibiting symptoms and signs of confusion can make a critical difference to their overall health and ability to function independently.

In the community, about 5 percent of those older than 65, and close to 20 percent of those older than 75, have some degree of clinically detectable impairment of cognitive function. As more people live into the tenth decade of life, the chance that they will develop some form of dementia approaches one in three. In nursing homes, 50 to 80 percent of those older than 65 have some degree of cognitive impairment (Gurland and Cross, 1982; Rovner et al., 1986). Between one-third and one-half of elderly patients admitted to acute care medical and surgical services will also exhibit varying degrees of confusion (Gillick et al., 1982; Warshaw et al., 1982).

Misdiagnosis and inappropriate management of these patients

can cause substantial morbidity among the patients and hardship to their families and result in millions of dollars in health care expenditure.

This chapter provides a practical framework for diagnosing and managing elderly patients who appear confused. Details of the anatomy, biochemistry, and pathophysiology of these disorders can be found in the Suggested Readings list at the end of this chapter.

DEFINING CONFUSION

Imprecise definition of the abnormalities of cognitive function in elderly patients labeled as "confused" has led to problems in the diagnosis and management of these patients. *Confusion* has been defined as a "mental state in which reactions to environmental stimuli are inappropriate; a state in which the person is bewildered or perplexed or unable to orientate himself" (*Stedman's Medical Dictionary,* 1976). This type of definition, although descriptive, is too broad and imprecise to be clinically useful. Thus, labels such as "confused" or "confused at times" should be avoided. Descriptions such as "impairment of mental function" or "cognitive impairment" coupled with careful documentation of specific abnormalities will yield more precise and clinically useful information. Such documentation is best accomplished by means of a standard mental status examination.

A thorough mental status examination has several components (Table 4-1). In evaluating an elderly patient who appears confused,

Table 4-1   Key Aspects of Mental Status Examinations

State of consciousness
General appearance and behavior
Orientation
Memory (short- and long-term)
Language
Intelligence, perception, and other cognitive functions (e.g., calculations)
Insight and problem-solving ability
Judgment
Thought content
Mood and affect

attention should focus on each of these components in a systematic manner. Recording observations in each of these areas is critical to recognizing and evaluating changes over time. Standardized and validated measures of cognitive function such as the ones shown in Chapter 3 can be helpful screening tools in these assessments as well as in subsequent monitoring. However, none of these is sufficiently sensitive or specific to be used as the only evidence for a specific diagnosis. Prior educational level or poor baseline intellectual function can make the interpretation of standardized test results difficult. Thus, scores on one or more of these tests should not be used to replace a more comprehensive examination including all the components listed in Table 4-1.

Important information can be gleaned unobtrusively from simply observing and interacting with the patient during the history. Is the patient alert? Does the patient respond appropriately to questions? How is the patient groomed? Are the patient's clothes soiled? Orientation to person, place, time, and situation can sometimes be assessed during the history as well.

Questions relating to specific areas of cognitive functioning should be introduced in a nonthreatening manner, because many patients with early deficits will respond defensively. Each of the three basic components of memory should be tested: immediate recall (e.g., repeating digits), recent memory (e.g., recalling three objects after a few minutes), and remote memory (e.g., ability to give details of early life). Language and other cognitive functions should be carefully evaluated. Is the patient's speech clear? Can the patient read (and understand) and write? Does there seem to be a good general fund of knowledge (e.g., current events)? Other cognitive functions that can be specifically tested include the ability to perform simple calculations and to copy diagrams. The ability to interpret proverbs abstractly is a sensitive indicator of cognitive function and is easy to test.

Judgment and insight can usually be assessed during the examination without asking specific questions, although input from family members or other care givers can be helpful and sometimes necessary. Any abnormal thought content should also be noted during the examination; bizarre ideas, mood-incongruent thoughts, and delusions (especially paranoid delusions) may be prominent in elderly patients with cognitive impairment and are important both diagnostically and therapeutically.

Throughout the examination, the patient's mood and affect should be assessed. Depression and emotional lability are common in elderly patients with cognitive impairment; failure to recognize these abnormalities can lead to improper diagnosis and management. In some patients, such as very intelligent or poorly educated or low-intelligence individuals and those in whom depression is suspected, more detailed neuropsychological testing by an experienced psychologist is helpful in more precisely defining abnormalities in cognitive function and in differentiating between the many and often interacting underlying causes (LaRue, 1982).

DIFFERENTIAL DIAGNOSIS OF CONFUSION IN THE ELDERLY

The causes of confusion in the elderly are myriad. Similar to many other disorders in elderly patients, confusion often results from multiple interacting processes, rather than a single causative factor. Accurate diagnosis depends on specifically defining abnormalities in mental status and cognitive function and on consistent definitions for clinical syndromes.

Several clinical entities are associated with cognitive impairment in the elderly (Table 4-2). These disorders can be broadly categorized into three groups:

1   Acute disorders, usually associated with acute illness, drugs, and environmental factors (i.e., delirium)
2   More slowly progressive impairment of cognitive function, as seen in most dementias, amnestic syndromes, and benign senescent forgetfulness
3   Impaired cognitive function associated with affective disorders and psychoses

Old age alone does not cause impairment of cognitive function of sufficient severity to render an individual dysfunctional. Mild, recent-memory loss and slowed thinking and reaction time are com-

Table 4-2   Disorders Associated with Cognitive Impairment in the Elderly

Delirium
Dementia
Depression (pseudodementia)
Paranoid states and other psychoses
Amnestic syndromes
Aging changes (e.g., "benign senescent forgetfulness")

mon. Elderly patients are often labeled "senile" because they are unable to answer a question, or because they are not given adequate time to respond. Other age-associated disorders such as impaired hearing can also lead to mislabeling an elderly patient as "confused" or "senile."

Three questions are helpful in making an accurate diagnosis:

1 Has the onset of the abnormalities been acute (i.e., over a few hours or a day)?
2 Are there physical factors (i.e., medical illness, sensory deprivation, drugs) that may be contributing to the abnormalities?
3 Are there psychological factors (i.e., depression and/or psychosis) contributing to or complicating the impairments in cognitive function?

These questions focus on identifying treatable conditions, which, when diagnosed and treated, might result in substantially improved cognitive function.

Major disorders causing impairment of cognitive function in the elderly are briefly discussed below. The Suggested Readings provide more detailed discussions of these disorders.

Delirium

Delirium is an acute or subacute alteration in mental status especially common in the elderly. In the past, a variety of labels have been used to describe delirious patients (including acute confusional state, acute brain syndrome, metabolic encephalopathy, and toxic psychosis). The *Diagnostics and Statistics Manual of Mental Disorders* (DSM III-R) (American Psychiatric Association, 1987) defines diagnostic cri-

teria for delirium (Table 4-3). The key features of this disorder
include:

- Disturbed cognition
- Disorder of attention
- Symptoms and signs developing over a short period of time
(hours to days)
- Fluctuation of the symptoms and signs, especially at night
- Interruption of normal sleep-wake cycle
- Abnormal psychomotor behavior
- Improvement of normalization of mental function after the
underlying condition has been appropriately treated

Table 4-3   Diagnostic Criteria for Delirium

A. Reduced ability to maintain attention to external stimuli (e.g., questions must
be repeated because attention wanders) and to appropriately shift attention to
new external stimuli (e.g., perseverates answer to a previous question)

B. Disorganized thinking, as indicated by rambling, irrelevant, or incoherent
speech

C. At least two of the following:
1. Reduced level of consciousness, e.g., difficulty keeping awake during
examination
2. Perceptual disturbances: misinterpretations, illusions, or hallucinations
3. Disturbance of sleep-wake cycle with insomnia or daytime sleepiness
4. Increased or decreased psychomotor activity
5. Disorientation to time, place, or person
6. Memory impairment, e.g., inability to learn new material, such as the names
of several unrelated objects after 5 min, or to remember past events, such
as history of current episode of illness

D. Clinical features develop over a short period of time (usually hours to days)
and tend to fluctuate over the course of a day

E. Either 1 or 2:
1. Evidence from the history, physical examination, or laboratory tests of a
specific organic factor (or factors) judged to be etiologically related to the
disturbance
2. In the absence of such evidence, an etiologic organic factor which can be
presumed if the disturbance cannot be accounted for by any nonorganic
mental disorder, e.g., manic episode accounting for agitation and sleep
disturbance

Source: American Psychiatric Association, 1987.

The disorder of attention (often referred to as "clouding of consciousness") with the suddenness of onset and the fluctuating cognitive status are the major features that distinguish delirium from other causes of impaired cognitive function. Delirium is characterized by difficulty in sustaining attention to external and internal stimuli, sensory misperceptions (e.g., illusions), and a fragmented or disordered stream of thought. Disturbances of psychomotor activity (such as restlessness, picking at bedclothes, attempting to get out of bed, sluggishness, drowsiness, and generally decreased psychomotor activity) and emotional disturbances (anxiety, fear, irritability, anger, apathy) are very common in delirious patients. Neurological signs (except asterixis) are uncommon in delirium.

Many factors predispose the elderly to the development of delirium, including impaired sensory functioning and sensory deprivation, sleep deprivation, immobilization, transfer to an unfamiliar environment, and psychosocial stresses such as bereavement. It is extremely important to recognize delirium rapidly because it is often related to other reversible conditions and its development may be a poor prognostic sign. It is also important to differentiate delirium from dementia because the latter is not immediately life-threatening, and inappropriately labeling a delirious patient as demented may delay the diagnosis of serious and treatable conditions. It is not possible to make the diagnosis of dementia when delirium is present in a patient with previously normal or unknown cognitive function; it must await the treatment of all of the potentially reversible causes of delirium discussed below. Table 4-4 shows some of the key clinical features that are helpful in differentiating delirium from dementia.

A complete list of conditions that can cause delirium in the elderly would be too long to be useful in a clinical setting. Table 4-5 lists some of the common causes of this disorder. Several of them deserve further attention.

Each elderly patient who becomes acutely "confused" should be evaluated to rule out treatable conditions such as metabolic disorders, infections, and causes for decreased cardiac output (i.e., dehydration, acute blood loss, heart failure).

Small cortical strokes, which do not produce focal symptoms or signs, can cause delirium. These events may be difficult or impossible to diagnose with certainty, but there should be a high index of suspi-

Table 4-4   Key Features Differentiating Delirium from Dementia

Feature	Delirium	Dementia
Onset	Acute, often at night	Insidious
Course	Fluctuating, with lucid intervals, during day; worse at night	Generally stable over course of day
Duration	Hours to weeks	Months or years
Awareness	Reduced	Clear
Alertness	Abnormally low or high	Usually normal
Attention	Hypoalert or hyperalert, distractible; fluctuates over course of day	Usually normal
Orientation	Usually impaired for time, tendency to mistake unfamiliar for familiar place and persons	Often impaired
Memory	Immediate and recent impaired	Recent and remote impaired
Thinking	Disorganized	Impoverished
Perception	Illusions and hallucinations (usually visual) relatively common	Usually normal
Speech	Incoherent, hesitant, slow, or rapid	Difficulty in finding words
Sleep-wake cycle	Always disrupted	Often fragmented sleep
Physical illness or drug toxicity	Either or both present	Often absent, especially in Alzheimer's disease

Source: After Lipkowski, 1987.

cion for this diagnosis in certain subgroups of elderly patients—especially in those with a history of hypertension, previous strokes, transient ischemic attacks, or cardiac arrhythmias. If delirium recurs, a source for emboli should be sought and associated conditions (such as hypertension) should be treated optimally.

Drugs are a major cause of acute, as well as chronic, impairment of cognitive function in elderly patients (Larson et al., 1986, 1987). Table 4-6 lists commonly prescribed drugs that can cause or contribute to delirium (as well as dementia). Every attempt should be made

Table 4-5   Common Causes of Delirium

Metabolic disorders
   Electrolyte abnormalities
   Acid-base disturbances
   Hypoxia
   Hypercarbia
   Hypo- or hyperglycemia
   Azotemia
Infections
Decreased cardiac output
   Dehydration
   Acute blood loss
   Acute myocardial infarction
   Congestive heart failure
Stroke (small cortical)
Drugs (see Table 4-6)
Intoxication (alcohol, other)
Hypo- or hyperthermia
Acute psychoses
Transfer to unfamiliar surroundings (especially when sensory input is diminished)
Other
   Fecal impaction
   Urinary retention

to avoid or discontinue any medication that may be worsening cognitive function in a delirious elderly patient.

Environmental factors, especially rapid changes in location (such as being hospitalized, going on a vacation, or entering a nursing home) and sensory deprivation, can precipitate delirium in many elderly persons. This is especially true of those with early forms of dementia (see below). The "sundowner syndrome" (confusion and agitation with the onset of evening) is a familiar example of this problem (Evans, 1987). Measures such as preparing elderly patients for changes in location, placing familiar objects in the new surroundings, and maximizing sensory input with lighting, clocks, and calendars may help prevent or manage delirium in some patients, although controlled trials of such interventions are lacking.

Fecal impaction and urinary retention, common in elderly patients (especially those in acute care hospitals), can have dramatic effects on cognitive function; the response to relief from these conditions can be just as impressive.

Table 4-6   Drugs That Can Cause or Contribute to Delirium and Dementia

Analgesics	Cardiovascular
Narcotic	Atropine
Codeine	Digitalis
Meperidine	Diuretics
Morphine	Lidocaine
Pentazocine	Hypoglycemics
Propoxyphene	Insulin
Nonnarcotic	Sulfonylureas
Indomethacin	Psychotropic drugs
Antihistamines	Antianxiety drugs
Diphenhydramine	Benzodiazepines
Hydroxyzine	Antidepressant drugs
Antihypertensives	Lithium
Clonidine	Tricyclics
Hydralazine	Antipsychotics
Methyldopa	Haloperidol
Propranolol	Thiothixene
Reserpine	Thioridazine
Antimicrobials	Chlorpromazine
Gentamicin	Hypnotics
Isoniazid	Barbiturates
Antiparkinsonism drugs	Benzodiazepines
Amantadine	Chloral hydrate
Bromocriptine	Others
Carbidopa	Cimetidine
L-Dopa	Steroids
Trihexyphenidyl and other anticholinergics	

Dementia

Dementia is a clinical syndrome involving loss of intellectual functions and memory of sufficient severity to cause dysfunction in daily living. Its key features include:

- A gradually progressing course (usually over months to years)
- No disorder of alertness (i.e., normal consciousness)

Imprecise definitions and incomplete differential diagnoses have led to the underdiagnosis, misdiagnosis, and overdiagnosis of this syndrome in many clinical settings (especially acute care hospitals and nursing homes). Given the present state of knowledge, an attempt should be made to diagnose these patients more accurately. Tables 4-7 and 4-8 list the diagnostic criteria for dementia, and for the most common form of dementia, Alzheimer's disease. With the use of these definitions and a careful history, physical examination, and selected laboratory tests, an accurate diagnosis should be made in over 90 percent of patients with impaired cognitive functioning.

Table 4-7 Diagnostic Criteria for Dementia

I. Criteria for dementia
  A. Demonstrable evidence of impairment in short- and long-term memory. Impairment in short-term memory (inability to learn new information) may be indicated by inability to remember three objects after 5 min; long-term memory impairment (inability to remember information that was known in the past) may be indicated by inability to remember past personal information (e.g., what happened yesterday, birthplace, occupation) or facts of common knowledge (e.g., past presidents, well-known dates)
  B. At least one of the following:
    1. Impairment in abstract thinking, as indicated by inability to find similarities and differences between related words, difficulty in defining words and concepts, and other similar tasks
    2. Impaired judgment, as indicated by inability to make reasonable plans to deal with interpersonal, family, and job-related problems and issues
    3. Other disturbances of higher cortical function, such as aphasia (disorder of language), apraxia (inability to carry out motor activities despite intact comprehension and motor function), agnosia (failure to recognize or identify objects despite intact sensory function), and "constructional difficulty" (e.g., inability to copy three-dimensional figures, assemble blocks, or arrange sticks in specific designs)
    4. Personality change, i.e., alteration or accentuation of premorbid traits
  C. The disturbance in A and B significantly interferes with work or usual social activities or relationships with others
  D. Not occurring exclusively during the course of delirium (see Tables 4-3 and 4-4)
  E. Either 1 or 2:
    1. There is evidence from the history, physical examination, or laboratory tests of a specific organic factor (or factors) judged to be etiologically related to the disturbance
    2. In the absence of such evidence, an etiologic organic factor can be presumed if the disturbance cannot be accounted for by a nonorganic mental disorder, e.g., major depression accounting for cognitive impairment

Table 4-7   Diagnostic Criteria for Dementia (*Continued*)

II. Criteria for primary degenerative dementia of the Alzheimer's type (see also Table 4-8)
   A. Dementia (IA–E)
   B. Insidious onset with a generally progressive deteriorating course
   C. Exclusion of all other specific causes of dementia by history, physical examination, and laboratory tests
III. Criteria for multi-infarct dementia
   A. Dementia (IA–E)
   B. Stepwise deteriorating course with "patchy" distribution of deficits (i.e., affecting some functions but not others) early in the course
   C. Focal neurological signs and symptoms (e.g., exaggeration of deep tendon reflexes, extensor plantar response, pseudobulbar palsy, gait abnormalities, weakness of an extremity)
   D. Evidence from history, physical examination, or laboratory tests of significant cerebrovascular disease (recorded on Axis III) that is judged to be etiologically related to the disturbance.
IV. Criteria for severity of dementia
   Mild: Although work or social activities are significantly impaired, the capacity for independent living remains, with adequate personal hygiene and relatively intact judgment
   Moderate: Independent living is hazardous, and some degree of supervision is necessary
   Severe: Activities of daily living are so impaired that continual supervision is required, e.g., inability to maintain minimal personal hygiene; largely incoherent or mute

Source: After American Psychiatric Association, 1987.

Aging itself does not cause dementia. Aging is associated with anatomic and biochemical changes in the central nervous system and, in some elderly people, detectable changes in memory ("benign senescent forgetfulness") and other psychomotor performance; however, these changes are not of sufficient severity to cause dysfunction in daily life. It is also important to recognize that dementia often coexists with delirium and depression, both treatable disorders.

Dementia in the elderly can be grouped into four broad categories:

Primary degenerative dementia	50–60%
Multi-infarct dementia	10–20%
Reversible or partially reversible dementias	20–30%
Other disorders (mainly neurologic)	5–10%

Table 4-8 NINCDS-ADRDA Criteria for Clinical Diagnosis of Alzheimer's Disease

I. The criteria for the clinical diagnosis of *probable* Alzheimer's disease include:
   A. Dementia established by clinical examination and documented by the Mini-Mental Test, Blessed Dementia Scale, or some similar examination, and confirmed by neuropsychological tests
   B. Deficits in two or more areas of cognition
   C. Progressive worsening of memory and other cognitive functions
   D. No disturbance of consciousness
   E. Onset between ages 40 and 90, most often after age 65
   F. Absence of systemic disorders or other brain diseases that in and of themselves could account for the progressive deficits in memory and cognition

II. The diagnosis of *probable* Alzheimer's disease is supported by:
   A. Progressive deterioration of specific cognitive functions such as language (aphasia), motor skills (apraxia), and perception (agnosia)
   B. Impaired activities of daily living and altered patterns of behavior
   C. Family history of similar disorders, particularly if confirmed neuropathologically
   D. Laboratory results of
      1. Normal lumbar puncture as evaluated by standard techniques
      2. Normal pattern or nonspecific changes in EEG, such as increased slow-wave activity
      3. Evidence of cerebral atrophy on CT with progression documented by serial observation

III. Other clinical features consistent with the diagnosis of *probable* Alzheimer's disease, after exclusion of causes of dementia other than Alzheimer's disease, including:
   A. Plateaus in the course of progression of the illness
   B. Associated symptoms of depression, insomnia, incontinence, delusions, illusions, hallucinations; catastrophic verbal, emotional, or physical outbursts; sexual disorders; and weight loss
   C. Other neurological abnormalities in some patients, especially with more advanced disease and including motor signs such as increased muscle tone, myoclonus, or gait disorder
   D. Seizures in advanced disease
   E. CT normal for age

IV. Features that make the diagnosis of *probable* Alzheimer's disease uncertain or unlikely include:
   A. Sudden, apoplectic onset
   B. Focal neurological findings such as hemiparesis, sensory loss, visual field deficits, and incoordination early in the course of the illness
   C. Seizures or gait disturbances at the onset or very early in the course of the illness

Table 4-8   NINCDS-ADRDA Criteria for Clinical Diagnosis of Alzheimer's Disease (*Continued*)

V. Clinical diagnosis of *possible* Alzheimer's disease:

   A. May be made on the basis of the dementia syndrome, in the absence of other neurological, psychiatric, or systemic disorders sufficient to cause dementia, and in the presence of variations in the onset, in the presentation, or in the clinical course

   B. May be made in the presence of a second systemic or brain disorder sufficient to produce dementia, which is not considered to be the cause of the dementia

   C. Should be used in research studies when a single, gradually progressive severe cognitive deficit is identified in the absence of other identifiable cause

VI. Criteria for diagnosis of *definite* Alzheimer's disease:

   A. The clinical criteria for probable Alzheimer's disease

   B. Histopathologic evidence obtained from a biopsy or autopsy

VII. Classification of Alzheimer's disease for research purposes should specify features that may differentiate subtypes of the disorder, such as:

   A. Familial occurrence

   B. Onset before age of 65

   C. Presence of trisomy-21

   D. Coexistence of other relevant conditions such as Parkinson's disease

Source: From McKhann et al., 1984 (report of the work group of the National Institute of Neurological and Communicative Disorders and Stroke and the Alzheimer's Disease and Related Disorders Association).

Table 4-9 lists the types and causes of dementia, classified after the 1987 NIH Consensus Conference (NIH, 1987).

Reversible Causes   It is especially important to rule out treatable and potentially reversible causes of dementia (Table 4-9). A mnemonic has been devised to help in identifying many of the potentially reversible causes of dementia (Lamy, 1980):

   D   Drugs

   E   Emotional disorders

   M   Metabolic or endocrine disorders

   E   Eye and ear dysfunctions

   N   Nutritional deficiencies

   T   Tumor and trauma

   I   Infections

   A   Arteriosclerotic complications (i.e., myocardial infarction, heart failure) and alcohol

Table 4-9 Types and Causes of Dementia in the Elderly

Potentially arrestable or reversible conditions*
  Intoxications (drugs, including alcohol; see Table 4-6)
  Infections of the central nervous system
  Metabolic disorders
  Nutritional disorders
  Vascular diseases (multi-infarct dementia, other)
  Space-occupying lesions
  Normal pressure hydrocephalus
  Depression ("depressive pseudodementia")
Progressive degenerative diseases
  With no other important neurological findings (other than dementia)
    Alzheimer's disease
    Pick's disease
  With other prominent neurological signs
    Parkinson's disease
    Huntington's disease
    Progressive supranuclear palsy
    Other rare degenerative diseases

*Many of these conditions are only partially arrestable or reversible; some may not be at all. See text for a helpful mnemonic.
Source: After NIH Consensus Conference, 1987.

These disorders can be detected by careful history, physical examination, and selected laboratory studies (see below). Drugs known to cause abnormalities in cognitive function (Table 4-6) should be discontinued whenever feasible. There should be a high index of suspicion regarding excessive alcohol intake in elderly patients. Although precise data are not available and the incidence will vary considerably in different populations, alcohol intake is easily missed in the elderly and can cause dementia as well as delirium, depression, falls, and other medical complications.

One particular disorder, depressive pseudodementia, deserves special emphasis. *Depressive pseudodementia* is a term that has been used to refer to patients who have reversible or partially reversible impairments of cognitive function caused by depression. Depression may coexist with dementia in over one-third of outpatients with dementia and an even greater proportion in nursing homes (Rovner et al., 1986; Lazarus et al., 1987; Merriam et al., 1988). The interrelationship between depression and dementia is very complex. Many patients with early forms of dementia become depressed. Sorting out how much of the cognitive impairment is caused by depression and how much by an organic factor(s) can be extremely difficult. Table 4-10 compares some clinical characteristics that can be helpful in differentiating a primary dementia from pseudodementia. In addition to these characteristics, detailed neuropsychological testing, performed by a psychologist or other health care professional skilled in the use of these tools, can be helpful in many patients (LaRue, 1982). At times, even after a complete assessment, uncertainty still exists regarding the role of depression in producing intellectual deficits. Under these circumstances, a careful trial of antidepressants (in rare instances, electroconvulsive therapy) is justified to facilitate the diagnosis and often helps improve overall (but not cognitive) functioning (Reifler et al., 1986).

Primary Degenerative Dementia   Primary degenerative dementia (also known as *Alzheimer's type of dementia*) is a disorder involving alterations in the number, structure, and function of neurons in certain areas of the cerebral cortex. (Pick's disease is a rare condition that can also cause primary degenerative dementia.) Although no primary cause has been identified for this disorder, current research has focused on abnormal proteins found in neurofibrillary tangles and neuritic plaques, alterations in cholinergic activity in specific areas of the brain, slow virus infections, chromosomal abnormalities, and environmental and genetic factors. (See Suggested Readings for greater detail on the potential causes of primary dementias.)

Primary degenerative dementia is a clinical diagnosis, made by excluding other disorders. Definitive diagnosis can be made only at autopsy or by brain biopsy, which cannot currently be justified for purely diagnostic purposes. It is important to recognize that cortical atrophy on CT scan or MRI scan is *not* diagnostic nor specific for primary degenerative dementia, for its also occurs with aging and other specific disease processes.

Multi-infarct Dementia   The other major cause of dementia in the elderly, multi-infarct dementia, can occur alone or in combination

Table 4-10   Dementia versus Depressive Pseudodementia: Comparison of Clinical Characteristics

Characteristics	Dementia	Depressive pseudodementia
A. History		
1. Onset can be dated with some precision	Unusual	Usual
2. Duration of symptoms before physician consulted	Long	Short
3. Rapid progression of symptoms	Unusual	Usual
4. Patient's complaints of cognitive loss	Variable (minimized in later stages)	Emphasized
5. Patient's description of cognitive loss	Vague	Detailed
6. Family aware of dysfunction and severity	Variable (usual in later stages)	Usual
7. Loss of social skills	Late	Early
8. History of psychopathology	Uncommon	Common
B. Examination		
1. Memory loss for recent versus remote events	Greater	About equal
2. Specific memory loss ("patchy" deficits)	Uncommon	Common
3. Attention and concentration	Often poor	Often good
4. "Don't know" answers	Uncommon	Common
5. "Near miss" answers	Variable (common in later stages)	Uncommon
6. Performance on tasks of similar difficulty	Consistent	Variable
7. Patient's emotional reaction to symptoms	Variable (unconcerned in later stages)	Great distress
8. Patient's affect	Labile, blunted, or depressed	Depressed
9. Patient's efforts in attempting to perform tasks	Great	Small
10. Patient's efforts to cope with dysfunction	Maximal	Minimal

Source: After Small et al., 1981.

with other disorders that cause dementia. Multi-infarct dementia results when a patient has sustained recurrent cortical or subcortical strokes. Many of these strokes are too small to cause permanent or residual focal neurological deficits or CT scan evidence of strokes. Magnetic resonance imaging scanning may be more sensitive in detecting small infarcts, but there has been a tendency to overinterpret some of these findings as more MRI scans are being done (Cutler et al., 1984). Table 4-11 identifies characteristics of patients likely to

Table 4-11   Primary Degenerative Dementia versus Multi-infarct Dementia: Comparison of Clinical Characteristics

Characteristics	Primary degenerative dementia	Multi-infarct dementia
A. Demographic		
1. Sex	Women more commonly affected	Men more commonly affected
2. Age	Generally over age 75	Generally over age 60
B. History		
1. Time course of deficits	Gradually progressive	Stuttering or episodic, with stepwise deterioration
2. History of hypertension	Less common	Common
3. History of stroke(s), transient ischemic attack(s), or other focal neurological symptoms	Less common	Common
C. Examination		
1. Hypertension	Less common	Common
2. Focal neurological signs	Uncommon*	Common
3. Signs of atherosclerotic cardiovascular disease or peripheral vascular disease	Less common	Common
4. Emotional lability	Less common	More common

*Pathological reflexes, such as grasp, palmomental, and other cortical release signs may be seen in patients with primary degenerative dementia. (See text.)

have multi-infarct dementia and compares the clinical characteristics of primary degenerative and multi-infarct dementia. The modified Hachinski ischemia score (Table 4-12) provides a useful means to sum key clinical characteristics in making the differential diagnosis. The differentiation between Alzheimer's and multi-infarct types of dementia may, however, be very difficult even with the data in Table 4-11 and the Hachinski score, and many patients probably have elements of both. Another form of vascular-related dementia has been described, termed *senile dementia of the Binswanger type,* which may be impossible to differentiate clinically from multi-infarct dementia (Roman, 1987). Both of these vascular forms of dementia often have clinical features of what has been described as "subcortical dementia" (Cummings and Benson, 1983). As research yields more precise definitions of the underlying pathophysiology involved in dementia, and hopefully more specific treatments, differentiating multi-infarct and other vascular forms of dementia from the other causes of dementia will become increasingly important.

Neurological Disorders Specific (and generally less common or rare) neurological disorders account for the remainder of dementias in the elderly. Of these, Parkinson's disease, Huntington's chorea, and normal-pressure hydrocephalus are probably the most common. Parkinson's disease and its management are discussed in Chapter 8. Normal-pressure hydrocephalus is an uncommon disorder involving a relatively rapidly progressing dementia associated with

Table 4-12   Modified Hachinski Ischemia Score

Characteristic	Point score
Abrupt onset	2
Stepwise deterioration	1
Somatic complaints	1
Emotional incontinence	1
History or presence of hypertension	1
History of strokes	2
Focal neurological symptoms	2
Focal neurological signs	2

Note: This tool has been validated on a small number of demented patients by autopsy findings (Rosen et al., 1980). A score of 4 or more is consistent with multi-infarct dementia.

gait disturbance and urinary incontinence. This is important to remember, because if it is diagnosed early, surgery to shunt cerebrospinal fluid may yield improvement in cognitive function. The diagnosis should be suspected when the CT scan or MRI scan shows ventricular enlargement out of proportion to the degree of cortical atrophy. Considerable controversy remains regarding the precise diagnosis of this condition and the indications for and the efficacy of surgical treatments. These forms of dementia usually exhibit the clinical features of subcortical dementias, including abnormalities of posture and gait, abnormal movements, and the appearance of depression (Cummings and Benson, 1983).

Amnestic Syndromes and Benign Senescent Forgetfulness

Because of the clinical and social implications, dementia should be differentiated from two other related disorders: amnestic syndromes and benign senescent forgetfulness. In these disorders the predominant feature is memory impairment, whereas in dementia other areas of intellectual function are affected. Amnestic syndromes are characterized by recent-memory loss and are usually caused by (1) thiamine deficiency (often associated with alcohol abuse), (2) lesions of the median temporal structure of the brain (such as anoxia or trauma), and (3) transient global ischemia from cerebrovascular insufficiency.

Benign senescent forgetfulness involves minor degrees of memory loss that are not progressive and do not cause dysfunction in daily living, and probably falls within the spectrum of age-related changes in cognitive functioning. The memory loss is recognized by the patients and their families and friends, often because the patient continually repeats questions or accounts of events. The only way to distinguish this disorder from early dementia is to observe the patient over several months. If the memory difficulties progress and other areas of intellectual function are affected, a diagnosis of dementia can then be considered. Patients with benign senescent forgetfulness and their families need reassurance about the natural history of the disorder and practical advice about how to manage the condition. Similar to patients with early forms of dementia, these patients generally do well if tasks that stress their memories are avoided and if aids to memory are employed (e.g., signs, notes, chalkboards). Families and friends should be advised that the patient's cognitive function may suddenly worsen if the patient is moved to unfamiliar surroundings, becomes physically or emotionally ill, or is treated with certain medications.

EVALUATION

The evaluation of dementia includes a careful history, physical examination, and selected diagnostic studies. Important aspects of the history are outlined in Table 4-13. Because many physical illnesses and drugs can cause cognitive dysfunction (see Tables 4-6 and 4-9), active medical problems and use of prescription and nonprescription drugs (including alcohol) should be reviewed.

The nature and severity of the symptoms should be characterized in detail. What are the deficits? Does the patient admit to them, or is a family member describing them? How is the patient reacting to the problems? The responses to these questions can be helpful in

Table 4-13 Evaluating Dementia: The History

Summarize active medical problems and current physical complaints
List drugs (including over-the-counter preparations and alcohol)
Cardiovascular and neurological history (see Table 14-11)
Characterize the symptoms
    Nature of the deficits (memory vs. other cognitive functions)
    Onset and rate of progression
    Associated psychological symptoms
      Depression
      Anxiety or agitation
      Paranoid ideation
      Psychotic thought processes (delusions and/or hallucinations)
Assess the social situation
    Living arrangements
    Social supports
    Basic and instrumental activities of daily living
Ask about special problems
    Wandering (and getting lost)
    Disruptive or self-endangering behaviors
    Incontinence

differentiating between dementia and depressive pseudodementia (see Table 4-10).

The onset of symptoms and the rate of progression are particularly important. Although precise time units vary, the sudden onset of cognitive impairment (over a few days) should prompt a search for one of the underlying causes of delirium listed in Table 4-5. Primary degenerative dementia, multi-infarct dementia, and dementia resulting from other neurological disorders generally progress over months to years. As noted in Tables 4-11 and 4-12 and illustrated in Figure 4-1, irregular, stepwise decrements in cognitive functions (as opposed to a more even and gradual loss) favor a diagnosis of multi-infarct dementia. Patients with dementia are often brought for evaluation at a time of sudden worsening of cognitive function (as illustrated by the dotted line in Figure 4-1) and may even meet the criteria for delirium. These sudden changes may be triggered by a number of acute events (a small stroke without focal signs, acute physical illness, drugs, changes in environment, or personal loss such as the death or departure of a relative). Only a careful history (or familiarity with the patient) will help determine when an acute event has been superimposed on a preexisting dementia. Appropriate management of the

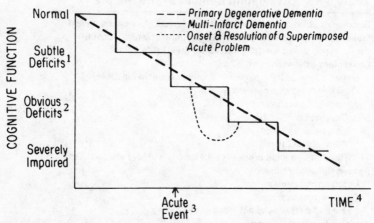

Figure 4-1 Primary degenerative dementia versus multi-infarct dementia: comparison of time courses. [1]Recognized by patient, but only detectable on detailed testing. [2]Deficits recognized by family and friends. [3]See text for explanation. [4]Exact time courses are variable; see text.

acute event will, in many instances, result in improvement in cognitive function (Figure 4-1, dotted line).

Early symptoms of dementia, especially Alzheimer's disease, usually occur insidiously and may include forgetfulness, a tendency to misplace things, and repetition of words or actions. Social and conversational ability may be maintained. As the dementia worsens, deficits become more obvious and patients may fail at work, be unable to handle their financial affairs, and get lost. Psychological symptoms such as depression, anxiety, restlessness, apathy, and paranoia should be sought because they can contribute to the cognitive impairment and may need specific treatment. Often these symptoms will be elicited from family, friends, or other care givers rather than from the patient.

A social history is especially important in elderly patients with dementia. Living arrangements, other social supports, and functional status (see Chapter 3) should be assessed. These factors play a major role in the management of patients with dementia and are of critical importance in determining the necessity for institutionalization. A patient with dementia and weak social supports may require institutionalization at a higher level of function than will a patient with strong social supports (Figure 4-2).

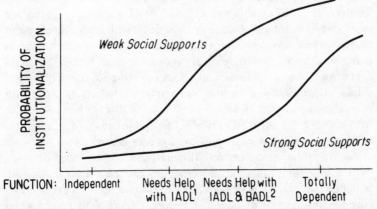

Figure 4-2   Effect of social supports on the probability of institutionalization in patients with dementia. [1]Instrumental activities of daily living. [2]Basic activities of daily living.

The history should also include specific questions about common problems requiring special attention in patients with dementia (especially the more advanced forms). These problems may include wandering, disruptive behavior (e.g., physical aggression and nighttime agitation), and incontinence. They require careful management and most often substantial involvement of family or other care givers.

A general physical examination should focus particularly on blood pressure, cognitive status, and neurological assessment. Focal neurological signs (such as unilateral weakness or sensory deficit, hemianopsia, Babinski reflex) favor a diagnosis of multi-infarct dementia.

Pathological reflexes (such as glabellar sign, grasp, snout, and palmomental reflexes) are nonspecific and occur in many forms of dementia as well as in a small proportion of normal aged persons. These frontal lobe release signs, as well as impaired stereognosis or graphesthesia, gait disorder, and abnormalities on cerebellar testing, are significantly more common in patients with Alzheimer's disease than in age-matched controls (Huff et al., 1987). Signs of Parkinson's disease (tremor, bradykinesia, muscle rigidity) should be sought because specific treatment can be instituted.

Selected diagnostic studies are especially useful in ruling out treatable forms of dementia (Table 4-14). Most of these studies have been recommended by a National Institutes of Health Consensus Conference (1987). Although CT and MRI scans of the head are expensive, they should be done in all patients with dementia of recent onset in whom no other clinical findings explain the dementia and in patients with focal neurological signs or symptoms. Recall that cerebral atrophy on one of these scans does not establish the diagnosis of primary degenerative dementia (Alzheimer's type); it can occur with normal aging as well as with several specific disease processes. The scan is thus recommended to rule out treatable causes (e.g., subdural hematoma, tumors, normal-pressure hydrocephalus).

Certain diagnostic studies, although not recommended for standard use in the evaluation of dementia, can be helpful in certain patients. Electroencephalographic (EEG) abnormalities are not specific for any type of dementia; however, seizure activity and focal abnormalities can be detected. Although age-related changes in EEG

Table 4-14   Evaluating Dementia: Diagnostic Studies

Blood studies:
    Complete blood count
    Glucose
    Urea nitrogen
    Electrolytes
    Calcium and phosphorous
    Liver function tests
    Thyroid function tests
    Vitamin B_{12} and folate
    Human immunodeficiency antibodies*
    VDRL
Radiographic studies:
    Chest films
    Computerized axial tomography (or magnetic resonance imaging) of the head*
Other studies:
    Electrocardiogram (possibly Holter monitor)
    Urinalysis
    Electroencephalogram*
    Neuropsychological testing*
    Lumbar puncture*

*These studies are not recommended for routine screening, but they may be helpful in some instances.
Source: After NIH Consensus Conference, 1987.

patterns occur (Raskin and Jarvik, 1979) and EEG findings are not specific for the diagnosis of dementia, most patients with clinically significant primary degenerative dementia (as well as delirium) have abnormal EEGs (usually diffuse slowing). A normal EEG in a patient with substantial cognitive dysfunction should thus raise suspicion of the potential reversible causes of dementia rather than a disease of the cerebral cortex. Lumbar puncture should be done only to rule out specific diagnoses such as tertiary syphilis and fungal meningitis. Detailed neuropsychological testing can be helpful in patients in whom depression or delirium is suspected, in very intelligent patients in whom early dementia is suspected, and in patients in whom the findings are ambiguous and a baseline documentation of deficits is important.

An example of a form useful in evaluating patients suspected of having dementia is shown in the Appendix.

MANAGEMENT

Although complete cure is not available for most forms of dementia, optimal management can provide improvements in the ability of these patients to function, as well as in their overall well-being (and that of their families and other care givers). Key principles for management of dementia are outlined in Table 4-15.

If causes of reversible or partially reversible forms of dementia are identified (Table 4-9), they should be specifically treated. Small strokes (lacunar infarcts), which can cause further deterioration of cognitive function, may be prevented by controlling hypertension; thus hypertension should be more aggressively treated in patients with dementia as long as side effects can be avoided (see Chapter 9). Other specific diseases such as Parkinson's disease (see Chapter 8) should be optimally managed. The treatment of these and other medical conditions is especially challenging because the treatment (usually drugs) may have adverse effects on cognitive function.

Problems such as insomnia, depression, anxiety, agitation, paranoid delusions, and other forms of psychosis should be treated. Depression and insomnia are discussed further in Chapter 5, and other psychotropic drugs are discussed in Chapter 14. In many instances, supportive measures can be used successfully, thus obviating the need for drug treatment. Drugs should not be used as chemical restraints in these patients. They should be used only when anxiety, agitation, or insomnia is distressing to the patient or disruptive to the environment and nonpharmacologic interventions are unsuccessful or impractical. Training family and institutional care givers about appropriate interactional and behavioral management techniques may help avoid the overuse of psychotropic drugs.

Many drugs (such as cerebral vasodilators, various cholinergic agents, and vitamins) have been recommended for the treatment of dementia. None have as yet been shown to yield improvements in cognitive abilities substantial enough to improve the overall function of these patients in daily life. Many of the drugs are expensive and have disturbing side effects. Until further controlled clinical trials are done, these drugs should not be routinely prescribed.

A variety of supportive measures and other management techniques are useful in improving the overall function and well-being of

Table 4-15   Key Principles in the Management of Dementia

Optimize the patient's function
  Treat underlying medical conditions (e.g., hypertension, Parkinson's disease)
  Avoid use of drugs with CNS side effects (unless required for management of
    psychological or behavioral disturbances—see Chapter 14)
  Assess the environment and suggest alterations, if necessary
  Encourage physical and mental activity
  Avoid situations stressing intellectual capabilities; use memory aids whenever
    possible
  Prepare the patient for changes in location
  Emphasize good nutrition
Identify and manage complications
  Wandering and other hazards
  Behavioral disorders
  Depression (see Chapter 5)
  Agitation or aggressiveness
  Incontinence (see Chapter 6)
Provide ongoing care
  Reassessment of cognitive and physical function
  Treatment of medical conditions
Provide medical information to patient and family
  Nature of the disease
  Extent of impairment
  Prognosis
Provide social service information to patient and family
  Community health care resources (day centers, homemakers, home health
    aides)
  Legal and financial counseling
Provide family counseling for:
  Identification and resolution of family conflicts
  Handling anger and guilt
  Decisions on respite or institutional care
  Legal concerns
  Ethical concerns (see Chapter 18)

patients with dementia and their families (Table 4-15). These interventions range from specific recommendations such as alterations in the physical environment, the use of memory aids, the avoidance of stressful tasks, and preparation for changes in living setting to more general techniques such as providing information and counseling to the patient's family. Many long-term-care facilities are now establishing specialized dementia units, with optimally designed environments, trained staff, and intensive activities programming.

Providing ongoing care is especially important in the management of these patients. They are often abandoned by health professionals who find their problems uninteresting and difficult to manage. Reassessment of the patient's cognitive abilities can be helpful in identifying potentially reversible causes for deteriorating function and in making specific recommendations to family and other care givers.

The family is the primary target of strategies to help manage dementia patients in noninstitutional settings. Information on the disease itself and the extent of impairment, and on community resources helpful in managing these patients can be of critical importance to family and care givers. Anticipating and teaching family members strategies to cope with common behavioral problems associated with dementia, such as wandering, incontinence, day-night reversal and nighttime agitation can be of critical importance. Wandering may be especially hazardous for the dementia patient's safety and is associated with falls in this patient population (Buchner and Larson, 1987). Incontinence is common and often very difficult for families to manage (see Chapter 6). Books providing information and suggestions for family management techniques are very useful (Mace and Rabins, 1981; Jarvik and Small, 1988). Support groups for families of patients with Alzheimer's disease are available in many cities. Family counseling can be helpful in dealing with a variety of issues such as anger, guilt, and decisions on institutionalization, on handling the patient's assets, and on terminal care. Dementia patients and their families should also be encouraged to discuss and document their wishes, using a durable power of attorney for health care or equivalent mechanism, early in the cause of the illness (see Chapter 18). Often a multidisciplinary group of primary care givers made up of a physician, a nurse, a social worker, and, when needed, rehabilitation therapists, a lawyer, and a clergy member must coordinate efforts to manage these patients and provide support to family and care givers.

Further details on the management of patients with dementia are provided in the Suggested Readings section. Information on the disease and resources helpful in its management can be obtained from the Alzheimer's Disease and Related Disorders Association (ADRDA), a national organization with many local branches.

REFERENCES

American Psychiatric Association: *Diagnostic and Statistical Manual of Mental Disorders* (3d ed revised). Washington, DC, 1987.

Buchner DM, Larson EB: Falls and fractures in patients with Alzheimer-type dementia. *JAMA* 257:1492–1495, 1987.

Cummings JL, Benson FD: *Dementia: A Clinical Approach.* Boston, Butterworths, 1983.

Cutler NR, Duara R, Creasey H, et al: Brain imaging: Aging and dementia. *Ann Intern Med* 101:355–369, 1984.

Evans LK: Sundown syndrome in institutionalized elderly. *J Am Geriatr Soc* 35:101–108, 1987.

Gillick MR, Serrell NA, Gillick LS: Adverse consequences of hospitalization in the elderly. *Soc Sci Med* 16:1033–1038, 1982.

Gurland BJ, Cross PS: Epidemiology of psychopathology in old age: Some implications for clinical services. *Psychiatr Clin North Am* 5:11–26, 1982.

Huff JF, Boller F, Lucchelli F, et al: The neurologic examination in patients with probable Alzheimer's disease. *Arch Neurol* 44:929–932, 1987.

Jarvik LF, Small GW: *Parentcare.* New York, Crown, 1988.

Lamy PP: *Prescribing for the Elderly.* Littleton, MA, PSG Publishing, 1980.

Larson EB, Reifler BV, Sumi SM, et al: Diagnostic tests in the evaluation of dementia: A prospective study of 200 elderly outpatients. *Arch Intern Med* 146:1917–1922, 1986.

Larson EB, Kukull WA, Buchner D, et al: Adverse drug reactions associated with global cognitive impairment in elderly persons. *Ann Intern Med* 107:169–173, 1987.

LaRue A: Memory loss and aging: Distinguishing dementia from benign senescent forgetfulness and depressive pseudodementia. *Psychiatr Clin North Am* 5:89–104, 1982.

Lazarus LW, Newton N, Cohler B, et al: Frequency and presentation of depressive symptoms in patients with primary degenerative dementia. *Am J Psychiatr* 144:41–45, 1987.

Lipowski ZJ: Delirium (acute confusional states). *JAMA* 258:1789–1792, 1987.

Mace NL, Rabins PV: *The 36-Hour Day: A Family Guide to Caring for Persons with Alzheimer's Disease, Related Dementing Illnesses, and*

Memory Loss in Later Life. Baltimore, Johns Hopkins University Press, 1981.

McKhann G, Drachman D, Folstein M, et al: Clinical diagnosis of Alzheimer's disease: Report of the NINCDS-ADRDA work group under the auspices of Department of Health and Human Services Task Force on Alzheimer's disease. *Neurology* 34:939–944, 1984.

Merriam AR, Aronson MK, Gaston P, et al: The psychiatric symptoms of Alzheimer's disease. *J Am Geriatr Soc* 36:7–12, 1988.

NIH Consensus Conference: Differential diagnosis of dementing diseases. *JAMA* 258:3411–3416, 1987.

Raskin A, Jarvik LF (eds): *Psychiatric Symptoms and Cognitive Loss in the Elderly: Evaluation and Assessment Techniques*. New York, Hemisphere, 1979.

Reifler BV, Larson E, Teri L, et al: Dementia of the Alzheimer's type and depression. *J Am Geriatr Soc* 34:855–859, 1986.

Roman GC: Senile dementia of the Binswanger type: A vascular form of dementia in the elderly. *JAMA* 258:1780–1788, 1987.

Rosen WG, Terry RD, Fuld PA, et al: Pathological verification of ischemic score in differentiation of dementia. *Ann Neurol* 7:486–488, 1980.

Rovner BW, Kafonek S, Filipp L, et al: Prevalence of mental illness in a community nursing home. *Am J Psychiatr* 143:1446–1449, 1986.

Small GW, Liston EH, Jarvik LF: Diagnosis and treatment of dementia in the aged. *West J Med* 135:469–481, 1981.

Stedman's Medical Dictionary (23d ed). New York, Williams & Wilkins, 1976.

Warshaw GA, Moore JT, Friedman SW, et al: Functional disability in the hospitalized elderly. *JAMA* 248:847–850, 1982.

SUGGESTED READINGS

Beck JC, Benson DF, Schiebel AB, et al: Dementia in the elderly: The silent epidemic. *Ann Intern Med* 97:231–241, 1982.

Cohen-Mansfield J, Billig N: Agitated behaviors in the elderly: I. A conceptual review. *J Am Geriatr Soc* 34:711–721, 1986.

Cummings JL, Benson FD: Dementia of the Alzheimer type: An inventory of diagnostic clinical features. *J Am Geriatr Soc* 34:12–19, 1986.

Habot B, Libow LS: The interrelationship of mental and physical status and its assessment in the older adult: Mind-body interaction, in Birren JE, Sloane RB (eds): *Handbook of Mental Health and Aging*. Englewood Cliffs, NJ: Prentice-Hall, 1980.

Katzman R: Alzheimer's disease. *N Engl J Med* 314:964–973, 1986.

Larson EB, Reifler BV, Sumi SM, et al: Diagnostic evaluation of 200 elderly outpatients with suspected dementia. *J Gerontol* 40:536–543, 1985.

Liston EH: Delirium in the aged. *Psychiatr Clin North Am* 5:49–66, 1982.

Teri L, Larson EB, Reifler BV: Behavioral disturbance in dementia of the Alzheimer's type. *J Am Geriatr Soc* 36:1–6, 1988.

Wells ED (ed): *Dementia* (2d ed). Philadelphia, Davis, 1977.

Chapter 5

Diagnosis and Management of Depression

Depression is probably the most common example of the nonspecific and atypical presentation of illness in the elderly. The signs and symptoms can be the result of a variety of treatable physical illnesses or the presenting manifestations of depression or a related condition that requires specific diagnosis and management by a psychiatrist. Frequently depression and physical illness(es) coexist in elderly patients. Thus, it is not surprising that treatable depressions are often overlooked in elderly patients with physical illness, and that treatable physical illnesses are often not managed optimally in elderly patients diagnosed as having a depression.

Sorting out the complex interrelationships between symptoms and signs of depression caused by physical illnesses and those caused primarily by an affective disorder or related psychiatric diagnosis challenges those caring for the elderly. This chapter addresses these issues from the perspective of the nonpsychiatrist, recognizing that the optimal management of most of these patients should involve psychiatrists and psychologists experienced with and interested in the elderly. The Suggested Readings offer more extensive discussions of this topic from the perspective of psychiatrists and psychologists.

AGING AND DEPRESSION

Symptoms and signs of depression are common in the elderly population. Over 10 percent of community-dwelling elderly persons express sadness or feel ill at ease (dysphoric mood), and close to 5 percent have a clinically diagnosable depression (Gurland and Cross, 1982). The prevalence of these conditions is even higher among the elderly in acute care hospitals and nursing homes. Suicide is disturbingly common in the elderly; elderly white males have the highest rate of suicide—three to four times that in the general population (Osgood, 1985).

Several biological, physical, psychological, and sociological factors predispose elderly persons to depression (Table 5-1). Aging changes in the central nervous system such as increased monoamine oxidase activity and decreased neurotransmitter concentrations (especially catecholaminergic neurotransmitters) may play a role in the development of depression in the elderly (Lipton and Nemeroff, 1978). Although these aging changes alone probably do not cause depression, when combined with other factors, they could increase the susceptibility to a depressive episode.

Table 5-1   Factors Predisposing the Elderly to Depression

Biological
  Family history (genetic predisposition)
  Prior episode(s) of depression
  Aging changes in neurotransmission
Physical
  Specified diseases (see Table 5-5)
  Chronic medical conditions (especially with pain or loss of function)
  Exposure to drugs (see Table 5-6)
  Sensory deprivation (loss of vision or hearing)
Psychological
  Unresolved conflicts (e.g., anger, guilt)
  Memory loss and dementia
  Personality disorders
Social
  Losses of family and friends (bereavement)
  Isolation
  Loss of job
  Loss of income

The incidence of several specific diseases associated with symptoms of depression, the prevalence of chronic medical conditions, and the frequency of medication usage increase with age. Each of these factors can predispose the elderly to depression.

Losses are common among the elderly. Physical losses can mean a reduction in the abilities for self-care, often leading to loss of independence; markedly reduced sensory capacities (especially vision and hearing) can result in isolation and sensory deprivation. Both can play a role in the development of depression. Memory loss and loss of other intellectual functions (dementia) are frequently associated with depression in the elderly (see Chapter 4). Losses of job, income, and social supports (especially the death of family and friends) increase with age. Bereavement can turn into isolation and depression.

Given the many factors that predispose the elderly to depression, it is surprising that the prevalence of symptoms and signs of this disorder is not higher. Suicide, the most serious yet preventable consequence of depression, has an alarmingly high rate among the elderly. The highest suicide rate is, in fact, among elderly males. Among males over age 80 the rate approaches 50 per 100,000, as compared to 10 per 100,000 for the general population (Osgood, 1985). Several factors have been associated with suicide in the elderly (Table 5-2). Although none have been shown to be highly predictive, it is essential for clinicians to keep these factors in mind and have a high index of suspicion for impending suicide attempts when one or more are present.

SYMPTOMS AND SIGNS OF DEPRESSION

Many common symptoms and signs in the elderly can represent depression. Several factors may make these difficult to interpret:

- Aging changes, as well as several common medical conditions, can lead to the physical appearance of depression—even when depression is not present.
- Nonspecific physical symptoms (such as fatigue, weakness, anorexia, diffuse pain) may represent a variety of treatable medical illnesses, as well as depression.

Table 5-2   Factors Associated with Suicide in the Elderly

Factor	High risk	Low risk
Sex	Male	Female
Religion	Protestant	Catholic or Jewish
Race	White	Nonwhite
Marital status	Widowed or divorced	Married
Occupational background	Blue-collar, low-paying job	Professional or white-collar job
Current employment status	Retired or unemployed	Employed full or part time
Living environment	Urban	Rural
	Living alone	Living with spouse or other relatives
	Isolated	
	Recent move	Living in close-knit neighborhood
Physical health	Poor health	Good health
	Terminal illness	
	Pain and suffering	
Mental health	Depression (current or previous)	Happy and well adjusted
	Alcoholism	Positive self-concept and outlook
	Low self-esteem	Sense of personal control over life
	Loneliness	
	Feeling rejected, unloved	
Personal background	Broken home	Intact family of origin
	Dependent personality	Independent, assertive, flexible personality
	History of poor interpersonal relationships	History of close friendships
	Family history of mental illness	No family history of mental illness
	Poor marital history	No previous suicide attempts
	Poor work record	No history of suicide in family
		Good marital history
		Good work record

Source: After Osgood, 1985, p. 12.

• Specific physical symptoms, relating to every major organ system, can represent depression rather than physical illness in the elderly.

• Depression can exacerbate symptoms of coexisting physical illnesses.

The physical appearance of elderly patients suspected of being depressed should be interpreted cautiously. Aging changes such as graying and loss of hair, wrinkled skin, loss of teeth (with altered facial architecture), stooped posture, and slowed gait can present an image of depression. Several medical conditions can further the physical appearance of depression. Parkinson's disease, which manifests itself by masked facies, bradykinesia, and stooped posture, can be misinterpreted as depression. Patients with presbycusis may appear withdrawn and disinterested simply because they cannot hear enough of normal conversation to actively participate and withdraw out of frustration. The psychomotor retardation of hypothyroidism may offer the physical appearance of depression. Paradoxically, hyperthyroidism can also cause apathy and withdrawal (apathetic thyrotoxicosis). Systemic illnesses, such as disseminated tuberculosis, malignancy, and malnutrition (alone or resulting from a medical condition) can produce a depressed appearance. Moreover, true depression commonly accompanies many of these medical conditions in the elderly.

Symptoms must also be interpreted very cautiously. Many different symptoms can represent depression, physical illness, or a combination of both. Table 5-3 lists several examples of somatic symptoms that may actually represent, or be exacerbated by, depression in the elderly. Depression presenting primarily with physical symptoms, termed *masked depression,* is especially common in the elderly for several reasons. Many of today's elderly were raised in an atmosphere that inhibited the expression of emotion. Finding direct expression of feelings of sadness, guilt, and anger difficult, they may somatasize these emotions and complain of physical symptoms. In addition, many elderly persons with diminished sensory input from losses of vision, hearing, or touch may overrespond to internal cues (such as their heartbeat and gastrointestinal motility) and focus on these concerns when anxious and depressed.

Insomnia is an example of a very common, yet nonspecific, symptom in the elderly. Although it is one of the key symptoms in diagnosing different forms of depression, a variety of factors may underlie this complaint (Table 5-4). In addition to depression, insomnia may be caused by other psychiatric disorders as well as several types of medical problems. For example, orthopnea and nocturia caused by congestive heart failure, abdominal discomfort from reflux esophagitis or ulcer disease, or anxiety and restlessness from hyperthyroidism could underlie the complaint of insomnia. A careful history should help identify these and other medical conditions that

Table 5-3   Examples of Physical Symptoms That Can Represent Depression

System	Symptom
General	Fatigue
	Weakness
	Anorexia
	Weight loss
	Anxiety
	Insomnia (see Table 5-4)
	"Pain all over"
Cardiopulmonary	Chest pain
	Shortness of breath
	Palpitations
	Dizziness
Gastrointestinal	Abdominal pain
	Constipation
Genitourinary	Frequency
	Urgency
	Incontinence
Musculoskeletal	Diffuse pain
	Back pain
Neurological	Headache
	Memory disturbance
	Dizziness
	Paresthesias

might be contributing to the problem. Insomnia can also be caused by the effects of (or withdrawal from) several types of drugs and alcohol. As more elderly patients with sleep disturbances have undergone detailed analysis (including continuous observation during sleep and monitoring by polysomnography), other conditions have been detected, including sleep apnea syndromes and nocturnal myoclonus. As many as one-third of the elderly population may have a specific sleep disorder (Dement et al., 1982). Obstructive sleep apnea is the most common of these disorders and results not only in complaints of insomnia but also in nighttime hypoxia with associated risks for cardiac arrhythmias and myocardial and cerebral infarction. Specific symptoms, which are often elicited from the bed partner, should prompt consideration for referral to a sleep center because hypnotics

Table 5-4   Key Factors in Evaluating the Complaint of Insomnia

Sleep disturbance should be carefully characterized
  Delayed sleep onset
  Frequent awakenings
  Early-morning awakenings
Physical symptoms can underlie insomnia (from patient and bed partner)
  Symptoms of physical illnesses
    Pain from musculoskeletal disorders
    Orthopnea, paroxysmal nocturnal dyspnea or cough
    Nocturia
    Gastroesophageal reflux
  Symptoms suggestive of nocturnal myoclonus
    Periodic leg movements
  Symptoms suggestive of sleep apnea
    Loud or irregular snoring
    Awakening sweating, anxious, tachycardiac
    Excessive movement
    Morning drowsiness
Aging changes occur in sleep patterns
  Increased sleep latency
  Decreased time in deeper stages of sleep
  Increased awakenings
Behavioral factors can affect sleep patterns
  Daytime naps
  Earlier bedtime
Medications can affect sleep
  Hypnotic withdrawal
  Alcohol causes sleep fragmentation

may exacerbate the conditions and other more specific treatments are available, including nasal continuous positive airway pressure and uvulopalatopharyngeoplasty. Aging itself is associated with changes in sleep pattern, such as daytime naps, early bedtime, increased time until onset of sleep, decreases in the absolute and relative amounts of the deeper stages of sleep, and increased periods of wakefulness which could contribute to the complaint of insomnia. Thus there is a lengthy differential diagnosis of insomnia in the elderly, and the complaint should not be attributed simply to aging or depression and treated with a sedating antidepressant or hypnotic before other potential causes are considered. The Suggested Readings section at the end of this chapter contains an excellent source of more detailed information on sleep disturbances.

Health care professionals should be keenly aware of the potentially deceiving nature of signs and symptoms of depression in the elderly discussed above. Awareness of these factors will help avoid the underdiagnosis (and in some instances, overdiagnosis) of depressions in this population.

DEPRESSION ASSOCIATED WITH MEDICAL CONDITIONS

Symptoms and signs of depression are associated with medical conditions in the elderly in several ways:

- Some diseases can result in the physical appearance of depression, even when depression is not present (e.g., Parkinson's disease).
- Many diseases can either directly cause depression or elicit a reaction of depression. The latter is especially true of conditions that cause fear of or produce chronic pain, disability, and dependence.
- Drugs used to treat medical conditions can cause symptoms and signs of depression (Table 5-5).
- The environment (factors such as isolation, sensory deprivation, forced dependency) in which medical conditions are treated can predispose to depression.

A wide variety of physical illnesses can present with, or be accompanied by, symptoms and signs of depression (Table 5-6). Any medical condition associated with systemic involvement and metabolic disturbances can have profound effects on mental function and affect in elderly patients. The most common among these are fever, dehydration, decreased cardiac output, electrolyte disturbances, and hypoxia. Hyponatremia (whether from disease process or drugs) and hypercalcemia (associated especially with malignancy) may also cause an elderly patient to appear depressed.

Systemic diseases, especially malignancies and endocrine disorders, are often associated with symptoms of depression in the elderly. Depression, accompanied by anorexia, weight loss, and back pain, is

Table 5-5   Drugs That Can Cause Symptoms of Depression

Antihypertensives	Cardiovascular preparations
Reserpine	Digitalis
Methyldopa	Diuretics
Propranolol	Lidocaine
Clonidine	Hypoglycemic agents
Hydralazine	Psychotropic agents
Guanethidine	Sedatives
Analgesics	Barbiturates
Narcotic	Benzodiazepines
Morphine	Meprobamate
Codeine	Antipsychotics
Meperidine	Chlorpromazine
Pentazocine	Haloperidol
Propoxyphene	Thiothixene
Nonnarcotic	Hypnotics
Indomethacin	Chloral hydrate
Antiparkinsonism drugs	Flurazepam
Levodopa	Steroids
Antimicrobials	Corticosteroids
Sulfonamides	Estrogens
Isoniazid	Others
	Cimetidine
	Cancer chemotherapeutic
	agents
	Alcohol

Sources: After Hall, 1980; Levenson and Hall, 1981.

commonly present in patients with cancer of the pancreas. These patients often lack the feelings of guilt, agitation, delusions, memory impairment, and suicidal thoughts that can accompany depression in later years. Among the endocrine disorders, thyroid and parathyroid conditions are most commonly accompanied by symptoms of depression. Of hypothyroid patients, 80 to 90 percent manifest psychomotor retardation, irritability, or depression (Brown, 1975). Hyperthyroidism may also present as withdrawal and depression in the elderly—so called apathetic thyrotoxicosis (Thomas et al., 1970). Hyperparathyroidism, with attendant hypercalcemia, can simulate depression and is often manifest by apathy, fatigue, bone pain, and constipation. Other systemic physical conditions, such as infectious diseases, ane-

Table 5-6   Medical Illnesses Associated with Depression

Metabolic disturbances
   Dehydration
   Azotemia, uremia
   Acid-base disturbances
   Hypoxia
   Hypo- and hypernatremia
   Hypo- and hyperglycemia
   Hypo- and hypercalcemia
Endocrine
   Hypo- and hyperthyroidism
   Hyperparathyroidism
   Diabetes mellitus
   Cushing's disease
   Addison's disease
Infections
   Viral
      Pneumonia
      Encephalitis
   Bacterial
      Pneumonia
      Urinary tract infection
      Meningitis
      Endocarditis
   Other
      Tuberculosis
      Fungal meningitis
      Neurosyphilis
Cardiovascular
   Congestive heart failure
   Myocardial infarction
Pulmonary
   Chronic obstructive lung disease
   Malignancy
Gastrointestinal
   Malignancy (especially pancreatic)
   Irritable bowel
   Other (e.g., ulcer, diverticulosis)
Genitourinary
   Urinary incontinence
Musculoskeletal
   Degenerative arthritis
   Osteoporosis with vertebral compression or hip fracture
   Polymyalgia rheumatica
   Paget's disease

Table 5-6   Medical Illnesses Associated with Depression (*Continued*)

Neurological
   Cerebrovascular disease
      Transient ischemic attacks
      Strokes
   Dementia (all types)
   Intracranial mass
      Primary or metastatic tumors
   Parkinson's disease
Other
   Anemia (of any cause)
   Vitamin deficiencies
   Hematologic or other systemic malignancy

Sources: After Hall, 1980; Levenson and Hall, 1981.

mia, and vitamin deficiencies, can also have prominent manifestations of depression in the elderly.

Because cardiovascular and nervous system diseases are among the most threatening and potentially disabling, they can precipitate symptoms of depression. Myocardial infarction, with attendant fear of shortened life span and restricted life-style, commonly precipitates depression. Stroke is often accompanied by depression, but the depression may not always correlate with the extent of physical disability. Patients in whom stroke has produced substantial disability (e.g., hemiparesis, aphasia) can become depressed in response to their loss of function; others whose stroke has produced only minor degrees of physical disability (but in theory may have affected areas of the brain controlling emotion) can also become depressed. Other causes of brain damage, especially in the frontal lobes, such as tumors and subdural hematomas, can also be associated with depression. Elderly individuals with dementia, both primary degenerative (Alzheimer's type) and multi-infarct dementia, may have prominent symptoms of depression. (The relationship between depression and dementia is discussed in greater detail in Chapter 4.) Patients with Parkinson's disease also have a high incidence of clinically diagnosed depression (Mindham, 1970).

Depression that develops in response to the chronic pain, loss of function and self-esteem, dependence, and fear of death that accompany physical illness can become severe. Many elderly individuals who commit suicide have an active physical illness at the time of death. The relationship between physical illness and suicide has been shown to be especially prominent in elderly men and after surgery (Dorpat et al., 1968).

Several sets of factors determine emotional responses to physical illness in the elderly (Verwoerdt, 1976). The first set of factors relates to the illness: its time course, severity, and organ system involvement. A slowly developing illness may leave more time for the individual to adjust, thereby producing fewer psychological complications. Acute illness, associated with more intense symptoms, can result in an abrupt loss of function and more dramatic psychological responses. Illnesses associated with prominent changes in body image (such as amputations, stroke, and gait disturbances necessitating assistive devices) and those illnesses that provoke greater anticipation of disability and death (such as malignancy and myocardial infarction) also tend to produce more intense psychological responses. A second set of factors relates to the patient: his or her prior experiences and premorbid personality structure. Those elderly individuals who have remained free of major psychological problems may have more energy and greater flexibility in coping with physical illness. Some individuals may welcome physical illness as a good excuse to regress and play the dependent sick role; overly self-reliant individuals may become agitated and depressed and rebel against their care givers. The final set of factors influencing emotional responses to physical illness involves the illness situation—the responses to hospitalization or other changes in environment, the effects of the illness on family relationships, and the effectiveness of the physician-patient relationships. These multiple and highly individual factors account for the complex and heterogeneous emotional responses to physical illnesses seen in the elderly population.

Symptoms of depression are often caused not only by, and in response to, physical illness but also by the treatment of medical conditions. A variety of psychological responses to hospitalization (including depression) have been observed in the elderly. Isolation, sensory deprivation, and immobilization, common in elderly patients hospitalized with physical illness, can cause or contribute to depressive symptoms. Iatrogenic complications such as fecal impaction and urinary retention or incontinence can also cause psychological symptoms, including those of depression.

Drugs are the most common cause of treatment-induced symptoms and signs of depression. Although a wide variety of pharmacologic agents can produce symptoms of depression (Table 5-5), antihypertensive agents and sedatives are probably the most common drugs that cause symptoms and signs of depression in the elderly. The mechanisms by which various drugs cause these effects differ and are poorly understood in many instances. Some drugs such as alcohol, sedatives, antipsychotics, and antihypertensives have direct effects on the central nervous system (probably mediated by influencing central neurotransmitters and their receptors); others have toxicity (such as dehydration from diuretics or hypoglycemia from insulin or sulfonylurea overdose) that produce these symptoms and/or signs. Thus, depressive symptoms, especially new symptoms, should raise a high index of suspicion about the role of drugs. Whenever possible, drugs that can potentially produce these symptoms should be discontinued.

DIAGNOSING DEPRESSION

In view of the prevalence of symptoms and signs of depression in the elderly, aging changes that may complicate the diagnosis, and the interrelationship between depression and its signs and symptoms, medical illnesses, and treatment effects, how is the diagnosis of depression made?

Several general principles can be helpful:

- Nonspecific or multiple somatic symptoms that are suggestive of depression should not be diagnosed as such until physical illnesses (especially treatable physical illnesses) have been excluded.
- Somatic symptoms unexplained by physical findings or diagnostic studies, especially those of relatively sudden onset in an elderly person who is not usually hypochondriacal, should raise the suspicion of depression.
- Drugs used to treat medical illnesses (Table 5-5), sedatives, hypnotics, and alcohol should be considered as potential causes for symptoms and signs of depression.

• Standard diagnostic criteria should be the basis for diagnosing various forms of depression in the elderly, but several differences may distinguish depressions in the elderly compared with those in younger patients.

• Major depressive episodes should be differentiated from other diagnoses such as uncomplicated bereavement, bipolar disorder, dysthymic disorder, and adjustment disorders with a depressed mood.

• Consultation with psychiatrists and/or psychologists experienced with the elderly should be obtained whenever possible to help diagnose and manage depressive disorders.

• Whenever there is uncertainty about the diagnosis, a judicious (but adequate) therapeutic trial of an antidepressant can be very helpful.

The revised *Diagnostic and Statistical Manual of Mental Disorders* of the American Psychiatric Association (DSM III-R) (American Psychiatric Association, 1987a) lists several classifications and diagnoses that are useful to describe depressions in the elderly (Table 5-7). The most common clinical problem is differentiating major depressive episodes from other forms of depression. Table 5-8 shows the diagnostic criteria for a major depressive episode. Several differences in the presentation of depressions in the elderly can make the diagnosis much more challenging and difficult (Table 5-9). Some of the key features that distinguish major depression from other forms of depression are shown in Table 5-10.

Attention has recently focused on the potential for certain neuroendocrine abnormalities to be useful in diagnosing depression. For example, a substantial proportion of depressed individuals fail to suppress cortisol secretion after a dose of dexamethasone (Carroll et al., 1981). Unfortunately, the sensitivity, specificity, and predictive values of the dexamethasone suppression test for diagnosis of depression in the elderly are unknown. In addition, many medical conditions and even dementia appear to produce false-positive tests (Spar and Gerner, 1982, American Psychiatric Association, 1987b). Thus, the clinical usefulness of tests such as the dexamethasone suppression test in the elderly is uncertain, and these tests should not be used routinely.

Because of the overlap of symptoms and signs of depression and physical illness and the close association between many medical con-

Table 5-7   Diagnostic Classification of Various Forms of Depression

Affective disorders
  Major affective disorders
    Major depression
      Single episode
      Recurrent
    Bipolar disorder
      Mixed
      Manic
      Depressed
  Other
    Cyclothymic disorder
    Dysthymic disorder (depressive neurosis)
    Atypical bipolar disorder
    Atypical depression
Organic mental disorders
  Dementia with depression
  Organic mood syndrome
Adjustment disorders
  Adjustment disorder with depressed mood
Other
  Uncomplicated bereavement

Source: After American Psychiatric Association, 1987a.

ditions and depression, elderly patients presenting with what appears to be a depression should have physical illnesses carefully excluded. This can almost always be accomplished by a thorough history, physical examination, and basic laboratory studies (Table 5-11). Other diagnostic studies can provide helpful objective data in patients with persistent somatic symptoms that are difficult to distinguish from psychosomatic complaints (e.g., masked depression). For example, exercise testing echocardiography and radionucleotide cardiac scans (thallium, multiple gated acquisition) can help rule out organic heart disease as a basis for chest pain, fatigue, and dyspnea. Pulmonary function tests can exclude intrinsic lung disease as a cause for chronic shortness of breath. A new complaint of constipation may be related to depression but may also be caused by hypothyroidism or colonic disease; thus a test for occult blood in the stool, barium enema or colonoscopy, and thyroid function tests can be helpful in the evaluation of this symptom (Table 5-11).

Table 5-8   Diagnostic Criteria for Major Depressive Episode

A. At least five of the following symptoms have been present during the same 2-week period and represent a change from previous functioning; at least one of the symptoms is either (1) depressed mood or (2) loss of interest or pleasure. (Do not include symptoms that are clearly due to a physical condition, mood-incongruent delusions or hallucinations, incoherence, or marked loosening of associations.)

  1. Depressed mood most of the day, nearly every day, as indicated either by subjective account or observation by others

  2. Markedly diminished interest or pleasure in all, or almost all, activities most of the day, nearly every day (as indicated either by subjective account or observation by others of apathy most of the time)

  3. Significant weight loss or weight gain when not dieting (e.g., >5% of body weight in a month), or decrease or increase in appetite nearly every day

  4. Insomnia or hypersomnia nearly every day

  5. Psychomotor agitation or retardation nearly every day (observable by others, not merely subjective feelings of restlessness or being slowed down)

  6. Fatigue or loss of energy nearly every day

  7. Feelings of worthlessness or excessive or inappropriate guilt (which may be delusional) nearly every day (not merely self-reproach or guilt about being sick)

  8. Diminished ability to think or concentrate, or indecisiveness, nearly every day (either by subjective account or as observed by others)

  9. Recurrent thoughts of death (not just fear of dying), recurrent suicidal ideation without a specific plan, or a suicide attempt or a specific plan for committing suicide

B. 1. Cannot be established that an organic factor initiated and maintained the disturbance

  2. Disturbance not a normal reaction to the death of a loved one (uncomplicated bereavement)*

C. At no time during the disturbance have there been delusions or hallucinations for as long as 2 weeks in the absence of prominent mood symptoms (i.e., before the mood symptoms developed or after they have remitted)

D. Not superimposed on schizophrenia, schizophreniform disorder, delusional disorder, or psychotic disorder

*Morbid preoccupation with worthlessness, suicidal ideation, marked functional impairment of psychomotor retardation, or prolonged duration suggest bereavement complicated by major depression.

Source: After American Psychiatric Association, 1987a.

Table 5-9   Some Differences in the Presentation of Depression in the Elderly, Compared with Younger Population

Somatic complaints, rather than psychological symptoms, often predominate in the clinical picture

Elderly patients often deny having a dysphoric mood

Apathy and withdrawal are common

Feelings of guilt are less common

Loss of self-esteem is prominent

Inability to concentrate, with resultant impairment of memory and other cognitive functions, is common (see Chapter 4)

MANAGEMENT

Several treatment modalities are available to manage depressed elderly persons (Table 5-12). The choice of treatment(s) for an individual patient depends on many factors, including the primary disorder causing the depression, the severity of symptoms, the availability and practicality of the various treatment modalities, and underlying conditions that might contraindicate a specific form of treatment (e.g., disorders of vision and hearing that make psychotherapy difficult or severe cardiovascular disease that precludes the use of certain antidepressants).

When a specific active medical condition or drug is suspected as the cause for the symptoms and signs of depression (e.g., an organic affective syndrome), these factors should be attended to before other therapies are initiated, unless the depression is severe enough to warrant immediate treatment (e.g., the patient is delusional or suicidal). Treatment of the medical condition should be optimized, and all drugs that could be worsening the depression should be discontinued, if medically feasible.

Supportive measures such as those listed in Table 5-12 and psychotherapy are often ignored and can be very helpful in managing mildly depressed patients; they may also be useful adjuncts to other treatments for patients with more severe depressions. Little information is available on the efficacy of the myriad forms of psychotherapy with the elderly, and very few health professionals have experience and interest in these techniques. Many depressed patients have hearing impairments, other physical disabilities, or cognitive impairment

Table 5-10 Major Depression versus Other Forms of Depression

Diagnostic classification	Key features distinguishing from major depression
Bipolar disorders	The patient may meet, or have met in the past, criteria for major depression, but is having or has had one or more manic episodes; the latter are characterized by distinct periods of a relatively persistent elevated or irritable mood, and other symptoms such as increased activity, restlessness talkativeness, flight of ideas, inflated self-esteem, and distractibility
Cyclothymic disorder	There are numerous periods during which symptoms of depression and mania are present but not of sufficient severity or duration to meet the criteria for a major depressive or manic episode; in addition to a loss of interest and pleasure in most activities, the periods of depression are accompanied by other symptoms such as fatigue, insomnia or hypersomnia, social withdrawal, pessimism, and tearfulness
Dysthymic disorder	Patient usually exhibits a prominently depressed mood, marked loss of interest or pleasure in most activities, and other symptoms of depression; the symptoms are not of sufficient severity or duration to meet the criteria for a major depressive episode, and the periods of depression may be separated by up to a few months of normal mood
Adjustment disorder with depressed mood	The patient exhibits a depressed mood, tearfulness, hopelessness, or other symptoms in excess of a normal response to an identifiable psychosocial or physical stressor; the response is not an exacerbation of another psychiatric condition, occurs within 3 months of the onset of the stressor, eventually remits after the stressor ceases (or the patient adapts to the stressor), and does not meet the criteria for other forms of depression or uncomplicated bereavement
Uncomplicated bereavement	This is a depressive syndrome that arises in response to the death of a loved one—its onset is not more than 2 to 3 months after the death, and the symptoms last for variable periods of time; the patient generally regards the depression as a normal response—guilt and thought of death refer directly to the loved one; morbid preoccupation with worthlessness, marked or prolonged functional impairment, and marked psychomotor retardation are uncommon and suggest the development of major depression
Dementia with depression	See Chapter 4
Organic mood syndrome	This is a disturbance in mood that resembles a depressive (or in some instances a manic) episode that is usually caused by a toxic or metabolic factor; at least two of the symptoms associated with depression are present (see A in Table 5-8), there is no clouding of consciousness, and evidence of a specific organic factor can be etiologically related to the mood disturbance

Note: The DMS IIIR (American Psychiatric Association, 1987a) contains the formal diagnostic criteria for these disorders.

Table 5-11   Diagnostic Studies Helpful in Evaluating Apparently Depressed Elderly Patients with Somatic Symptoms

Basic evaluation
History
Physical examination
Complete blood count
Erythrocyte sedimentation rate
Serum electrolytes, glucose, and calcium
Renal function tests
Liver function tests
Thyroid function tests

Examples of other helpful studies*	
Symptom or sign	**Diagnostic study**
Pain	Appropriate radiological procedure (e.g., bone film, bone scan, GI series)
Chest pain	ECG, noninvasive cardiovascular studies (e.g., exercise stress test, echocardiography, radionucleotide scans)
Shortness of breath	Chest films, pulmonary function tests, arterial blood gases
Constipation	Test for occult blood in stool, barium enema, thyroid function tests
Focal neurological signs or symptoms	CT or MRI scan EEG

*These studies are not recommended for all patients with these symptoms. They are helpful if the symptoms are new or to exclude physical illness when depression is thought to underlie the complaint.

that can make psychotherapy difficult. In general, psychoanalytically oriented and insight psychotherapies are less useful with elderly patients; more direct interventions such as behavior modification and cognitive techniques may be more successful.

Elderly patients with depressions caused by uncomplicated bereavement, adjustment disorders related to a psychosocial stress (retirement, family conflicts, etc.) or physical conditions (myocardial infarction, stroke, hip fracture, etc.), and dysthymic disorders may respond well to supportive measures and psychotherapeutic approaches.

Table 5-12   Treatment Modalities for Depression in the Elderly

Supportive measures
  Information and encouragement
  Environmental alterations
  Activities (physical and mental)
  Involvement of family and friends
  Ongoing interest and care
Psychotherapy
  Individual
  Group
Drugs
  Antidepressants
  Tricyclics and related drugs (see Table 5-13)
  Lithium
  Methylphenidate
  Monoamine oxidase inhibitors
Sedatives for associated anxiety or agitation (see Chapter 14)
Antipsychotics for associated psychoses (see Chapter 14)
Electroconvulsive therapy

When symptoms and signs of depression are of sufficient severity and duration to meet the criteria for major depression (Table 5-8), or if the depression is producing marked functional disability or interfering with recovery from other illnesses, drug treatment should be considered. Several types of drugs can be used to treat depression in the elderly, including tri- and tetracyclic antidepressants and some other newer agents (e.g., trazodone, maprotiline, fluoxetine) (Table 5-13), stimulants (e.g., methylphenidate), monoamine oxidase inhibitors, and lithium.

Tricyclic antidepressants have been the most widely used in the elderly. In general, those patients who respond best to these agents have

- More prominent "endogenous" symptoms: weight loss, early-morning awakening, diurnal variation in mood, and psychomotor retardation or agitation
- More pervasive symptoms and decreased functional capacity
- Prior history of depression or response to tricyclic drugs
- Family history of depression or response to tricyclic drugs

Table 5-13 Characteristics of Selected Antidepressant Drugs

Drug	Level of sedation	Anticholinergic activity	Usual young-adult dosage, mg/day	Recommended geriatric dosages, mg/day*	Elimination half-life†
Tricyclic teriary amines					
Amitriptyline (Elavil, Endep, Amitril, etc.)	Very high	Very high	100–300	25–150	Intermediate
Doxepin (Sinequan, Adapin)	High	High	100–300	25–150	Intermediate
Imipramine (Tofranil, SK-Pramine)	Middle	Middle	100–300	25–150	Long
Tricyclic secondary amines					
Desipramine (Norpramin, Pertofrane)	None	Low	100–300	25–150	Long
Protriptyline (Vivactil)	None	Middle	20–70	5–30	Very long
Nortriptyline (Aventyl, Pamelor)	Low	Middle	25–100	10–35	Long
Other amines					
Amoxapine (Asendin)	Middle	Middle	100–300	25–150	Intermediate
Maprotiline (Ludiomil)	Middle	Middle	100–300	25–150	Very long
Other drugs					
Trazodone (Desyrel)	Middle	Very low	150–400	50–200	Short
Fluoxetine (Prozac)	Very low	Very low	20–80	10–40	Very long

Note: Other antidepressant drugs are discussed in the text.

*Some elderly patients may require higher dosages than those recommended (see text).

†May be longer and more variable in the elderly; Short = <8 h; Intermediate = 8–20 h; Long = 20–30 h; Very long = >30 h.

Source: Based on Richelson, 1984.

All the tricyclics have the potential to produce bothersome and sometimes disabling side effects (Table 5-14), although there are some differences among the drugs (Table 5-13). Patients with psychomotor agitation, prominent anxiety, and insomnia may do better with a more sedating drug such as doxepin or trazodone (which has less cardiotoxicity than tricyclics); patients with more prominent psychomotor retardation may respond better to a less sedating drug such as desipramine or nortriptyline. Nortriptyline offers some advantage in that blood levels are readily available and correlate with therapeutic efficacy (Katz et al., 1988), and it does not appear to have significant negative inotropic effects on cardiac function (Roose et al., 1986). Newer agents such as maprotiline and fluoxetine have not been well tested in the elderly.

In general, elderly patients may respond to lower doses than the usual adult dosages (Table 5-13), and clinical response can take from 2 to 4 weeks. Some elderly patients require and can tolerate dosages similar to those used in younger adults. Divided dosages may help

Table 5-14   Potential Side Effects of Tricyclic Antidepressants

Anticholinergic
   Dry mouth
   Blurred vision (impairment of lens accommodation)
   Acute angle-closure glaucoma (unusual)
   Constipation, fecal impaction, incontinence
   Reflux esophagitis (diminished esophageal sphincter tone)
   Urinary retention, overflow incontinence
   Tachycardia
   Psychosis ("anticholinergic crisis")
Cardiovascular
   Postural hypotension
   Decreased myocardial contractility
   Prolonged cardiac conduction
   Tachycardia
   Exacerbation of angina or heart failure
Central nervous system
   Sedation
   Cognitive impairment
   Psychosis

minimize side effects, although compliance can become a problem. In patients with sleep disturbances, a single bedtime dose can be used to take advantage of the sedative effects; however, these patients should be carefully instructed about the potential for postural hypotension in order to avoid falls in the middle of the night. Tricyclic blood levels, especially for nortriptyline, may be helpful in patients who are not responding or who develop side effects at low dosages. If the levels are therapeutic or high in a patient who has not responded after 2 to 4 weeks of treatment, switching to another antidepressant is probably indicated.

Tricyclic antidepressants may be unsuccessful or contraindicated in some patients (such as those with heart blocks, heart disease that could be exacerbated by tachycardia or hypotension, closed-angle glaucoma, or urinary retention). Methylphenidate (Ritalin) in small doses (10 mg one to three times a day) has been effective and safe in some elderly patients with retarded depressions and cardiovascular disease (Katon and Raskind, 1980). Its effects may diminish over time, and anorexia can be a side effect. Monoamine oxidase inhibitors (such as isocarboxazid, phenelzine, tranylcypromine) have been used in the elderly but require a relatively strict diet (avoidance of tyramine-rich foods) and can cause prominent hypotension. Although some feel that these drugs should be first-line agents in geriatric depression, they probably should be reserved for patients in whom other drugs have failed and who can be followed very closely.

For patients with bipolar disorder, lithium is useful in treating the manic phase of the illness and in preventing recurrent depression. It may also enhance the effects of other antidepressants in treating unipolar depression. Lithium has a very narrow therapeutic-toxic ratio and must be used very carefully in the elderly; its renal clearance is diminished, and it can interact adversely with diuretics. Blood levels should be monitored once or twice each week until a stable dosage is achieved, and then at least once a month thereafter. Dosages of 150 to 300 mg three times a day generally yield adequate blood levels in the elderly (0.3 to 0.6 meq per liter for maintenance). The elderly are especially susceptible to lithium toxicity, especially delirium. Hypothyroidism can occur in patients on lithium, and thyroid function tests should be monitored periodically in patients on chronic therapy.

Depressed elderly patients with psychotic features (paranoid and other types of delusions, hallucinations) may also require antipsychotic drug treatment. These drugs, as well as sedative and hypnotic agents (which are also useful in some depressed elderly patients with prominent anxiety or psychomotor agitation), are discussed in Chapter 14. Further details on the drug treatment of depression in the elderly can be found in the Suggested Readings at the end of this chapter.

If drug treatment fails or is contraindicated by medical conditions, or if rapid relief from depression is desired (such as might be the case in delusional, suicidal, or extremely vegetative patients), electroconvulsive therapy (ECT) should be considered. Despite its recent loss of popularity in many areas, ECT is relatively safe and can be highly effective in the elderly. Certain added precautions are necessary in elderly patients with hypertension and cardiac arrhythmias (such as close cardiac monitoring, diminished doses of pretreatment atropine), and cardiology consultation is advisable in these situations. Adequate pretreatment muscle relaxation will help avoid musculoskeletal complications, which are of special concern in those patients with osteoporosis. Posttreatment confusion and memory loss is usually mild and improves as the depression subsides. Many experts recommend unilateral ECT for the elderly, feeling that it may cause fewer problems with memory and have the same clinical effectiveness. The Suggested Readings cite several sources of more detailed information on ECT.

REFERENCES

American Psychiatric Association: *Diagnostic and Statistical Manual of Mental Disorders* (3d ed, revised). Washington, DC, American Psychiatric Association, 1987a.

American Psychiatric Association: Task Force on Laboratory Tests in Psychiatry. *Am J Psychiatr* 144:1253–1262, 1987b.

Brown GM: Psychiatric and neurologic aspects of endocrine disease. *Hosp Pract* 71–79, August 1975.

Carroll BJ, Feinberg M, Greden JF, et al: A specific laboratory test for the diagnosis of melancholia. *Arch Gen Psychiatr* 38:15–22, 1981.

Dement WC, Miles LE, Carkson MA: White paper on sleep and aging. *J Am Geriatr Soc* 30:25–50, 1982.

Dorpat TL, Anderson WF, Ripley HS: The relationship of physical illness to suicide, in Resnik H (ed): *Suicidal Behaviors*. Boston, Little Brown, 1968.

Gurland BJ, Cross PS: Epidemiology of psychopathology in old age: Some implications for clinical services. *Psychiatr Clin North Am* 5:11–26, 1982.

Hall RCW (ed): *Psychiatric Presentations of Medical Illness—Somatopsychic Disorders*. New York, SP Medical & Scientific Books, 1980.

Katon W, Raskind M: Treatment of depression in the medically ill with methylphenidate. *Am J Psychiatr* 137:963–965, 1980.

Katz IR, Curlit S, Lesher EL: Use of antidepressants in the frail elderly—when, why and how. *Clin Geriatr Med* 4:203–222, 1988.

Levenson AJ, Hall RCW (eds): *Neuropsychiatric Manifestation of Physical Disease in the Elderly*. New York, Raven Press, 1981.

Lipton MA, Nemeroff CB: The biology of aging and its role in depression, in Usdin G, Jofling CJ (eds): *Aging: The Process and the People*. New York, Brunner/Mazel, 1978.

Mindham RHS: Psychiatric symptoms in parkinsonism. *J Neurol Neurosurg Psychiatr* 33:188–191, 1970.

Osgood NJ: *Suicide in the Elderly*. Rockville, Aspen, Maryland, 1985.

Richelson E: Psychotropics and the elderly: Interactions to watch for. *Geriatrics* 39(12):30–42, 1984.

Roose SP, Glassman AH, Giardina EV, et al: Nortriptyline in depressed patients with left ventricular impairment. *JAMA* 256:3253–3257, 1986.

Spar JF, Gerner R: Does the dexamethasone suppression test distinguish dementia from depression? *Am J Psychiatr* 139:238–239, 1982.

Thomas FB, Mazzaferi EL, Skillman TG: Apathetic thyrotoxicosis: A distinctive clinical and laboratory entity. *Ann Intern Med* 72:679, 1970.

Verwoerdt A: Psychological responses to physical illness, in Verwoerdt A (ed): *Clinical Geropsychiatry*. Baltimore, Williams & Wilkins, 1976.

SUGGESTED READINGS

General

Blazer DG (ed): *Depression in Late Life*. St Louis, Mosby, 1982.

Busse EW, Blazer DG (eds): *Handbook of Geriatric Psychiatry*. New York, Van Nostrand Reinhold, 1980.

Hall RCW (ed): *Psychiatric Presentations of Medical Illness—Somato-psychic Disorders.* New York, SP Medical Scientific Books, 1980.

Salzman C, Shader RI: Clinical evaluation of depression in the elderly, in Raskin A, Jarvik LF (eds): *Psychiatric Symptoms and Cognitive Loss in the Elderly.* New York, Wiley, 1979.

Insomnia

Dement WC: Rational basis for the use of sleeping pills. *Pharmacology* 27(suppl 2):3–38, 1983.

Knight H, Millman RP, Gur RC, et al: Clinical significance of sleep apnea in the elderly. *Am Rev Resp Dis* 136:845–850, 1987.

Antidepressants

Bressler R: Antidepressant agents, in Conrad KA, Bressler R (eds): *Drug Therapy for the Elderly.* St Louis, Mosby, 1982.

Jarvik LF, Kakkar PR: Aging and response to antidepressants, in Jarvik LF, Greenblatt DG, Harman D (eds): *Clinical Pharmacology and the Aged Patient.* New York, Raven Press, 1981.

Richardson JW: Antidepressants: A clinical update for medical practitioners. *Mayo Clin Proc* 59:330–337, 1984.

Risch SC, Groom GP, Janowsky DS: Interfaces of psychopharmacology and cardiology: Parts I and II. *J Clin Psychol* 42:23–34, 47–59, 1981.

Electroconvulsive Therapy

Fraser RM, Glass IB: Unilateral and bilateral ECT in elderly patients. *Acta Psychiatr Scand* 62:13–31, 1980.

Salzman C: Electroconvulsive therapy in the elderly patient. *Psychiatr Clin North Am* 5:191–197, 1982.

Weiner RD: The psychiatric use of electronically induced seizures. *Am J Psychiatr* 136:1507–1517, 1979.

Chapter 6

Incontinence

Incontinence is a common, disruptive, and potentially disabling condition in the elderly. It is defined as the involuntary loss of urine (or stool) in sufficient amount or frequency to constitute a social and/or health problem. The prevalence of urinary incontinence increases with age, is slightly higher in females, and is more common in the elderly in acute care hospitals and nursing homes than in those dwelling in the community (Figure 6-1) (Mohide, 1986; Diokno et al., 1986). Incontinence is a very heterogeneous condition, ranging in severity from occasional episodes of dribbling small amounts of urine to continuous urinary incontinence with concomitant fecal incontinence. Incontinent elderly persons are not always severely demented, bedridden, and in nursing homes. Many, both in institutions and in the community, are ambulatory and have good mental function.

Physical health, psychological well-being, social status, and the costs of health care can all be adversely affected by incontinence (Table 6-1). Urinary incontinence is curable in many elderly patients, especially those who have adequate mobility and mental functioning.

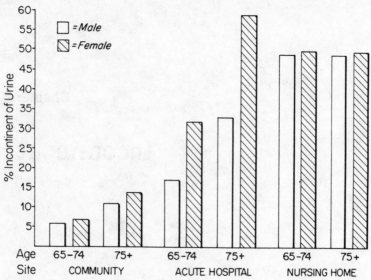

Figure 6-1 Prevalence of urinary incontinence by age and site (*From Harris, 1986; Sier et al., 1986; Ouslander et al., 1982.*)

Table 6-1   Potential Adverse Effects of Urinary Incontinence

Physical health
  Skin breakdown
  Recurrent urinary tract infections
Psychological health
  Isolation
  Depression
  Dependency
Social consequences
  Stress on family, friends, and care givers
  Predisposition to institutionalization
Economic costs
  Supplies (padding, catheters, etc.)
  Laundry
  Labor (nurses, housekeepers)
  Management of complications

Even when not curable, incontinence can always be managed in a manner that will keep patients comfortable, make life easier for care givers, and minimize costs of caring for the condition and its complications. Since many elderly patients are embarrassed and frustrated by their incontinence and either deny it or do not discuss it with a health professional, it is essential that specific questions about incontinence be included in periodic assessments and that incontinence be noted as a problem when detected in institutional settings.

This chapter briefly reviews the pathophysiology of incontinence in the elderly and provides detailed information on the evaluation and management of this condition. Although most of the chapter focuses on urinary incontinence, much of the pathophysiology also applies to fecal incontinence, which is briefly addressed at the end of the chapter.

NORMAL URINATION

Continence requires effective functioning of the lower urinary tract, adequate cognitive and physical functioning, motivation, and an appropriate environment (Table 6-2). Thus, the pathophysiology of

Table 6-2 Requirements for Continence

Effective lower urinary tract function
  Storage
    Accommodation by bladder of increasing volumes of urine under low pressure
    Closed bladder outlet
    Appropriate sensation of bladder fullness
    Absence of involuntary bladder contractions
  Emptying
    Bladder capable of contraction
    Lack of anatomic obstruction to urine flow
    Coordinated lowering of outlet resistance with bladder contractions
Adequate mobility and dexterity to use toilet or toilet substitute and to manage clothing
Adequate cognitive function to recognize toileting needs and to find a toilet or toilet substitute
Motivation to be continent
Absence of environmental and iatrogenic barriers such as inaccessible toilets or toilet substitutes, unavailable care givers, or drug side effects

incontinence in the elderly can relate to the anatomy and physiology of the lower urinary tract, as well as to functional psychological and environmental factors. Several anatomic components participate in normal urination (Figure 6-2). At the most basic level, urination is governed by a reflex centered in the sacral micturition center. Affer-

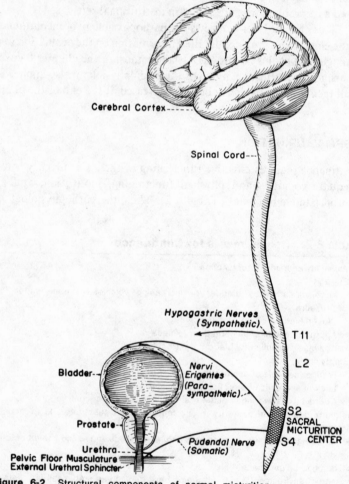

Figure 6-2 Structural components of normal micturition.

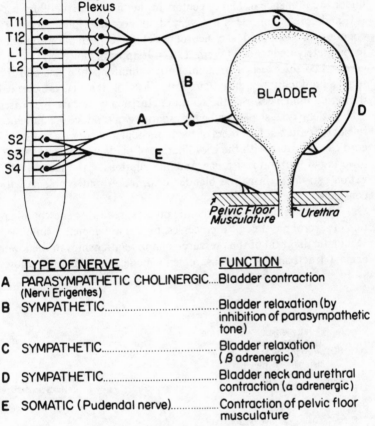

	TYPE OF NERVE	FUNCTION
A	PARASYMPATHETIC CHOLINERGIC (Nervi Erigentes)	Bladder contraction
B	SYMPATHETIC	Bladder relaxation (by inhibition of parasympathetic tone)
C	SYMPATHETIC	Bladder relaxation (β adrenergic)
D	SYMPATHETIC	Bladder neck and urethral contraction (α adrenergic)
E	SOMATIC (Pudendal nerve)	Contraction of pelvic floor musculature

Figure 6-3   Peripheral nerves involved in micturition.

ent pathways (via somatic and autonomic nerves) carry information on bladder volume to the spinal cord as the bladder fills. Motor output is adjusted accordingly (Figure 6-3). Thus, as the bladder fills, sympathetic tone closes the bladder neck, relaxes the dome of the bladder, and inhibits parasympathetic tone; somatic innervation maintains tone in the pelvic floor musculature (including striated muscle around the urethra). When urination occurs, sympathetic and somatic tones diminish, and parasympathetic cholinergically mediated impulses cause the bladder to contract. All these processes are under the influence of higher centers in the brainstem, cerebral cortex, and cerebellum. This is a very simplified description of a very complex process, and the neurophysiology of urination remains incompletely understood (Wein, 1987). It appears, however, that the cerebral cortex exerts a predominantly inhibitory influence and the brainstem facilitates urination. Thus, loss of the central cortical inhibiting influences over the sacral micturition center from diseases such as dementia, stroke, and parkinsonism can produce incontinence in elderly patients. Disorders of the brainstem and suprasacral spinal cord can interfere with the coordination of bladder contractions and lowering of urethral resistance, and interruptions of the sacral innervation can cause impaired bladder contraction and problems with continence.

Normal urination is a dynamic process, requiring the coordination of several physiological processes. Figure 6-4 depicts a simplified schematic diagram of the pressure-volume relationships in the lower urinary tract, similar to measurements made in urodynamic studies

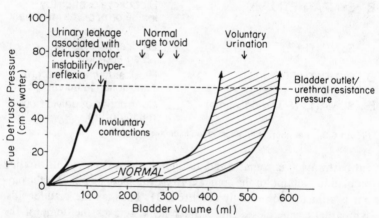

Figure 6-4   Simplified schematic diagram of pressure-volume relationships during bladder filling depicting the normal relationship and involuntary contractions (detrusor motor instability or hyperreflexia). True detrusor pressure is measured by subtracting intraabdominal pressure from total intravesical pressure, as would be done during a multichannel cystometrogram (see text).

(which are discussed later in this chapter). Under normal circumstances, as the bladder fills, pressure remains low (<15 cmH₂O). The first urge to void is variable but generally occurs between 150 and 350 ml, and normal bladder capacity is 300 to 600 ml. When normal urination is initiated, true detrusor pressure (bladder pressure minus intraabdominal pressure) increases until it exceeds urethral resistance, and urine flow occurs. If at any time during bladder filling total intravesical pressure (which includes intraabdominal pressure) exceeds outlet resistance, urinary leakage will occur. This will happen if, for example, intraabdominal pressure rises *without* a rise in true detrusor pressure by coughing or sneezing in someone with low outlet or urethral sphincter weakness. This would be defined as *genuine stress incontinence* in urodynamic terminology. Alternatively, the bladder can contract involuntarily and cause urinary leakage. This would be defined as *detrusor motor instability,* or *detrusor hyperreflexia* in patients with neurological disorders (International Continence Society, 1984).

CAUSES AND TYPES OF INCONTINENCE

Basic Causes

There are four basic categories of causes for urinary incontinence in the elderly (Figure 6-5). Determining the cause(s) is essential to proper management. It is very important to distinguish between urologic and neurological disorders that cause incontinence and other problems (such as diminished mobility and/or mental function, inaccessible toilets, and psychological problems) that can cause or contribute to the condition. As is the case for a number of other common geriatric problems discussed in this text, multiple disorders often interact to cause urinary incontinence, as depicted in Figure 6-5.

Aging alone does *not* cause urinary incontinence. Several age-related changes can, however, contribute to its development.

In general, with age, bladder capacity declines, residual urine increases, and involuntary bladder contractions are common (Figure 6-4). These contractions are found in 40 to 75 percent of elderly incontinent patients and 10 to 20 percent of elderly people with no or minimal urinary symptoms (Leach and Yip, 1986; Staskin, 1986). Combined with impaired mobility, these contractions may account

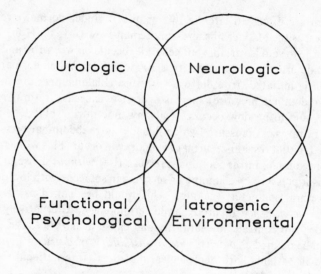

Figure 6-5   Basic underlying causes of geriatric urinary incontinence.

for a substantial proportion of incontinence in elderly functionally disabled patients.

Aging is also associated with a decline in bladder outlet and urethral resistance pressure in females. This decline, which is related to diminished estrogen influence and laxity of pelvic structures in females associated with prior childbirths, surgeries, and deconditioned muscles, predisposes to the development of stress incontinence (Figure 6-6). Decreased estrogen can also cause atrophic vaginitis and urethritis, which can, in turn, cause symptoms of dysuria and urgency and predispose to the development of urinary infection and urge incontinence. In men, prostatic enlargement is associated with decreased urine flow rates and detrusor motor instability and can lead to urge and/or overflow types of incontinence (see below).

Acute (Reversible) versus Persistent Incontinence

The distinction between acute, reversible forms of incontinence and persistent incontinence is clinically important. *Acute incontinence* refers to those situations in which the incontinence is of sudden onset,

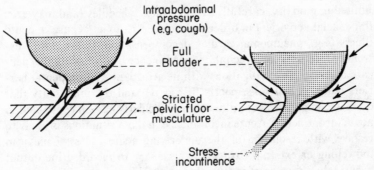

Figure 6-6 Simplified schematic diagram depicting age-associated changes in pelvic floor muscle, bladder, and urethra-vesical position predisposing to stress incontinence. Normally (left), the bladder and outlet remain anatomically inside the intraabdominal cavity and rises in pressure contribute to bladder outlet closure. Age-associated changes (e.g., estrogen deficiency, surgeries, childbirth) can weaken the structures maintaining bladder position (right); in this situation, increases in intraabdominal pressure can cause urine loss (stress incontinence).

usually related to an acute illness or an iatrogenic problem, and subsides once the illness or medication problem has been resolved. *Persistent incontinence* refers to incontinence that is unrelated to an acute illness and persists over time.

The causes of acute and reversible forms of urinary incontinence can be remembered by the acronym "DRIP" (Table 6-3), which was developed after another similar acronym for reversible causes of incontinence ("DIAPPERS"; Resnick, 1984). Many elderly persons, because of urinary frequency and urgency, especially when they are

Table 6-3   Causes of Acute and Reversible Forms of Urinary Incontinence

D	Delirium
R	Restricted mobility, retention
I	Infection,* inflammation,* impaction (fecal)
P	Polyuria,† pharmaceuticals‡

*Acute symptomatic urinary tract infection, atrophic vaginitis or urethritis.
†Hyperglycemia, volume-expanded states causing excessive nocturia (e.g., CHF, venous insufficiency).
‡See Table 6-4.

limited in mobility, carefully arrange their schedules (and may even limit social activities) in order to be close to a toilet. Thus, an acute illness (e.g., pneumonia, cardiac decompensation, stroke, lower extremity fracture) can precipitate incontinence by disrupting this delicate balance. Hospitalization, with its attendant environmental barriers (such as bed rails, poorly lit rooms), and the immobility that often accompanies acute illnesses in the elderly can all contribute to acute incontinence. Acute incontinence in these situations is likely to resolve with resolution of the underlying acute illness. Unless an indwelling or external catheter is necessary to record urine output accurately, this type of incontinence should be managed by environmental manipulations, scheduled toiletings, the appropriate use of toilet substitutes and pads, and careful attention to skin care. In a substantial proportion of patients incontinence may persist for several weeks after hospitalization and should be evaluated as for persistent incontinence (see below) (Sier et al., 1987).

Fecal impaction is a common problem in both acutely and chronically ill elderly patients. Its role in and mechanism of producing urinary incontinence are unclear. Possibilities include mechanical obstruction of the bladder outlet with overflow-type incontinence and reflex bladder contractions induced by rectal distension. Whatever the underlying mechanism, relief of a fecal impaction can lead to resolution of the urinary incontinence.

Urinary retention with overflow incontinence should be considered in any patient who suddenly develops urinary incontinence. Immobility; anticholinergic, narcotic, and beta-adrenergic drugs; and fecal impaction can all precipitate overflow incontinence in an elderly patient. In addition, this condition may be a manifestation of an underlying process causing spinal cord compression presenting acutely.

Although the relationship of bacteriuria and pyuria to the pathogenesis of incontinence is unclear (see below), any acute inflammatory condition in the lower urinary tract that causes frequency and urgency can precipitate incontinence. Treatment of an acute cystitis or urethritis can restore continence.

Conditions that cause polyuria, including hyperglycemia and hypercalcemia, as well as diuretics (especially the rapid-acting loop diuretics), can precipitate acute incontinence. Patients with volume-expanded states, such as congestive heart failure and lower extremity venous insufficiency, may have polyuria at night which can contribute to nocturia and nocturnal incontinence. Similar to many other conditions discussed throughout this text, a wide variety of medications can play a role in the development of incontinence in elderly patients (Table 6-4). Whether the incontinence is acute or persistent, the potential role of these medications in causing or contributing to the patients' incontinence should be considered. Whenever feasible, stopping the medication, switching to an alternative, or modifying the dosage schedule can be an important component (and possibly the only one necessary) of the treatment for incontinence.

Persistent forms of incontinence can be classified clinically into four basic types (Figure 6-7). As depicted, these types can overlap with each other and an individual patient may have more than one type simultaneously. While this classification is not in complete agreement with others described in the literature (Williams and Pannill, 1982; Resnick and Yalla, 1985; Wein, 1981) and does not

Table 6-4 Medications That Can Potentially Affect Continence

Type of medication	Potential effects on continence
Diuretics	Polyuria, frequency, urgency
Anticholinergics	Urinary retention, overflow incontinence, impaction
Psychotropics	
Antidepressants	Anticholinergic actions, sedation
Antipsychotics	Anticholinergic actions, sedation, rigidity, immobility
Sedatives and hypnotics	Sedation, delirium, immobility, muscle relaxation
Narcotic analgesics	Urinary retention, fecal impaction, sedation, delirium
Alpha-adrenergic blockers	Urethral relaxation
Alpha-adrenergic agonists	Urinary retention
Beta-adrenergic agonists	Urinary retention
Calcium channel blockers	Urinary retention
Alcohol	Polyuria, frequency, urgency, sedation, delirium, immobility

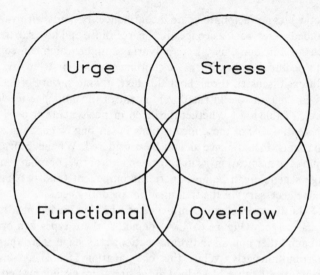

Figure 6-7   Basic types of persistent geriatric urinary incontinence.

include all the neurophysiological abnormalities associated with incontinence (such as reflex incontinence), it is helpful in approaching the clinical assessment and treatment of incontinence in the elderly.

Three of these types—stress, urge, and overflow—result from one or a combination of two basic abnormalities in lower genitourinary tract function:

1 Failure to store urine, caused by a hyperactive or poorly compliant bladder or by diminished outflow resistance
2 Failure to empty bladder, caused by a poorly contractile bladder or by increased outflow resistance

The clinical definitions and common causes of persistent urinary incontinence are shown in Table 6-5. Stress incontinence is common in elderly women, especially in ambulatory clinic settings (Ouslander et al., 1986b; Wells et al., 1987a; Diokno et al., 1987). It may be

Table 6-5   Basic Types and Causes of Persistent Urinary Incontinence

Type	Definition	Common causes
Stress	Involuntary loss of urine (usually small amounts) with increases in intraabdominal pressure (e.g., cough, laugh, or exercise)	Weakness and laxity of pelvic floor musculature Bladder outlet or urethral sphincter weakness
Urge	Leakage of urine (usually larger volumes) because of inability to delay voiding after sensation of bladder fullness is perceived	Detrusor motor and/or sensory instability, isolated or associated with one or more of the following: Local genitourinary condition such as cystitis, urethritis, tumors, stones, diverticuli, and outflow obstruction CNS disorders such as stroke, dementia, parkinsonism, suprasacral spinal cord injury or disease*
Overflow	Leakage of urine (usually small amounts) resulting from mechanical forces on an overdistended bladder or from other effects of urinary retention on bladder and sphincter function	Anatomic obstruction by prostate, stricture, cystocele Acontractile bladder associated with diabetes mellitus or spinal cord injury Neurogenic (detrusor-sphincter dyssynergy), associated with multiple sclerosis and other suprasacral spinal cord lesions
Functional	Urinary leakage associated with inability to toilet because of impairment of cognitive and/or physical functioning, psychological unwillingness, or environmental barriers	Severe dementia and other neurological disorders Psychological factors such as depression, regression, anger, and hostility

*When detrusor motor instability is associated with a neurological disorder, it is termed "detrusor hyperreflexia" by the International Continence Society.

infrequent and involve very small amounts of urine and need no specific treatment in women who are not bothered by it. On the other hand, it may be so severe and/or bothersome that it requires surgical correction. It is most often associated with weakened supporting tissues surrounding the bladder outlet and urethra caused by lack of estrogen and/or previous vaginal deliveries or surgery (Figure 6-6). Obesity and chronic coughing can also contribute. Stress incontinence is unusual in men, but can occur after transurethral surgery and/or radiation therapy for lower urinary tract malignancy when the anatomic sphincters are damaged.

Urge incontinence can be caused by a variety of lower genitourinary and neurological disorders (Table 6-5). It is most often, but not always, associated with detrusor motor instability or detrusor hyperreflexia (Figure 6-4). Some patients have a poorly compliant bladder without involuntary contractions (e.g., radiation or interstitial cystitis, both unusual conditions in the elderly). Other patients have symptoms of urge incontinence but do not exhibit detrusor motor instability on urodynamic testing. This is sometimes termed "sensory instability" or "hypersensitive bladder"; it is likely that some of these patients do have detrusor motor instability in their everyday lives, which is not documented at the time of the urodynamic study. On the other hand, there are some patients with neurologic disorders, who do have detrusor hyperreflexia on urodynamic testing, but may not have urgency and have incontinence without any warning symptoms. Almost all of the above-described patients are generally treated as if they have urge incontinence if they empty their bladders and do not have other correctable genitourinary pathology (see below). Recently, a subgroup of very elderly incontinent patients with detrusor hyperreflexia have been described who also have impaired bladder contractility—emptying less than one-third of their bladder volume with involuntary contractions on urodynamic testing (Resnick and Yalla, 1987). The implications of this urodynamic finding for the pathophysiology and treatment of incontinence in the elderly are unclear and currently under investigation.

Urinary retention with overflow incontinence can result from anatomic or neurogenic outflow obstruction, a hypotonic or acontractile bladder, or both. The most common causes include prostatic enlargement, diabetic neuropathic bladder, and urethral stricture.

Low spinal cord injury and anatomic obstruction in females (caused by pelvic prolapse and urethral distortion) are less common causes of overflow incontinence. Several types of drugs can also contribute to this type of persistent incontinence (Table 6-4). Some patients with suprasacral spinal cord lesions (e.g., multiple sclerosis) develop detrusor-sphincter dyssynergy and consequent urinary retention, which must be treated in a similar manner as overflow incontinence; in some instances a sphincterotomy is necessary.

Stress, urge, and overflow incontinence can occur in combination. Thus, a woman with stress incontinence or a man with obstruction may also have urge incontinence and detrusor motor instability or hyperreflexia. The coexistence of these disorders can have important therapeutic implications (see below).

Functional incontinence results when an elderly person is unable or unwilling to reach a toilet on time. Distinguishing this type of incontinence from other types of persistent incontinence is critical to appropriate management. Factors that cause functional incontinence (such as inaccessible toilets and psychological disorders) can also exacerbate other types of persistent incontinence. Patients with incontinence that appears to be predominantly related to functional factors may also have abnormalities of the lower genitourinary tract, such as detrusor hyperreflexia. In some patients it can be very difficult to determine whether the functional factors or the genitourinary factors predominate without a trial of specific types of treatment.

EVALUATION

In patients with the sudden onset of incontinence (especially when associated with an acute medical condition and hospitalization), the causes of acute incontinence (Table 6-3) can be ruled out by a brief history, physical examination, postvoid residual determination, and basic laboratory studies (urinalysis, culture, serum glucose or calcium).

Table 6-6 shows the basic components of the evaluation of persistent urinary incontinence. The history should focus on the characteristics of the incontinence, on current medical problems and medications, and on the impact of the incontinence on the patient and care givers (Table 6-7). The incontinence should be carefully characterized in terms of onset; frequency, timing, and amount of leakage;

Table 6-6   Basic Components of the Diagnostic Evaluation of Persistent Urinary Incontinence

All patients
History
Physical examination
Urinalysis
Urine culture
Simple tests of lower urinary tract function (see Table 6-9)
Selected patients*
Gynecologic evaluation
Urologic evaluation
Cystoscopy
Voiding cystourethrography
Urodynamic tests
Urine flowmetry
Cystometrogram
Pressure flow study
Urethral pressure profilometry
Sphincter electromyography

*See text and Table 6-10.

bladder sensation; symptoms of urge versus stress incontinence; and associated genitourinary symptoms such as dysuria and hematuria; and symptoms of voiding difficulty, including hesitancy, intermittent stream, and straining to void. Although these symptoms are generally not specific for the different types of incontinence, a careful history is essential in targeting the important parts of the evaluations and treatment. This history must be taken carefully; for example, women who actually have stress incontinence may report "leaking on the way to the toilet" after they stand up, which may sound on superficial questioning like urge incontinence. Reliably reported symptoms of voiding difficulty, especially if confirmed on clinical assessment, are an indication to consider referral for further evaluation (see below). Bladder records such as those shown in Figures 6-8 (for outpatients) and 6-9 (for institutionalized patients) can be helpful in characterizing symptoms as well as in following the response to treatment.

Physical examination should focus on abdominal, rectal, and genital examinations and an evaluation of lumbosacral innervation (Table 6-8). During the history and physical examination, special

Table 6-7   Key Aspects of an Incontinent Patient's History

Active medical conditions, especially
  Neurological disorders, diabetes mellitus, congestive heart failure, venous
    insufficiency
Medications (see Table 6-4)
Fluid intake pattern
  Type and amount of fluid (especially before bedtime)
Past genitourinary history, especially:
  Childbirth, surgery, dilatations, urinary retention, radiation, recurrent urinary
    tract infections
Symptoms of incontinence
  Onset and duration
  Type—stress vs. urge vs. mixed vs. other
  Frequency, timing, and amount of incontinence episodes and of continent voids
    (see Figures 6-8 and 6-9)
Other lower urinary tract symptoms
  Irritative—dysuria, frequency, urgency, nocturia
  Voiding difficulty—hesitancy, slow or interrupted stream, straining, incomplete
    emptying
  Other—hematuria, suprapubic discomfort
Other symptoms
  Neurological (indicative of stroke, dementia, parkinsonism, normal pressure
    hydrocephalus, spinal cord compression, multiple sclerosis)
  Psychological (depression)
  Bowel (constipation, stool incontinence)
  Symptoms suggestive of volume-expanded state (e.g., lower extremity edema,
    shortness of breath while horizontal or with exertion)
Perceptions of incontinence
  Patient's concerns or ideas about underlying cause(s)
  Interference with daily life
  Severity (e.g., Is it enough of a problem for you to consider surgery?)
Environmental factors
  Location and structure of bathrooms
  Availability of toilet substitutes

attention should be given to factors such as mobility, mental status, medications, and accessibility of toilets that may either be causing the incontinence or interacting with urologic and neurological disorders to worsen the condition.

Urinalysis and urine culture are the next steps in the evaluation of incontinence, although there is controversy about how this is best

BLADDER RECORD

Day:_____   Date:_____/_____.

month   day

1NSTRUCTIONS:

1) In the 1st column make a mark every time during the 2—hour period you urinate into the toilet

2) Use the 2nd column to record the amount you urinate (if you are measuring amounts)

3) In the 3rd or 4th column, make a mark every time you accidentally leak urine

Time Interval	Urinated in Toilet	Amount	Leaking Accident	or	Large Accident	Reason for Accident *
6—8 am						
8—10 am						
2—4 pm						
4—6 pm						
6—8 pm						
8—10 pm						
10—12 pm						
Overnight						

Number of pads used today: _____

* For example, if you coughed and have a leaking accident, write "cough".
   If you had a large accident after a strong urge to urinate, write "urge".

Figure 6-8   Example of a bladder record for ambulatory care settings.

done and how the results relate to incontinence. The following considerations are important:

1   Clean urine specimens are often difficult to obtain, especially in elderly women. The risk of inducing infection by a single sterile catheterization is small, probably less than 2 percent (Kunin, 1987); because it yields a clean bladder specimen and minimizes false positives, and because other valuable information can be obtained with the catheter in place, it is probably worth the risk.

INCONTINENCE MONITORING RECORD

INSTRUCTIONS: EACH TIME THE PATIENT IS CHECKED:
1) Mark *one* of the circles in the BLADDER section at the hour closest to the time the patient is checked.
2) Make an X in the BOWEL section if the patient has had an incontinent or normal bowel movement.

| ⬤ = Incontinent, small amount | ∅ = Dry | X = Incontinent BOWEL |
| ⬤ = Incontinent, large amount | ⬠ = Voided correctly | X = Normal BOWEL |

PATIENT NAME _____ ROOM # _____ DATE _____

| | BLADDER | | | BOWEL | | | |
	INCONTINENT OF URINE	DRY	VOIDED CORRECTLY	INCONTINENT X	NORMAL X	INITIALS	COMMENTS
12 am	● ●	○	△ cc ___				
1	● ●	○	△ cc ___				
2	● ●	○	△ cc ___				
3	● ●	○	△ cc ___				
4	● ●	○	△ cc ___				
5	● ●	○	△ cc ___				
6	● ●	○	△ cc ___				
7	● ●	○	△ cc ___				
8	● ●	○	△ cc ___				
9	● ●	○	△ cc ___				
10	● ●	○	△ cc ___				
11	● ●	○	△ cc ___				
12 pm	● ●	○	△ cc ___				
1	● ●	○	△ cc ___				
2	● ●	○	△ cc ___				
3	● ●	○	△ cc ___				
4	● ●	○	△ cc ___				
5	● ●	○	△ cc ___				
6	● ●	○	△ cc ___				
7	● ●	○	△ cc ___				
8	● ●	○	△ cc ___				
9	● ●	○	△ cc ___				
10	● ●	○	△ cc ___				
11	● ●	○	△ cc ___				
TOTALS:							

Figure 6-9 Example of a record to monitor bladder and bowel functions in institutional settings. This type of record is especially useful for implementing and following the results of various training procedures and other treatment protocols. (*From Ouslander et al., 1986a.*)

Table 6-8   Key Aspects of an Incontinent Patient's Physical Examination

Mobility and dexterity
   Functional status compatible with ability to self-toilet
   Gait disturbance (parkinsonism, normal-pressure hydrocephalus)
Mental status
   Cognitive function compatible with ability to self-toilet
   Motivation
   Mood and affect
Neurological
   Focal signs (especially in lower extremities)
   Signs of parkinsonism
   Sacral arc reflexes
Abdominal
   Bladder distension
   Suprapubic tenderness
   Lower abdominal mass
Rectal
   Perianal sensation
   Sphincter tone (resting and active)
   Impaction
   Masses
   Size and contour of prostate
Pelvic
   Perineal skin condition
   Perineal sensation
   Atrophic vaginitis (friability, inflammation, bleeding)
   Cystourethrocele / pelvic prolapse
   Pelvic mass
   Other anatomic abnormality
Other
   Lower extremity edema or signs of congestive heart failure (if nocturia is a
    prominent complaint)

2   Although there is a clear relationship between acute symptomatic urinary tract infection and incontinence, the relationship between "asymptomatic" bacteriuria and incontinence is controversial. Because the prevalence of bacteriuria and incontinence roughly parallel each other in the elderly, and because the bacteriuria may resolve spontaneously and does not appear related to symptoms (Boscia et al., 1986a, 1986b), it is difficult to make clear recommendations. To add to the controversy, recent controlled studies of treating asymptomatic bacteriuria (including patients with incontinence), especially in nursing home settings, have not favored treatment (Nicolle et al., 1983, 1987; Boscia et al., 1987). Although hard data are lacking, it would still seem reasonable when evaluating persistent incontinence in an individual patient to eradicate the bacteriuria once and observe the effect on the incontinence.

3 Catheterization, in addition to yielding a clean urine specimen, allows other information to be obtained by performing the simple tests of lower urinary tract function described below.

Most authors, including ourselves, do not recommend that all incontinent elderly patients undergo a urologic, gynecologic, or complex urodynamic evaluation as listed in Table 6-6 (Abrams et al., 1983; Williams and Pannill, 1982; Resnick and Yalla, 1985; Diokno et al., 1987; Ouslander et al., 1988a). Complex urodynamic testing as outlined in Table 6-6, cystoscopy and radiological evaluations should be reserved for patients with specific indications, for whom irreversible therapy (i.e., surgical intervention) is being contemplated, and for whom these evaluations will alter the treatment approach.

Several algorithms have been described which attempt to determine the appropriate treatment approach without the need for more complex evaluations and to identify patients who would benefit from further evaluation (Hilton and Stanton, 1981; Abrams et al., 1983, Resnick et al., 1986, Ouslander, 1986). Some of these strategies depend on clinical history and physical examination alone; others include bladder catheterizations or simplified urodynamic procedures. None have been tested prospectively in sufficiently large populations of elderly incontinent patients to make definitive recommendations about the most cost-effective diagnostic strategy.

We recommend the use of a series of simple tests of lower urinary tract function which can be carried out in a clinic, hospital, nursing home, or even home setting (Table 6-9), in conjunction with information obtained from the history and physical examination and a series of criteria for referral for further evaluation (Table 6-10).

The simple tests are generally easy to perform and interpret after becoming experienced in a few patients with different types of incontinence. They take 15 to 20 minutes to complete, can in many patients be performed by a single examiner (although an extra pair of hands is usually helpful), and require less than $10 to $15 of equip-

Table 6-9 Procedures for Simple Tests of Lower Urinary Tract Function

Procedure	Observations	Interpretation
1. Stress maneuvers If possible, start the tests when the patient feels fullness in the bladder; ask the patient to cough forcefully 3 times in the standing position with a small pad over the urethral area	a. Timing (coincident or after stress) and amount (drops or larger volumes) of any leakage	Leakage of urine coincident with stress maneuver confirms presence of stress incontinence
2. Normal voiding Ask the patient to void privately in his or her normal fashion into a commode containing a measuring "hat" after a standard prep for clean urine specimen collection	a. Signs of voiding difficulty (hesitancy, straining, intermittent stream) b. Voided volume	Signs of voiding difficulty may indicate obstruction or bladder contractility problem
3. Postvoid residual determination A 14-French straight catheter is inserted into the bladder using sterile technique 5 to 10 minutes after the patient voids	a. Ease of catheter passage b. Postvoid residual volume	If there is great difficulty passing the catheter, obstruction may be present If the residual volume is elevated (e.g., >100 ml) after a normal void, obstruction or a bladder contractility problem may be present

4. Bladder filling

For females, position a fracture pan under their buttocks, and for males, have a urinal available to measure any leakage during filling

A 50-ml catheter tip syringe without the piston is attached to the catheter and used as a funnel to fill the bladder; the bladder is filled with room-temperature sterile water, 50 ml at a time, by holding the syringe so that it is approximately 15 cm above the pubic symphysis (bladder pressure should not normally exceed 15 cm of water during filling) until the patient feels the urge to void, and 25-ml increments until bladder capacity is reached (an involuntary contraction, or "I would rush to the toilet now, I can't hold it anymore"); then remove the catheter

a. First urge to void ("I'm starting to feel a little full")

b. Presence or absence of involuntary bladder contractions—detected by continuous upward movement of the column of fluid (sometimes accompanied by leaking around or expulsion of the catheter) in the absence of abdominal straining, which the patient cannot inhibit

c. Amount lost with involuntary contraction and subsequent bladder emptying

d. Bladder capacity—amount instilled before either an involuntary contraction or the strong urge to void is perceived

Involuntary contractions or severe urgency at relatively low bladder volume (e.g., <250–300 ml) suggest urge incontinence, especially if consistent with the patient's presenting symptoms

5. Repeat stress maneuvers

Ask the patient to cough forcefully 3 times in the supine and standing positions

a. Timing (coincident or after stress) and amount (drops or larger volumes) of any leakage

See above

Stress maneuvers with a full bladder are more sensitive for detecting stress incontinence

6. Bladder emptying

Ask the patient to empty the bladder again privately into the commode with the measuring "hat"

a. Signs of voiding difficulty (see above)

b. Voided volume

c. Calculated postvoid residual (amount instilled minus amount voided)

See above

Calculated postvoid residual may be more valid if patient did not feel full at beginning of tests

161

Table 6-10 Criteria for Referral of Elderly Incontinent Patients for Urologic, Gynecologic, or Urodynamic Evaluation

Criteria	Definition	Rationale
A. History		
1. Recent history of lower urinary tract or pelvic surgery or irradiation	Surgery or irradiation involving the pelvic area or lower urinary tract within the past 6 months	A structural abnormality relating to the recent procedure should be sought
2. Relapse or rapid recurrence of a symptomatic urinary tract infection	Onset of dysuria, new or worsened irritative voiding symptoms, fever, suprapubic or flank pain associated with growth of $> 10^5$ colony forming units of a urinary pathogen; symptoms and bacteriuria return within 4 weeks of treatment	A structural abnormality or pathological condition in the urinary tract predisposing to infection should be excluded
B. Physical examination		
1. Marked pelvic prolapse*	Pronounced uterine descensus to or through the introitus, or a prominent cystocele that descends the entire height of the vaginal vault with coughing during speculum examination	Anatomic abnormality may underlie the pathophysiology of the incontinence and may require surgical repair
2. Stress incontinence*†	Stress incontinence demonstrated standing or supine; urine, generally drops or small volumes, leaks coincident with increasing abdominal pressure by vigorous coughing	Bladder neck suspension procedures are generally well tolerated and successful in properly selected elderly women who have stress incontinence that responds poorly to more conservative measures

3. Marked prostatic enlargement and/or suspicion of cancer

Gross enlargement of the prostate on digital exam; prominent induration or asymmetry of the lobes

An evaluation to exclude prostate cancer that requires curative or palliative therapy should be undertaken

4. Severe hesitancy, straining, and/or interrupted urinary stream

Straining to begin voiding and a dribbling or intermittent stream at a time the patient's bladder feels full

Signs suggestive of obstruction or poor bladder contractility

C. Postvoid residual

1. Difficulty passing a 14-French straight catheter

Catheter passage is impossible or requires considerable force, or a larger, more rigid catheter

Anatomic blockage of the urethra or bladder neck may be present

2. Postvoid residual volume >100 ml

Volume of urine remaining in the bladder within 5-10 min after the patient voids spontaneously in as normal a fashion as possible‡

Anatomic or neurogenic obstruction, or poor bladder contractility may be present

D. Urinalysis

1. Hematuria

Greater than 5 red blood cells per high-power field on microscopic exam in the absence of infection

A pathological condition in the urinary tract should be excluded

2. Uncertain diagnosis

After the history, physical exam, simple tests of lower urinary tract function and urinalysis, none of the other referral criteria are met, and the results are not consistent with predominantly functional, urge, and/or stress incontinence

A formal urodynamic evaluation may better help to define and reproduce the symptoms associated with the patient's incontinence and target treatment

---

*If medical conditions precluded surgery, or if the patient is adamantly opposed to considering surgical intervention, the patient should not be referred.

†Stress incontinence that is a prominent, bothersome symptom which has not responded to nonsurgical treatment. Men with stress incontinence who are candidates for an artificial sphincter should also be referred.

‡For patients who cannot void at the time of the evaluation, postvoid residual can be calculated after filling the bladder (see Table 6-9).

ment. Bladder capacity and stability as determined by the procedure outlined in Table 6-9 have been shown to be highly correlated with results of formal multichannel cystometrograms (Ouslander, 1988a). In some settings, relatively inexpensive simple cystometric equipment and noninvasive methods of measuring urine flow rate may be available which can enhance the accuracy of the assessment. The bladder filling procedure may be unnecessary to make a reasonable treatment plan in some elderly patients, such as women who have sterile urine, no atrophic vaginitis, meet none of the criteria in Table 6-10 and who (1) reliably give a history of stress incontinence without irritative or obstructive voiding symptoms, leak with stress maneuvers, and empty their bladders completely (they can be treated for stress-type incontinence); or (2) reliably give a history of urge incontinence without symptoms of stress incontinence or voiding difficulty, and empty their bladders completely (they can be treated for urge-type incontinence).

The criteria for referral for further evaluation in Table 6-10 are liberal and in preliminary studies have been shown to be reasonably sensitive, but not very specific for identifying patients who require further evaluation for appropriate treatment.

Figure 6-10 summarizes the above outlined approach to the diagnostic evaluation of incontinent elderly patients. The Appendix contains a form intended to assist in such evaluations.

MANAGEMENT

Several therapeutic modalities are used in managing incontinent patients (Table 6-11). Although few of them have been studied in well-controlled trials in the elderly population, they can be especially helpful if specific diagnoses are made and attention is paid to all factors that may be contributing to the incontinence in a given patient. Even when cures are not possible, the comfort and satisfaction of both patients and care givers can almost always be enhanced.

Special attention should be given to the management of acute forms of incontinence, which are most common in elderly patients in acute care hospitals. These forms of incontinence are often transient if managed appropriately; on the other hand, inappropriate management may lead to a permanent problem. The most common approach

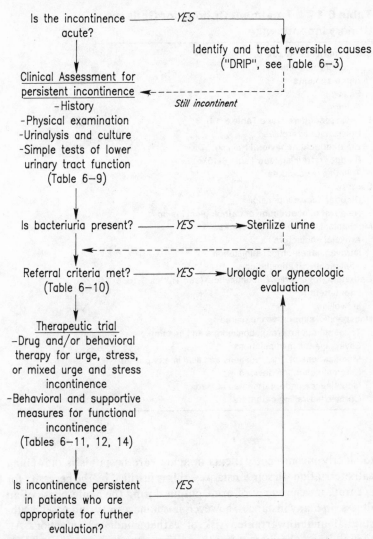

Is the incontinence acute? ———— YES ————

Identify and treat reversible causes ("DRIP", see Table 6–3)

Clinical Assessment for persistent incontinence ←- - - - - - - - - - - - - -
- History
- Physical examination
- Urinalysis and culture
- Simple tests of lower urinary tract function (Table 6–9)

Still incontinent

Is bacteriuria present? ———— YES ————→ Sterilize urine

Referral criteria met? ———— YES ————→ Urologic or gynecologic
(Table 6–10) evaluation

Therapeutic trial
- Drug and/or behavioral therapy for urge, stress, or mixed urge and stress incontinence
- Behavioral and supportive measures for functional incontinence
(Tables 6–11, 12, 14)

Is incontinence persistent in patients who are appropriate for further evaluation?

YES

Figure 6-10 Summary of assessment of geriatric urinary incontinence (see referenced tables and text for details).

Table 6-11   Treatment Options for Geriatric Urinary Incontinence

---

Drugs (see Table 6-13)
   Bladder relaxants
   Alpha agonists
   Estrogen
   Others
Training procedures (see Table 6-14)
   Pelvic floor exercises
   Biofeedback, behavioral training
   Bladder retraining (see Table 6-15)
   Toileting procedures
Surgery
   Bladder neck suspension
   Removal of obstruction or pathological lesion
Mechanical and electrical devices
   Artificial sphincters
   Intravaginal electrical stimulation
   Anal electrical stimulation
Catheters (for Overflow Incontinence) (see Tables 6-16, 6-17)
   Intermittent
   Indwelling
Nonspecific, supportive measures
   Toilet substitutes (e.g., commodes and urinals)
   Environmental manipulations
   Modifications of drug regimens and fluid intake pattern
   External collection devices
   Incontinence undergarments and pads
   Chronic indwelling catheters

---

to elderly incontinent patients in acute care hospitals is indwelling catheterization. In some instances, this is justified by the necessity for accurate measurement of urine output during the acute phase of an illness. In many instances, however, it is unnecessary and poses a substantial and unwarranted risk of catheter-induced infection. Although it may be more difficult and time-consuming, making toilets and toilet substitutes accessible combined with some form of scheduled toileting is probably a more appropriate approach in patients who do not require indwelling catheterization. Newer launderable or disposable and highly absorbent bed pads and undergarments may also be helpful in managing these patients. These products may be more costly than catheters, but probably result in less morbidity (and, therefore, overall cost) in the long run. All of the factors that can cause or contribute to reversible form of incontinence (Table 6-3) should be attended to in order to maximize the potential for regaining continence.

Supportive measures are critical in managing all forms of incontinence and should be used in conjunction with other more specific treatment modalities. A positive attitude, environmental manipulations, the appropriate use of toilet substitutes, avoidance of iatrogenic contributions to incontinence, modifications of diuretic and fluid intake patterns, and good skin care are all important.

Specially designed incontinence undergarments and pads can be very helpful in many patients, but must be used appropriately. They are now being marketed on television and are readily available in retail stores. Although they can be effective, several caveats should be raised:

1 Garments and pads are a nonspecific treatment. They should not be used as the first response to incontinence, or before some type of diagnostic evaluation is done.

2 Many patients are curable if treated with specific therapies, and some have potentially serious factors underlying their incontinence which must be diagnosed and treated.

3 Pants and pads can interfere with attempts at certain types of behaviorally oriented therapies designed to restore a normal pattern of voiding and continence (see below).

To a large extent the optimal treatment of persistent incontinence depends on identifying the type(s). Table 6-12 outlines the primary treatments for the basic types of persistent incontinence in the geriatric population. Each treatment modality is briefly discussed below.

Drug Treatment

Table 6-13 lists the drugs used to treat various types of incontinence. The efficacy of drug treatment has not been as well studied in the elderly as it has been in younger populations (Ouslander and Sier,

Table 6-12   Primary Treatments for Different Types of Geriatric Urinary Incontinence

Type of incontinence	Primary treatments
Stress	Pelvic floor (Kegel) exercises
	Alpha-adrenergic agonists
	Estrogen
	Biofeedback, behavioral training
	Surgical bladder neck suspension
Urge	Bladder relaxants
	Estrogen (if vaginal atrophy present)
	Training procedures (e.g., biofeedback, behavioral therapy)
	Surgical removal of obstructing or other irritating pathological lesions
Overflow	Surgical removal of obstruction
	Intermittent catheterization (if practical)
	Indwelling catheterization
Functional	Behavioral therapies (e.g., habit training, scheduled toileting)
	Environmental manipulations
	Incontinence undergarments and pads
	External collection devices
	Bladder relaxants (selected patients)*
	Indwelling catheters (selected patients)†

*Many patients with functional incontinence also have detrusor hyperreflexia, and some may benefit from bladder relaxant drug therapy (see text).

†See Table 6-16.

1986), but for many patients, especially those with urge or stress incontinence, drug treatment may be very effective. Drug treatment can be prescribed in conjunction with one or more of the behaviorally oriented training procedures discussed in the section that follows. There are no data on the relative efficacy of drug versus behavioral versus combination treatment in the elderly. Thus, until controlled trials are conducted, treatment decisions should be individualized and will depend in large part on the characteristics and preferences of the patient and the preference of the health care professional.

For urge incontinence, drugs with anticholinergic and bladder smooth muscle relaxant properties are used. All of them can have bothersome systemic anticholinergic side effects, especially dry mouth, and they can precipitate urinary retention in some patients. Men with some degree of outflow obstruction, diabetics, and patients with impaired bladder contractility (Resnick and Yalla, 1987) may be at the highest risk for developing urinary retention and should be followed carefully when these drugs are prescribed. Patients with Alzheimer's disease must be followed for the development of drug-induced delirium, which is unusual. Oxybutynin, starting in half the usual recommended dose (i.e., 2.5 mg three times per day) may offer some advantage over other drugs with more pronounced systemic anticholinergic side effects (Ouslander et al., 1988b) and does not have the potentially serious effects on blood pressure and cardiac conduction of imipramine. The latter drug has also been associated with hip fractures in the elderly (Ray et al., 1987), possibly because of the side effect of postural hypotension. Calcium channel blockers have been used for urge incontinence in Europe, but none have been studied or are approved for this indication as yet in the United States. Several studies suggest that cognitive and physical functional impairment are associated with poor responses to bladder relaxant drug therapy (Castleden et al., 1985; Zorzitto et al., 1986; Tobin and Brocklehurst, 1986a; Ouslander et al., 1988c). The results of these studies should not, however, preclude a treatment trial in this patient population. Some patients may respond, especially in conjunction with scheduled toileting or prompted voiding (see below). The *goal* of treatment in these patients may not be to cure the incontinence, but to reduce its severity and prevent discomfort and complications.

For stress incontinence drug treatment involves a combination of an alpha agonist and estrogen. Drug treatment is appropriate for motivated patients who (1) have mild to moderate degrees of stress incontinence, (2) do not have a major anatomic abnormality (e.g., large cystocele), and (3) do not have any contraindications to these drugs. These patients may also respond to behavioral treatments (see below), and preliminary data suggest that the two treatment modalities are roughly equivalent, with about three-quarters of patients reporting improvement (Wells et al., 1987b). A combination would also be a reasonable approach for some patients. Estrogen alone is not as effective as in combination with an alpha agonist for stress incontinence. If either oral or vaginal estrogen is used for a prolonged period of time (more than a few months), cyclic administration and the addition of a progestational agent should be considered (Lufkin et al.,

Table 6-13   Drugs Used to Treat Urinary Incontinence

Drugs	Dosages	Mechanisms of action	Types of incontinence	Potential adverse effects
Anticholinergic and antispasmodic agents				
Oxybutynin (Ditropan)	2.5–5.0 mg tid	Increase bladder capacity	Urge or stress with detrusor instability or hyperreflexia	Dry mouth, blurry vision, elevated intraocular pressure, delirium, constipation
Propantheline (Pro-Banthine)	15–30 mg tid			
Dicyclomine (Bentyl)	10–20 mg tid	Diminish involuntary bladder contractions		
Flavoxate (Urispas)	100–200 mg tid			
Imipramine (Tofranil)	25–50 mg tid			Above effects plus postural hypotension, cardiac conduction disturbances
Alpha-adrenergic agonists				
Pseudoephedrine (Sudafed)	15–30 mg tid	Increase urethral smooth muscle contraction	Stress incontinence with sphincter weakness	Headache, tachycardia, elevation of blood pressure
Phenylpropanolamine (Ornade)	75 mg tid			
Imipramine (Tofranil)	25–50 mg tid			All effects listed above

170

Conjugated estrogens* Oral (Premarin)	0.625 mg / day	Increased periurethral blood flow Strengthen periurethral tissues	Stress incontinence Urge incontinence associated with atrophic vaginitis	Endometrial cancer, elevated blood pressure, gallstones
Topical	0.5–1.0 g per application			
Cholinergic agonists† Bethanechol (Urecholine)	10–30 mg tid	Stimulate bladder contraction	Overflow incontinence with atonic bladder	Bradycardia, hypotension, bronchoconstriction, gastric acid secretion
Alpha-adrenergic antagonist Prazosin (Minipress)‡	1–2 mg tid	Relax smooth muscle of urethra and prostatic capsule	Overflow or urge incontinence associated with prostatic enlargement	Postural hypotension

*With prolonged use, cyclical administration with a progestational agent should be considered. Transdermal preparations are also available but have not been studied for treating incontinence.

†The efficacy of chronic bethanechol therapy in controversial (see text).

‡May provide some symptomatic relief in patients who are unwilling or unable to undergo prostatectomy (see text).

1988). Estrogen is also used, either chronically or on an intermittent basis (i.e., 1- to 2-month courses), for the treatment of irritative voiding symptoms and urge incontinence in women with atrophic vaginitis and urethritis.

Drug treatment for chronic overflow incontinence using a cholinergic agonist or an alpha-adrenergic antagonist is rarely highly efficacious. Bethanechol may be helpful when given for a brief period subcutaneously in patients with persistent bladder contractility problems after an overdistension injury, but is seldom effective when given long-term orally (Finkbeiner, 1985). Alpha-adrenergic blockers may be helpful in relieving symptoms associated with outflow obstruction in some patients but are probably not efficacious for long-term treatment of overflow incontinence in the elderly (Caine, 1986).

Many elderly women have symptomatically and urodynamically a combination of both urge and stress incontinence. A combination of estrogen and imipramine would, at least in theory, be appropriate for these patients because imipramine has both anticholinergic and alpha-adrenergic effects. If urge incontinence is the predominant symptom, a combination of estrogen and oxybutynin would be appropriate. Behavioral training procedures are also a reasonable approach to women with mixed incontinence.

Behaviorally Oriented Training Procedures

Many types of behavioral training procedures have been described for the management of urinary incontinence (Burgio and Burgio, 1986; Hadley, 1986). The nosology of these procedures has been somewhat confusing, and much of the literature has used the term *bladder training* to encompass a wide variety of techniques. It is very important to distinguish between procedures that are patient-dependent (i.e., require adequate function and motivation of the patient) in which the goal is to restore a normal pattern of voiding and continence, and procedures that are care giver-dependent and can be used for functionally disabled patients, in which the goal is to keep the patient and environment dry. Six of these procedures are discussed below according to the techniques used, the types of incontinence they are used for, and the characteristics of the patients for whom the techniques are most useful. This information is summarized in Table 6-14. All the patient-dependent procedures generally involve the patient's continuous self-monitoring using a record such as the one depicted in Figure 6-8, and the care giver-dependent procedures usually involve a record such as the one shown in Figure 6-9.

Pelvic floor (Kegel) exercises are used to treat stress incontinence in women, and occasionally in men. These exercises consist of repetitive contractions of the pelvic floor muscles. This procedure is taught by having the patient interrupt voiding to get a sense of the muscles being used or by having women squeeze the examiner's fingers during a vaginal examination (without doing a Valsalva maneuver, which is the opposite of the intended effect). Once learned, the exercises should be practiced many times throughout the day, both during voiding and at other times. Pelvic floor exercises may be done in conjunction with biofeedback procedures, which can be especially helpful for women who bear down (increasing intraabdominal pressure) when attempting to contract pelvic floor muscles.

Biofeedback procedures involve the use of bladder, rectal, or vaginal pressure or electrical activity recordings to train patients to contract pelvic floor muscles and relax the bladder. Studies have shown that these techniques can be very effective for managing both stress and urge incontinence, even in the elderly (Burgio et al., 1985). The use of biofeedback techniques may be limited by their requirements for equipment and trained personnel; in addition, some of these techniques are relatively invasive and require the use of bladder or rectal catheters, or both. Electrical stimulation, either vaginally or rectally, has also been used to help train muscles in the management of both stress and urge incontinence. Electrical stimulation techniques are not acceptable to many patients and have been not well studied or used to any great degree in the elderly in this county.

Other forms of patient-dependent training procedures include behavioral training and bladder retraining. Behavioral training involves the educational components taught during biofeedback, but without the use of biofeedback equipment. Patients are taught pelvic floor exercises, strategies to manage urgency, and to regularly use bladder records. There is some evidence that these techniques are as effective as biofeedback in a selected group of functional, motivated elderly patients (Burton et al., 1988). Bladder retraining as described here is similar to "bladder drill," which has been used successfully to treat urge incontinence in young women. An example of a bladder retraining protocol is shown in Table 6-15. This protocol is also appli-

Table 6-14 Examples of Behaviorally Oriented Training Procedures for Urinary Incontinence

Procedure	Definition	Types of incontinence	Comments
Patient-dependent			
Pelvic floor (Kegel) exercises	Repetitive contraction of pelvic floor muscles	Stress	Requires adequate function and motivation May be done in conjunction with biofeedback
Biofeedback	Use of bladder, rectal, or vaginal pressure recordings to train patients to contract pelvic floor muscles and relax bladder	Stress and urge	Requires equipment and trained personnel Relatively invasive Requires adequate cognitive and physical function and motivation
Behavioral training	Use of educational components of biofeedback, bladder records, pelvic floor and other behavioral exercises	Stress and urge	Requires trained therapist, adequate cognitive and physical functioning, and motivation
Bladder retraining*	Progressive lengthening or shortening of intervoiding interval,† with adjunctive techniques,† intermittent catheterization used in patients recovering from overdistension injuries with persistent retention	Acute (e.g., postcatheterization, with urge or overflow, poststroke)	Goal is to restore normal pattern of voiding and continence; requires adequate cognitive and physical function and motivation

174

Care giver-dependent Scheduled toileting and prompted voiding	Fixed toileting schedule with prompted voiding; adjunctive techniques may also be used	Urge and functional	Goal is to prevent wetting episodes Can be used in patients with impaired cognitive or physical functioning Requires staff or care giver availability and motivation
Habit training	Variable toileting schedule with positive reinforcement and adjunctive techniques†	Urge and functional	Goal is to prevent wetting episodes Can be used in patients with impaired cognitive or physical functioning Requires staff or care giver availability and motivation

*See Table 6-15.
†Techniques to trigger voiding (running water, stroking thigh, suprapubic tapping), completely empty bladder (bending forward, suprapubic pressure), and alterations of fluid or diuretic intake patterns.

Table 6-15 Example of a Bladder Retraining Protocol

Objective: To restore a normal pattern of voiding and continence after the removal of an indwelling catheter*

1. Remove the indwelling catheter (clamping the catheter before removal is not necessary)
2. Treat urinary tract infection if present†
3. Initiate a toileting schedule
   a. Begin by toileting the patient
      1. On awakening
      2. Q2h during the day and evening
      3. Before getting into bed
      4. Q4h at night
4. Monitor the patient's voiding and continence pattern with a record‡ that allows for the recording of
   a. Frequency, timing, and amount of continent voids
   b. Frequency, timing, and amount of incontinence episodes
   c. Fluid intake pattern
   d. Postvoid or intermittent catheter volume
5. If the patient is having difficulty voiding (complete urinary retention or very low urine outputs, e.g., <240 ml in an 8-h period while fluid intake is adequate):
   a. Perform in and out catheterization, recording volume obtained, q6–8h until residual values are <100 ml§
   b. Instruct the patient on techniques to trigger voiding (e.g., running water, stroking inner thigh, suprapubic tapping) and to help to completely empty bladder (e.g., bending forward, suprapubic pressure, double voiding)
6. If the patient is voiding frequently (i.e., >q2h)
   a. Perform postvoid residual determination to ensure the patient is completely emptying the bladder
   b. Encourage the patient to delay voiding as long as possible and instruct them to use techniques to help completely empty bladder (above)
7. If the patient continues to have frequency and nocturia, with or without urgency and incontinence, in the absence of infection
   a. Rule out other reversible causes (e.g., medication effects, hyperglycemia, congestive heart failure)
   b. Consider urologic referral to rule out bladder instability (unstable bladder, detrusor hyperreflexia)

---

*Indwelling catheters should be removed from all patients who do not have an indication for their acute or chronic use (see text and Table 6-16). Clamping routines have never been shown to be helpful and are not appropriate for patients who have had overdistended bladders.

†Significant bacteriuria with pyuria (>10 white blood cells per high-power field on a spun specimen).

‡See Figure 6-9.

§In patients who have been in urinary retention, it may take days or weeks for the bladder to regain normal function. If residuals remain high, urologic consultation should be considered before the patient is committed to a chronic indwelling catheter.

cable to patients who have had indwelling catheterization for monitoring of urinary output during a period of acute illness or for treatment of urinary retention with overflow incontinence. Such catheters should always be removed as soon as possible, and this type of bladder retraining protocol should enable most indwelling catheters to be removed from patients in acute care hospitals as well as some in long-term-care settings. A patient who continues to have difficulty voiding after 1 to 2 weeks of such a bladder retraining protocol should be examined for other potentially reversible causes of voiding difficulties, such as those mentioned in the preceding section on acute incontinence. When difficulties persist, a urologic referral should be considered in order to rule out correctable lower genitourinary pathology.

The goal of care giver-dependent procedures such as habit training and scheduled toileting is to prevent incontinence episodes rather than restore normal pattern of voiding and complete continence. Such procedures have also been referred to as "habit retraining," "prompted voiding," and "contingency management techniques." In its simplest form, scheduled toileting or prompted voiding involves toileting the patient at regular intervals, usually every 2 h during the day and every 4 h during the evening and night. Habit training involves a schedule of toiletings or prompted voidings that is modified according to the patient's pattern of continent voids and incontinence episodes as demonstrated by a monitoring record such as that shown in Figure 6-9. Positive reinforcement is offered for continent voids and neutral reinforcement, when incontinence occurs. Adjunctive techniques to prompt voiding (e.g., running tap water, stroking the inner thigh, or suprapubic tapping) and to facilitate complete emptying of the bladder (e.g., bending forward after completion of voiding) may be helpful in some patients. The success of habit training and scheduled toileting procedures is largely dependent on the knowledge and motivation of the care givers who are implementing them, rather than on the physical functional and mental status of the incontinent patient. These techniques may not be feasible in home settings without available care givers. In order for these types of training procedures to be feasible and cost-effective in the nursing home setting, the amount of time generally spent by the nursing staff in changing patients after incontinence episodes should not be exceeded by the time and effort necessary to implement such training procedures. Targeting of these procedures to selected patients, such as those with less frequent voiding and larger bladder capacities or voided volumes, may enhance their cost-effectiveness (Schnelle et al., 1988).

Surgery

Surgery should be considered for elderly women with stress incontinence that continues to be bothersome after attempts at nonsurgical treatment and in women with a significant degree of pelvic prolapse. As with many other surgical procedures, patient selection and the experience of the surgeon are critical to success. All women being considered for surgical therapy should have a thorough evaluation, including urodynamic tests, by an experienced surgeon before undergoing the procedure. Women with mixed stress incontinence and detrusor motor instability may also benefit from surgery (McGuire and Savastano, 1985), especially if the clinical history and urodynamic findings suggest that stress incontinence is the predominant problem. In some patients this may be difficult to determine, and a trial of medical therapy as discussed above would be appropriate. New modified techniques of bladder neck suspension can be done with minimal risks and are highly successful in achieving continence (Schmidbauer et al., 1986). Urinary retention can occur after surgery, but it is usually transient and can be managed by intermittent catheterization.

Surgery may be indicated in men in whom incontinence is associated with anatomically and/or urodynamically documented outflow obstruction. Men who have experienced an episode of complete urinary retention are likely to have another episode within a short period of time and should have a prostatic resection, as should men with incontinence associated with a sufficient amount of residual urine to be causing recurrent symptomatic infections or hydronephrosis. The decision about surgery in men who do not meet these criteria must be an individual one, weighing carefully the degree to which the symptoms bother the patient, the potential benefits of surgery (obstructive symptoms often respond better than irritative symptoms), and the risks of surgery (which may be minimal with newer prostate resection techniques). Several recent articles discuss these issues in detail (Barry et al., 1988; Fowler et al., 1988; Wennberg et al., 1988), and a Veterans Administration Cooperative Study involving a randomized trial of surgical versus medical follow-up for men with moderately symptomatic prostatic hyperplasia is currently under way.

A small number of elderly patients, especially men who have stress incontinence related to sphincter damage due to previous transurethral surgery, may benefit from the surgical implantation of an artificial urinary sphincter.

Catheters and Catheter Care

Three basic types of catheters and catheterization procedures are used for the management of urinary incontinence: external catheters, intermittent straight catheterization, and chronic indwelling catheterization. External catheters generally consist of some type of condom connected to a drainage system. Improvements in design and observance of proper procedure and skin care when applying the catheter will decrease the risk of skin irritation as well as the frequency with which the catheter falls off. Studies of complications associated with the use of these devices have been limited. Existing data suggest that patients with external catheters are at increased risk of developing symptomatic infection (Ouslander et al., 1987a). External catheters should only be used to manage intractable incontinence in male patients who do not have urinary retention and who are extremely physically dependent. As with incontinence undergarments and padding, these devices should not be used as a matter of convenience, since they may foster dependency. Contrary to popular belief, urine specimens can be collected from male patients with external catheters that accurately reflect bladder urine by simply cleaning the penis with betadine, applying a new catheter and collecting the first urine the patient voids (Ouslander et al., 1987b). Use of this simple technique will avoid false positive cultures and the discomfort of straight catheterization in patients suspected of having an infection. An external catheter for use in female patients is now commercially available, but its safety and effectiveness have not been well documented in the elderly.

Intermittent catheterization can help in the management of patients with urinary retention and overflow incontinence. The procedure can be carried out by either the patient or a care giver and involves straight catheterization two to four times daily, depending on residual urine volumes. In the home setting, the catheter should be kept clean (but not necessarily sterile). Studies conducted largely among younger paraplegics have shown that this technique is practical and reduces the risk of symptomatic infection as compared with chronic catheterization. Self-intermittent catheterization has also been shown to be feasible for elderly female outpatients who are functional, willing, and able to catheterize themselves (Bennett and Diokno, 1984). However, studies carried out in young paraplegics and elderly female outpatients cannot automatically be extrapolated to an elderly male or institutionalized population. The technique may be useful for certain patients in acute care hospitals or nursing homes, such as women who have undergone bladder neck suspension, or following removal of an indwelling catheter in a bladder retraining protocol (Table 6-15). However, the practicality and safety of this procedure in a long-term-care setting have never been documented. Elderly nursing home patients, especially men, may be difficult to catheterize, and the anatomic abnormalities commonly found in elderly patients' lower urinary tracts may increase the risk of infection due to repeated straight catheterizations. In addition, using this technique in an institutional setting (which may have an abundance of organisms relatively resistant to many commonly used antimicrobial agents) may yield an unacceptable risk of nosocomial infections, and using sterile catheter trays for these procedures would be very expensive; thus, it may be extremely difficult to implement such a program in a typical nursing home setting.

Chronic indwelling catheterization is overused in some settings, and when used for periods of up to 10 years, has been shown to increase the incidence of a number of complications, including chronic bacteriuria, bladder stones, periurethral abscesses, and even bladder cancer. Elderly nursing home patients, especially men, managed by this technique are at relatively high risk of developing symptomatic infections (Warren et al., 1987; Ouslander et al., 1987c; Kunin et al., 1987). Given these risks, it seems appropriate to recommend that the use of chronic indwelling catheters be limited to certain specific situations (Table 6-16). When indwelling catheterization is used, certain principles of catheter care should be observed in order to attempt to minimize complications (Table 6-17).

Table 6-16   Indications for Chronic Indwelling Catheter Use

Urinary retention that:
  Is causing persistent overflow incontinence, symptomatic infections, or renal
    dysfunction
  Cannot be corrected surgically or medically
  Cannot be managed practically with intermittent catheterization
Skin wounds, pressure sores, or irritations that are being contaminated by
  incontinent urine
Care of terminally ill or severely impaired for whom bed and clothing changes are
  uncomfortable or disruptive
Preference of patient or care giver when patient has failed to respond to more
  specific treatments

Table 6-17   Key Principles of Chronic Indwelling Catheter Care

1. Maintain sterile, closed, gravity drainage system
2. Avoid breaking the closed system
3. Use clean techniques in emptying and changing the drainage system; wash
   hands between patients in institutionalized setting
4. Secure the catheter to the upper thigh or lower abdomen to avoid perineal
   contamination and urethral irritation due to movement of the catheter
5. Avoid frequent and vigorous cleaning of the catheter entry site; washing with
   soapy water once per day is sufficient
6. Do not routinely irrigate
7. If bypassing occurs in the absence of obstruction, consider the possibility of
   a bladder spasm, which can be treated with a bladder relaxant
8. If catheter obstruction occurs frequently, increase the patient's fluid intake
   and acidify the urine if possible
9. Do not routinely use prophylactic or suppressive urinary antiseptics or
   antimicrobials
10. Do not do routine surveillance cultures to guide management of individual pa-
    tients because all chronically catheterized patients have bacteriuria (which
    is often polymicrobial) and the organisms change frequently
11. Do not treat infection unless the patient develops symptoms; symptoms may
    be nonspecific and other possible sources of infection should be carefully
    excluded before attributing symptoms to the urinary tract
12. If a patient develops frequent symptomatic urinary tract infections, a
    genitourinary evaluation should be considered to rule out pathology such as
    stones, periurethral or prostatic abscesses, and chronic pyelonephritis

FECAL INCONTINENCE

Fecal incontinence is less common than urinary incontinence. Its occurrence is relatively unusual in elderly patients who are continent with regard to urine; however, a large proportion (30 to 50 percent) of elderly patients with frequent urinary incontinence also have episodes of fecal incontinence (Ouslander et al., 1982; Ouslander and Fowler, 1985; Tobin and Brocklehurst, 1986b). This coexistence suggests common pathophysiological mechanisms.

Defecation, like urination, is a physiological process that involves smooth and striated muscles, central and peripheral innervation, coordination of reflex responses, mental awareness, and physical ability to get to a toilet. Disruption of any of these factors can lead to fecal incontinence.

The most common causes of fecal incontinence are problems with constipation and laxative use, neurological disorders, and colorectal disorders (Table 6-18). Constipation is extremely common in the elderly and, when chronic, can lead to fecal impaction and incontinence. The hard stool (or scybalum) of fecal impaction irritates the rectum and results in the production of mucus and fluid. This fluid leaks around the mass of impacted stool and precipitates incontinence. Constipation is difficult to define; technically it indicates less than three bowel movements per week, although many patients use the term to describe difficult passage of hard stools or a feeling of incomplete evacuation. Poor dietary and toilet habits, immobility,

Table 6-18   Causes of Fecal Incontinence

Fecal impaction
Laxative overuse or abuse
Neurological disorders
   Dementia
   Stroke
   Spinal cord disease
Colorectal disorders
   Diarrheal illness
   Diabetic autonomic neuropathy
   Rectal sphincter damage

and chronic laxative abuse are the most common causes of constipation in the elderly (Table 6-19).

Appropriate management of constipation will prevent fecal impaction and resultant fecal incontinence. The first step in managing constipation in the elderly is the identification of all possible contributory factors. If the constipation is a new complaint and represents a recent change in bowel habit, then colonic disease, endocrine or metabolic disorders, depression, or drug side effects should be considered (Table 6-19). Proper diet, including adequate fluid intake and bulk, is important in preventing constipation. Crude fiber in amounts of 4 to 6 g (equivalent to 3 or 4 tablespoons of bran) a day is generally recommended. Improving mobility, body positioning during toileting, and the timing and setting of toileting are all important in managing constipation. Defecation should optimally take place in a private, unrushed atmosphere and should take advantage of the gastrocolic reflex, which occurs a few minutes after eating. These factors are often overlooked, especially in nursing home settings.

A variety of drugs can be used to treat constipation (Table 6-20). These drugs are often overused; in fact, their overuse may cause an atonic colon and contribute to chronic constipation ("cathartic

Table 6-19   Causes of Constipation

Diet low in bulk and fluid
Poor toilet habits
Immobility
Laxative abuse
Colorectal disorders
   Colonic tumor, stricture, volvulus
   Painful anal and rectal conditions (hemorrhoids, fissures)
Depression
Drugs
   Anticholinergic
   Narcotic
Diabetic autonomic neuropathy
Endocrine or metabolic
   Hypothyroidism
   Hypercalcemia
   Hypokalemia

Table 6-20   Drugs Used to Treat Constipation

Type	Examples	Mechanism of action
Stool softeners and lubricants	Dioctyl sodium succinate Mineral oil	Soften and lubricate fecal mass
Bulk-forming agents	Bran Psyllium mucilloid	Increase fecal bulk and retain fluid in bowel lumen
Osmotic cathartics	Milk of Magnesia Magnesium sulfate/citrate	Poorly absorbed salts retain fluid in bowel lumen; increase net secretions of fluid in small intestine
Stimulants and irritants	Cascara Senna Bisacodyl Phenolphthalein	Alter intestinal mucosal permeability; stimulate muscle activity and fluid secretions
Enemas	Tap water Saline Sodium phosphate Oil	Induce reflex evacuations
Suppositories	Glycerin Bisacodyl	Cause mucosal irritation

colon"). Laxative drugs can also contribute to fecal incontinence. Rational use of these drugs requires knowing the nature of the constipation and quality of the stool. For example, stool softeners will not help a patient with a large mass of already soft stool in the rectum. These patients would benefit from a glycerin or irritant suppository. The use of osmotic and irritant laxatives should be limited to no more than three or four times a week.

Fecal incontinence from neurological disorders is sometimes amenable to biofeedback therapy (Whitehead et al., 1985), although many elderly demented patients are unable to cooperate. For those patients with end-stage dementia, a program of alternating constipating agents (if necessary) and laxatives on a routine schedule (such as giving laxatives and enemas three times a week) is effective in controlling defecation in many patients with fecal incontinence. Experience suggests that these measures should permit management of even severely disoriented patients. As a last resort, specially designed incontinence undergarments are sometimes helpful in managing fecal incontinence and preventing complications.

The Appendix offers a simple incontinence assessment form intended to assist in the evaluation of incontinent patients. Two organizations may serve as a resource for incontinent patients and their care givers:

The Simon Foundation   Help for Incontinent People (HIP)
Box 835   P. O. Box 544
Wilmette, Illinois 60091   Union, South Carolina 29379

REFERENCES

Abrams P, Fenely R, Torrens M: *Urodynamics,* New York, Springer-Verlag, 1983, Chapter 5.

Barry MJ, Mulley AG, Fowler FJ, et al: Watchful waiting vs immediate transurethral resection for symptomatic prostatism: The importance of patients' preferences. *JAMA* 259:3010–3017, 1988.

Bennett CJ, Diokno AC: Clean intermittent self-catheterization in the elderly. *Urology* 24:43–45, 1984.

Boscia JA, Kobasa WD, Levison ME, et al: Lack of association between bacteriuria and symptoms in the elderly. *Am J Med* 81:979–982, 1986a.

Boscia JA, Kobasa WD, Knight RA, et al: Epidemiology of bacteriuria in elderly ambulatory population. *Am J Med* 80:208–214, 1986b.

Boscia JA, Kobasa WD, Knight RA, et al: Therapy vs. no therapy for bacteriuria in elderly ambulatory nonhospitalized women. *JAMA* 257:1067–1071, 1987.

Burgio KL, Whitehead WE, Engel BT: Urinary incontinence in elderly—bladder-sphincter biofeedback and toilet skills training. *Ann Intern Med* 104:507–515, 1985.

Burgio KL, Burgio LD: Behavior therapies for urinary incontinence in the elderly. *Clin Geriatr Med* 2:809–827, 1986.

Burton JR, Pearce KL, Burgio KL, et al: Behavioral training for urinary incontinence in elderly patients. *J Am Geriatr Soc* 36:693–698, 1988.

Caine M: The present role of alpha-adrenergic blockers in the treatment of benign prostatic hypertrophy. *J Urol* 136:1–4, 1986.

Castleden CM, Duffin HM, Asher MJ, et al: Factors influencing outcome in elderly patients with urinary incontinence and detrusor instability. *Age and Ageing* 14:303–307, 1985.

Diokno AC, Brock BM, Brown MB, et al: Prevalence of urinary incontinence and other urological symptoms in the non-institutionalized elderly. *J Urol* 136:1022–1025, 1986.

Diokno AC, Wells TJ, Brink CA: Urinary incontinence in elderly women: Urodynamic evaluation. *J Am Geriatr Soc* 35:940–946, 1987.

Finkbeiner AE: Is bathanechol chloride clinically effective in promoting bladder emptying? A literature review. *J Urol* 134:443–449, 1985.

Fowler FJ, Wennbert JE, Timothy RP, et al: Symptom status and quality of life following prostatectomy. *JAMA* 259:3018–3022, 1988.

Hadley E: Bladder training and related therapies for urinary incontinence in older people. *JAMA* 256:372–379, 1986.

Harris T: Aging in the eighties: Prevalence and impact of urinary problems in individuals age 65 years and over. National Center for Health Statistics, Advance Data No. 121, 1986.

Hilton P, Stanton SL: Algorithmic method for assessing urinary incontinence in elderly women. *Br Med J* 282:940–942, 1981.

International Continence Society: *The Standardization of Terminology of Lower Urinary Tract Infection,* 1984.

Kunin CM: *Detection, Prevention and Management of Urinary Tract Infections.* Philadelphia, Lea & Febiger, 1987.

Kunin CM, Chin QF, Chambers S: Morbidity and mortality associated with indwelling urinary catheters in elderly patients in a nursing home—confounding due to the presence of associated diseases. *J Am Geriatr Soc* 35:1001–1006, 1987.

Leach GE, Yip CM: Urologic and urodynamic evaluation of the elderly population. *Clin Geriatr Med* 2:731–755, 1986.

Lufkin EG, Carpenter PC, Ory SJ, et al: Estrogen replacement therapy: Current recommendations. *Mayo Clin Proc* 63:453–460, 1988.

McGuire EJ, Savastano JA: Stress incontinence and detrusor instability/ urge incontinence. *Neurourol Urodynamics* 4:313–316, 1985.

Mohide EA: The prevalence and scope of urinary incontinence. *Clin Geriatr Med* 2:639–655, 1986.

Nicolle LE, Bjornson J, Harding GMK, et al: Bacteriuria in elderly institutionalized men. *N Engl J Med* 309:1420–1425, 1983.

Nicolle LE, Mayhew JW, Bryan L, et al: Prospective randomized comparison of therapy and no therapy for asymptomatic bacteriuria in institutionalized elderly women. *JAMA* 83:27–33, 1987.

Ouslander JG, Kane RL, Abrass IB: Urinary incontinence in elderly nursing home patients. *JAMA* 248:1194–1198, 1982.

Ouslander JG, Fowler E: Incontinence in VA Nursing Home Care Units. *J Am Geriatr Soc* 33:33–40, 1985.

Ouslander JG: Diagnostic evaluation of geriatric urinary incontinence. *Clin Geriatr Med* 2:715–730, 1986.

Ouslander JG, Sier HC: Drug therapy for geriatric incontinence. *Clin Geriatr Med* 2:789–807, 1986.

Ouslander JG, Uman GC, Urman HN: Development and testing of an incontinence monitoring record. *J Am Geriatr Soc* 34:83–90, 1986a.

Ouslander JG, Raz S, Hepps K, et al: Genitourinary dysfunction in a geriatric outpatient population. *J Am Geriatr Soc* 34:507–514, 1986b.

Ouslander JG, Greengold BA, Chen S: External catheter use and urinary tract infections among male nursing home patients. *J Am Geriatr Soc* 35:1063–1070, 1987a.

Ouslander JG, Greengold BA, Silverblatt FJ, et al: An accurate method to obtain urine for culture in men with external catheters. *Arch Intern Med* 147:286–288, 1987b.

Ouslander JG, Greengold BA, Chen S: Complications of chronic indwelling urinary catheters among male nursing home patients: A prospective study. *J Urol* 138:1191–1195, 1987c.

Ouslander JG, Leach G, Abelson S, et al: Simple vs. multichannel cystometry in the evaluation of bladder function in an incontinent geriatric population. *J Urol* (in press) 1988a.

Ouslander JG, Blaustein J, Connor A, et al: Pharmacokinetics and clinical effects of oxybutynin in geriatric patients. *J Urol* 140:47–50, 1988b.

Ouslander JG, Blaustein J, Connor A, et al: Habit training and oxybutynin for incontinence in nursing home patients. *J Am Geriatr Soc* 36:40–46, 1988c.

Ray WA, Griffin MR, Schaffner W, et al: Psychotropic drug use and the risk of hip fracture. *N Engl J Med* 316:363–369, 1987.

Resnick NM: Urinary incontinence in the elderly. *Med Grand Rounds* 3:281–289, 1984.

Resnick NM, Yalla SV: Management of urinary incontinence in the elderly. *N Engl J Med* 313:800–805, 1985.

Resnick NM, Yalla SV: Detrusor hyperactivity with impaired contractile function: An unrecognized but common cause of incontinence in elderly patients. *JAMA* 257:3076–3081, 1987.

Resnick NM, Yalla SV, Reilly CH: A previously uncharacterized but common cause of geriatric incontinence. *Gerontologist* 25:31, 1985.

Resnick NM, Yalla SV, Laurino E: An algorithmic approach to urinary incontinence in the elderly. *Clin Res* 34:832A, 1986.

Schmidbauer CP, Chiang H, Raz S: Surgical treatment for female geriatric incontinence. *Clin Geriatr Med* 2:759–776, 1986.

Schnelle JF, Sowell VA, Hu TW, et al: Reduction of urinary incontinence in nursing homes: Does it reduce or increase costs? *J Am Geriatr Soc* 36:34–39, 1988.

Sier H, Ouslander JG, Orzeck S: Urinary incontinence among geriatric patients in an acute care hospital. *JAMA* 257:1767–1771, 1987.

Staskin DR: Age-related physiologic and pathologic changes affecting lower urinary tract function. *Clin Geriatr Med* 2:701–710, 1986.

Tobin GW, Brocklehurst JC: The management of urinary incontinence in local authority residential homes for the elderly. *Age Ageing* 15:292–298, 1986a.

Tobin GW, Brocklehurst JC: Fecal incontinence in residential homes for the elderly: Prevalence, aetiology and management. *Age Ageing* 15:41–46, 1986b.

Warren JW: Catheters and catheter care. *Clin Geriatr Med* 2:857–872, 1986.

Wein AJ: Lower urinary tract function and pharmacologic management of lower urinary tract dysfunction. *Urol Clin* 14:273–296, 1987.

Wein AJ: Classification of neurogenic voiding dysfunction. *J Urol* 125:605–609, 1981.

Wells TJ, Brink CA, Diokno A, et al: Urinary incontinence in elderly women: Clinical findings. *J Am Geriatr Soc* 35:933–939, 1987a.

Wells T, Brink C, Diokno A, et al: Pelvic muscle exercise for stress urinary incontinence in elderly women. *Gerontologist* (special issue) 244A–245A, 1987b.

Wennberg JE, Mulley AG, Hanley D, et al: An assessment of prostatectomy for benign urinary tract obstruction: Geographic variations and the evaluation of medical care outcomes. *JAMA* 259:3027, 1988.

Whitehead WE, Burgio KL, Engel BT: Biofeedback treatment of fecal incontinence in geriatric patients. *J Am Geriatr Soc* 33:320–324, 1985.

Williams ME, Pannill PC: Urinary incontinence in the elderly. *Ann Intern Med* 97:895–907, 1982.

Zorzitto ML, Jewett MAS, Fernie GR, et al: Effectiveness of propantheline bromide in the treatment of geriatric patients with detrusor instability. *Neurourol Urodynamics* 5:133–140, 1986.

SUGGESTED READINGS

Bockus HL: Simple constipation, in Bocus HL (ed): *Gastroenterology*. Philadelphia, Saunders, 1974.

Brink CA, Wells TJ: Environmental support for geriatric incontinence: Toilets, toilet supplements and external equipment. *Clin Geriatr Med* 2:829–840, 1986.

Eastwood HDH, Smart CJ: Urinary incontinence in the disabled elderly male. *Age Ageing* 14:235–239, 1985.

Hilton P: Urinary incontinence in women. *Br Med J* 295:426–432, 1987.

Gartley C: *Managing Incontinence: A Guide to Living with the Loss of Bladder Control.* Ottowa, IL, Jameson Books, 1985.

Hu TW: The economic impact of urinary incontinence. *Clin Geriatr Med* 2:673–687, 1986.

McCormick KA, Scheve AAS, Leahy E: Nursing management of urinary incontinence in geriatric inpatients. *Nurs Clin NA* 23:231–264, 1988.

Mohr DN, Offord KP, Melton JL: Isolated asymptomatic microhematuria: A cross-sectional analysis of test-positive and test-negative patients. *J Gen Intern Med* 2:318–324, 1987.

Ory MG, Wyman JF, Yu L: Psychosocial factors in urinary incontinence. *Clin Geriatr Med* 2:657–672, 1986.

Ouslander JG, Kane RL: The costs of urinary incontinence in nursing homes. *Med Care* 22:69–79, 1984.

Ouslander JG: Urinary incontinence. *Clin Geriatr Med* 2:715–730, 1986.

Ouslander JG, Morishita L, Blaustein J, et al: Clinical, functional, and psychosocial characteristics of an incontinent nursing home population. *J Gerontol* 42:631–637, 1987.

Ouslander JG, Bruskewitz RC: Micturition in the aging patient, in Stollerman GH (ed): *Advances in Internal Medicine* (vol 34). Chicago, Year Book, 1989.

Smith RG: Fecal incontinence. *J Am Geriatr Soc* 31:694–697, 1983.

Thompson IM: The evaluation of microscopic hematuria: A population-based study. *J Urol* 138:1189–1190, 1987.

Thompson JH: Laxatives and cathartics, in Levenson AJ (ed): *Neuropsychiatric Side Effects of Drugs in the Elderly* (vol 9, *Aging*). New York, Raven Press, 1979.

Thompson WG: Laxatives: Clinical pharmacology and rational use. *Drugs* 19:49–58, 1980.

Yu LC: Incontinence stress index: Measuring psychological impact. *J Gerontol Nurs* 13:18–25, 1987.

Wyman JF, Harkins SW, Choi SC, et al: Psychosocial impact of urinary incontinence in women. *Obstet Gynecol* 70:378–381, 1987.

Chapter 7

Instability and Falls

Instability of gait and falls are common among the elderly, and falls are among the major causes of morbidity in this population. Falling is probably a marker for frailty in the elderly, and falls may be predictors of death as well as causes. Close to one-third of those aged 65 and older living at home suffer a fall each year, and about 1 in 40 of those will be hospitalized. Only about half of the elderly patients hospitalized as the result of a fall will be alive 1 year later. Among the elderly in nursing homes, as many as half suffer a fall each year; 10 to 25 percent have serious consequences. Accidents are the fifth leading cause of death in persons older than 65, and falls account for two-thirds of these accidental deaths. Of deaths from falls in the United States, over 70 percent occur in the 11 percent of the population over age 65 (Rubenstein et al., 1988).

Table 7-1 lists potential complications of falls. Fractures of the hip, femur, humerus, wrist, and ribs and painful soft tissue injuries are the most frequent physical complications. Many of these injuries

Table 7-1   Complications of Falls in the Elderly

Injuries
   Painful soft tissue injuries
   Fractures
     Hip
     Femur
     Humerus
     Wrist
     Ribs
   Subdural hematoma
Hospitalization
   Complications of immobilization (see Chapter 8)
   Risk of iatrogenic illnesses (see Chapter 13)
Disability
   Impaired mobility due to physical injury
   Impaired mobility from fear, loss of self-confidence, and restriction
    of ambulation
Risk of institutionalization
Death

will result in hospitalization, with the attendant risks of immobilization and iatrogenic illnesses (see Chapters 8 and 13). Fractures of the
hip and lower extremities often lead to prolonged disability because
of impaired mobility. A less common, but important, injury is subdural hematoma. Neurological symptoms and signs that develop days to
weeks after a fall should prompt consideration of this treatable problem. Even when the fall does not result in serious injury, substantial
disability may result from fear of falling, loss of self-confidence, and
restricted ambulation (either self-imposed or imposed by care givers).
Repeated falls and consequent injuries can be important factors in
the decision to institutionalize an elderly person.

    Falls and their attendant complications are often preventable.
Thus, an understanding of the causes of falls and a practical
approach to the evaluation and management of patients with instability and falls are important components of geriatric care. Similar to
many other conditions described throughout this text, the factors that
can contribute to or cause falls are multiple, and very often more than
one of these factors plays an important role (Figure 7-1).

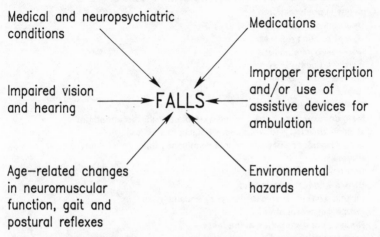

INTRINSIC FACTORS   EXTRINSIC FACTORS

Medical and neuropsychiatric
conditions

Medications

Impaired vision
and hearing

Improper prescription
and/or use of
assistive devices for
ambulation

FALLS

Age—related changes
in neuromuscular
function, gait and
postural reflexes

Environmental
hazards

Figure 7-1 Multifactorial causes and potential contributors to falls in the elderly.

AGING AND INSTABILITY

Several age-related factors contribute to instability and falls (Table 7-2). Most "accidental" falls are caused by one or a combination of these factors interacting with environmental hazards.

Aging changes in postural control and gait probably play a major role in many falls among the elderly. Increasing age is associated with diminished proprioceptive input, slower righting reflexes, diminished strength of muscles important in maintaining posture, and increased postural sway. All these changes can contribute to falling—especially the ability to avoid a fall after encountering an environmental hazard or an unexpected trip. Changes in gait also occur with increasing age. Although these changes may not be sufficiently prominent to be labeled truly pathological, they can increase susceptibility to falls. In general, elderly people do not pick their feet up as

**Table 7-2   Age-Related Factors Contributing
to Instability and Falls**

Changes in postural control
    Decreased proprioception
    Slower righting reflexes
    Decreased muscle tone
    Increased postural sway
    Orthostatic hypotension
Changes in gait
    Feet not picked up as high
    Men: develop flexed posture and wide-based, short-stepped gait
    Women: develop narrow-based, waddling gait
Increased incidence of pathological conditions relative to stability
    Degenerative joint disease
    Fractures of hip and femur
    Stroke with residual deficits
    Muscle weakness from disuse and deconditioning
    Peripheral neuropathy
    Diseases or deformities of the feet
    Impaired vision
    Impaired hearing
    Forgetfulness and dementia
    Other specific disease processes (e.g., cardiovascular disease,
      parkinsonism—see Table 7-3)

high, thus increasing the tendency to trip. Elderly men develop wide-based, short-stepped gaits; elderly women often walk with a narrow-based, waddling gait. Orthostatic hypotension (defined as a drop in systolic blood pressure of 20 mmHg or more when moving from a lying to a standing position) occurs in 11 to 30 percent of elderly persons (Johnson et al., 1965; Caird et al., 1973; Mader et al., 1987). Although not all elderly individuals with orthostatic hypotension are symptomatic, this impaired physiological response could play a role in causing instability and precipitating falls in a substantial proportion of patients.

    Several pathological conditions that increase in prevalence with increasing age can contribute to instability and falling. Degenerative joint disease (especially of the neck, the lumbosacral spine, and the lower extremities) can cause pain, unstable joints, muscle weakness, and neurological disturbances. Healed fractures of the hip and femur can cause an abnormal and less steady gait. Residual muscle weakness or sensory deficits from a recent or remote stroke can cause instability. Muscle weakness as a result of disuse and deconditioning (caused by pain and/or lack of exercise) can contribute to an unsteady gait and impair the ability to right oneself after a loss of balance. Diminished sensory input, such as in diabetic and other peripheral neuropathies, visual disturbances, and impaired hearing diminish cues from the environment that normally contribute to stability and thus predispose one to falls. Impaired cognitive function may result in the creation of, or wandering into, unsafe environments and may lead to falls. Podiatric problems (bunions, calluses, nail disease, joint deformities, etc.), which cause pain, deformities, and alterations in gait, are common, correctable causes of instability. Other specific disease processes common in the elderly (such as Parkinson's disease and cardiovascular disorders) can cause instability and falls and are discussed further below.

CAUSES OF FALLS IN THE ELDERLY

Table 7-3 outlines the multiple and often interacting causes of falls in the elderly. Frequently overlooked, environmental factors can increase susceptibility to falls and other accidents. Homes of elderly people are often full of environmental hazards (Table 7-4). Unstable furniture, rickety stairs with inadequate railings, throw rugs and frayed carpets, and poor lighting should be specifically sought on home visits. There are several factors associated with falls among the institutionalized elderly (Table 7-5). Awareness of these factors can help prevent morbidity and mortality in these settings. A checklist for the identification of hazards for falling is included in the Appendix.

Several factors can hinder precise identification of the specific causes for falls. These factors include lack of witnesses, inability of the elderly person to recall the circumstances surrounding the event, the transient nature of several causes [e.g., arrhythmia, transient ischemic attack (TIA), postural hypotension], and the fact that the majority of elderly people who fall do not seek medical attention. Somewhat more detailed information is available on the circumstances surrounding falls in institutionalized elderly (Table 7-5), but

Table 7-3   Causes of Falls

Accidents
   True accidents (trips, slips, etc.)
   Interactions between environmental hazards and factors increasing
    susceptibility (Table 7-2)
Syncope (sudden loss of consciousness)
Drop attacks (sudden leg weaknesses, without loss of consciousness)
Dizziness and/or vertigo
   Vestibular disease
   CNS disease
Orthostatic hypotension
   Hypovolemia or low cardiac output
   Autonomic dysfunction
   Impaired venous return
   Prolonged bed rest
   Drug-induced hypotension
Drug-related causes
   Diuretics
   Antihypertensives
   Tricyclic antidepressants
   Sedatives
   Antipsychotics
   Hypoglycemics
   Alcohol
Specific disease processes
   Acute illness of any kind ("premonitory fall")
   Cardiovascular
      Arrhythmias
      Valvular heart disease (aortic stenosis)
      Carotid sinus syncope
   Neurological causes
      Transient ischemic attack (TIA)
      Stroke (acute)
      Seizure disorder
      Parkinson's disease
      Cervical or lumbar spondylosis (with spinal cord or nerve root compression)
      Cerebellar disease
      Normal-pressure hydrocephalus (gait disorder)
      CNS lesions (e.g., tumor, subdural hematoma)
Idiopathic (no specific cause identifiable)

Table 7-4   Common Environmental Hazards

Old, unstable, and low-lying furniture
Beds and toilets of inappropriate height
Unavailability of grab bars
Uneven stairs and inadequate railing
Throw rugs, frayed carpets, cords, wires
Slippery floors and bathtubs
Inadequate lighting or glaring
Cracked and uneven sidewalks

these individuals represent a relatively low proportion and a highly select group among the total elderly population.

Close to half of all falls can be classified as accidental. Usually an accidental trip or a slip is precipitated by an environmental hazard, often in conjunction with factors listed in Table 7-2. Many of these falls are preventable if the patient and the patient's environment are carefully assessed. Over half of all falls are related to medically diagnosed conditions (Rubenstein et al., 1988), emphasizing the importance of a careful medical assessment for patients who fall (see below).

Syncope, "drop attacks," and "dizziness" are commonly cited causes of falls in the elderly. If there is a clear history of loss of consciousness, a cause for true syncope should be sought. Although the complete differential diagnosis is beyond the scope of this chapter, some of the more common causes of syncope in the elderly include vasovagal responses, cardiovascular disorders (such as brady- and tachyarrhythmias and aortic stenosis), acute neurological events

Table 7-5   Factors Associated with Falls among the Institutionalized Elderly

Recent admission
Certain activities (toileting, getting out of bed)
Psychotropic drugs causing daytime sedation
Low staff-patient ratio
Unsupervised activities
Unsafe furniture
Slippery floors

(such as TIA, stroke, or seizure), pulmonary embolus, and metabolic disturbances (e.g., hypoxia, hypoglycemia). Cardiovascular causes for syncope are more common in the elderly than in younger populations (Kapoor et al., 1986). A precise cause for syncope may remain unidentified in 40 to 60 percent of elderly patients (Kapoor et al., 1986; Lipsitz et al., 1983).

Drop attacks, described as sudden leg weakness causing a fall without loss of consciousness, are probably overdiagnosed in elderly people who fall. They are often attributed to vertebrobasilar insufficiency, frequently precipitated by a change in head position. Although a small proportion of elderly people who fall have truly had a drop attack, the underlying pathophysiology is poorly understood, and care should be taken to rule out other causes (Rubenstein et al., 1988).

Dizziness and unsteadiness are extremely common complaints among elderly people who fall (as well as those who don't). Very little careful research has examined the complaint of dizziness in the elderly (Belal and Glorig, 1986). A feeling of lightheadedness can be associated with several different disorders but is a nonspecific symptom and should be interpreted with caution. Patients complaining of lightheadedness should be carefully evaluated for postural hypotension and intravascular volume depletion. Vertigo (a sensation of rotational movement), on the other hand, is a more specific symptom and is probably an uncommon precipitant of falls in the elderly. It is most commonly associated with disorders of the inner ear, such as acute labyrinthitis, Ménière's disease, and benign positional vertigo. Vertebrobasilar ischemia and infarction and cerebella infarction can also cause vertigo. Patients with vertigo due to organic disorders often have nystagmus, which can be observed by having the patient quickly lie down and turning the patient's head to the side in one motion (Bárány's positional test). Many elderly patients with symptoms of dizziness and unsteadiness are anxious, depressed, and chronically afraid of falling, and the evaluation of their symptoms is quite difficult. Some patients, especially those with symptoms suggestive of vertigo, will benefit from a thorough otologic examination including auditory testing, which may help clarify the symptoms and differentiate inner-ear from CNS involvement.

As mentioned above, a substantial number (10 to 20 percent) of elderly persons have orthostatic hypotension. Orthostatic hypotension is best detected by taking the blood pressure and pulse in supine position, after 1 min in the sitting position, and after 1 min in the standing position. A drop of more than 20 mmHg in systolic blood pressure is generally considered to represent significant orthostatic hypotension. In many instances, this condition is asymptomatic; however, several conditions can cause orthostatic hypotension or worsen it to a severity sufficient to precipitate a fall (Mader et al., 1987). These conditions include low cardiac output from heart failure or hypovolemia, autonomic dysfunction (which can result from diabetes), impaired venous return (e.g., venous insufficiency), prolonged bed rest with deconditioning of muscles and reflexes, and several different drugs. Simply eating a full meal can precipitate a reduction in blood pressure in the elderly which may be worsened and precipitate a fall by standing up (Lipsitz et al., 1983).

Drugs that should be suspected of playing a role in falls include diuretics (hypovolemia), antihypertensives (hypotension), tricyclic antidepressants (postural hypotension), sedatives (excessive sedation), antipsychotics (sedation, muscle rigidity, postural hypotension), hypoglycemics (acute hypoglycemia), and alcohol (intoxication). Combinations of these drug types may greatly increase the risk of a fall. Psychotropic drugs are commonly prescribed and appear to substantially increase the risk of falls and hip fractures, especially in patients prescribed tricyclic antidepressants (Ray et al., 1987). One study in dementia patients documented an increased risk of both falls and fractures among those on psychotropic drugs (Buchner and Larson, 1987). Although the causes of the falls and fractures were not determined in this study, it is likely that psychotropic drugs were important factors through the mechanisms alluded to above.

Many disease processes, especially of the cardiovascular and neurological systems, can be associated with falls. Cardiac arrhythmias are common in ambulatory elderly persons and may be difficult to associate directly with a fall or syncope (Gibson and Heitzman, 1984). In general, cardiac monitoring should document a temporal association between a specific arrhythmia and symptoms (or a fall) before the arrhythmia is diagnosed (and treated) as the cause of falls. Syncope can be a symptom of aortic stenosis and is an indication of the need to evaluate a patient suspected of having significant aortic stenosis for valve replacement. Aortic stenosis is difficult to diagnose by physical examination alone, and all patients suspected of having this condition should have appropriate diagnostic tests (see below). Some elderly individuals have sensitive carotid baroreceptors and are susceptible to syncope resulting from reflex increase in vagal tone (caused by cough, straining at stool, micturition, etc.), which leads to bradycardia and hypotension. Carotid sinus sensitivity can be detected by bedside maneuvers (see below).

Cerebrovascular disease is often implicated as a cause or contributing factor for falls in the elderly. Although cerebral blood flow and cerebrovascular autoregulation may be diminished, these aging changes alone are not enough to cause unsteadiness or falls. They may, however, render the elderly person more susceptible to stresses such as diminished cardiac output, which will more easily precipitate symptoms. Acute strokes (caused by thrombosis, hemorrhage, or embolus) can cause, and may initially manifest themselves in, falls. TIAs of both the anterior and posterior circulations frequently last only minutes and are often poorly described. Thus, care must be taken in making these diagnoses. Anterior circulation TIAs may cause unilateral weakness and thus precipitate a fall. Vertebrobasilar (posterior circulation) TIAs may cause vertigo, but a history of transient vertigo alone is not sufficient basis for the diagnosis of a TIA. The diagnosis of posterior circulation TIA requires that one or more other symptoms (visual field cuts, dysarthria, ataxia, or limb weakness—which can be bilateral) be associated with vertigo. Vertebrobasilar insufficiency, as mentioned above, is often cited as a cause of drop attacks; in addition, mechanical compression of the vertebral arteries by osteophytes of the cervical spine when the head is turned has also been proposed as a cause of unsteadiness and falling. Both of these conditions have been poorly documented, are probably overdiagnosed, and should not be used as causes of a fall simply because nothing else can be found.

Other diseases of the brain and central nervous system can also cause falls. Parkinson's disease and normal-pressure hydrocephalus (Fisher, 1982) cause disturbances of gait, which lead to instability and falls. Cerebellar disorders, intracranial tumors, and subdural hematomas can cause unsteadiness, with a tendency to fall. A slowly progressive gait disability with a tendency to fall, especially in the presence of spasticity or hyperactive reflexes in the lower extremities, should prompt consideration of cervical spondylosis and spinal cord compression. It is especially important to consider these diagnoses because treatment may improve the condition before permanent disability ensues.

Despite this long list, the precise causes of many falls will remain unknown—even after a thorough evaluation.

EVALUATING THE ELDERLY PATIENT WHO FALLS

Elderly patients who report a fall (or recurrent falls) that is not clearly due to an accidental trip or slip should be carefully evaluated, even if the falls have not resulted in serious physical injury. A thorough evaluation consists of a detailed history, physical examination, gait and balance assessment, and, in certain instances, selected laboratory studies.

The history should focus on the general medical history and medications, the patient's thoughts about what caused the fall, the circumstances surrounding it, any premonitory or associated symptoms (such as palpitations caused by a transient arrhythmia or focal neurological symptoms caused by a TIA), and whether there was loss of consciousness (Table 7-6). A history of loss of consciousness after the fall (which is often difficult to document) is important information and should raise the suspicion of a cardiac event (transient arrhythmia or heart block) or a seizure (especially if there has been incontinence). Falls are often unwitnessed, and elderly patients may not recall any details of the circumstances surrounding the event. Detailed questioning can sometimes lead to identification of environmental factors that may have played a role in the fall and to symptoms that may lead to a specific diagnosis. Many elderly patients will not be able to give details about an unwitnessed fall and will simply report "I just fell down, I don't know what happened."

The skin, extremities, and painful soft tissue areas should be assessed to detect any injury that may have resulted from a fall. Several other aspects of the physical examination can be helpful in determining the cause(s) (Table 7-7). Because a fall can herald the onset of a variety of acute illnesses ("premonitory" falls), careful attention should be given to vital signs. Fever, tachypnea, tachycardia, and

Table 7-6   Evaluating the Elderly Patient Who Falls: Key Points in the History

General medical history
History of previous falls
Medications (especially antihypertensive and psychotropic agents)
Patient's thoughts on the cause of the fall
   Was patient aware of impending fall?
   Was it totally unexpected?
   Did patient trip or slip?
Circumstances surrounding the fall
  Location and time of day
  Witnesses
  Relationship to changes in posture, turning of head, cough, urination
Premonitory or associated symptoms
  Lightheadedness, dizziness, vertigo
  Palpitations, chest pain, shortness of breath
  Sudden focal neurological symptoms (weakness, sensory disturbance,
   dysarthria, ataxia, confusion, aphasia)
  Aura
  Incontinence of urine or stool
Loss of consciousness
  What is remembered immediately after the fall?
  Could the patient get up and, if so, how long did it take?
  Can loss of consciousness be verified by a witness?

hypotension should prompt a search for an acute illness (such as pneumonia or sepsis, myocardial infarction, pulmonary embolus, gastrointestinal bleeding). Postural blood pressure and pulse determinations taken supine, sitting, and standing (after 1 and 3 min) are critical in the diagnosis and management of falls in the elderly. As noted earlier, postural hypotension occurs in a substantial number of healthy, asymptomatic elderly persons, as well as in those who are deconditioned from immobility or have venous insufficiency. This finding can also be a sign of dehydration, acute blood loss (occult gastrointestinal bleeding), or a drug side effect. Visual acuity should be assessed for any possible contribution to instability and falls. The cardiovascular examination should focus on the presence of arrhythmias (many of which are easily missed during a brief examination) and signs of aortic stenosis. Since both of these conditions are potentially serious and treatable, yet difficult to diagnose by physical examina-

Table 7-7 Evaluating the Elderly Patient Who Falls: Key Aspects of the Physical Examination

Vital signs
   Fever, hypothermia
   Respiratory rate
   Pulse and blood pressure (lying, sitting, standing)
Skin
   Turgor
   Pallor
   Trauma
Eyes
   Visual acuity
Cardiovascular
   Arrhythmias
   Carotid bruits
   Signs of aortic stenosis
   Carotid sinus sensitivity
Extremities
   Degenerative joint disease
   Range of motion
   Deformities
   Fractures
   Podiatric problems (calluses; bunions; ulcerations; poorly fitted,
     inappropriate, or worn-out shoes)
Neurological
   Mental status
   Focal signs
   Muscles (weakness, rigidity, spasticity)
   Peripheral innervation (especially position sense)
   Cerebellar (especially heel-to-shin testing)
   Resting tremor, bradykinesia, other involuntary movements

tion, the patient should be referred for continuous monitoring and echocardiography if they are suspected. If the history suggests carotid sinus sensitivity, the carotid can be gently massaged for 5 s to observe whether this precipitates a profound bradycardia (>50% reduction in heart rate) or a long pause (>2 s). The extremities should be examined for evidence of deformities, limits to range of motion, or active inflammation that might underlie instability and cause a fall. Special attention should be given to the feet because deformities, painful lesions (calluses, bunions, ulcers), and poorly fitted, inappropriate, or worn-out shoes are common in the elderly and can contribute to instability and falls.

Neurological examination is also an important aspect of this physical assessment. Mental status should be assessed (see Chapter 4), with a careful search for focal neurological signs. Evidence of muscle weakness, rigidity, or spasticity should be noted, and signs of peripheral neuropathy (especially posterior column signs such as loss of position or vibratory sensation) should be ruled out. Abnormalities in cerebellar function (especially heel-to-shin testing) and signs of Parkinson's disease (such as resting tremor, muscle rigidity, and bradykinesia) should be sought.

Gait and balance assessments are a critical component of the examination and are probably more useful in identifying remediable problems than the standard neuromuscular exam (Tinetti and Ginter, 1988). Although sophisticated techniques have been developed to assess gait and balance, careful observation of a series of maneuvers is the most practical and useful assessment technique. The "get up and go" test and other practical performance-based balance and gait assessments have been developed (Mathias et al., 1986; Tinetti, 1986). Tables 7-8 and 7-9 provide examples of these types of assessment. Abnormalities on these assessments may be helpful in identifying patients who are likely to fall again and potentially remediable problems that might prevent future falls (Tinetti et al., 1986; Tinetti, 1986).

There is no specific laboratory workup for an elderly patient who falls (Rubenstein et al., 1988). Laboratory studies should be ordered based on information gleaned from the history and physical examination. If the cause of the fall is obvious (such as a slip or a trip) and no suspicious symptoms or signs are detected, laboratory studies are unwarranted. If the history or physical examination (especially vital signs) suggests an acute illness, appropriate laboratory studies (such as complete blood count, electrolytes, blood urea nitrogen, chest films, ECG) should be ordered. If a transient arrhythmia or heart block is suspected, ambulatory electrocardiographic monitoring should be done. Although the sensitivity and specificity of this procedure for determining the cause of falls in the elderly is unknown, and many elderly people have asymptomatic ectopy (Gibson and Heitzman, 1984), cardiac abnormalities detected on continuous monitor-

Table 7-8   Example of a Performance-Based Assessment of Gait

Components	Observation	
	Normal	**Abnormal**
Initiation of gait (patient asked to begin walking down hallway at a normal pace using any assistive device they normally walk with)	Begins walking immediately without observable hesitation; initiation of gait is single, smooth motion	Hesitates; multiple attempts; initiation of gait not a smooth motion
Step height (begin observing after first few steps: observe one foot, then the other; observe from side)	Swing foot completely clears floor but by no more than 1–2 in	Swing foot is not completely raised off floor (may hear scraping) or is raised too high (>1–2 in)
Step length (observe distance between toe of stance foot and heel of swing foot; observe from side; do not judge first few or last few steps; observe one side at a time)	At least the length of individual's foot between the stance toe and swing heel (step length usually longer but foot length provides basis for observation)	Step length less than described under normal
Step symmetry (observe the middle part of the path not the first or last steps; observe from side; observe distance between heel of each swing foot and toe of each stance foot)	Step length same or nearly same on both sides for most step cycles	Step length varies between sides or patient advances with same foot every step
Step continuity	Begins raising heel of one foot (toe off) as heel of other foot touches the floor (heel strike); no breaks or stops in stride; step lengths equal over most cycles	Places entire foot (heel and toe) on floor before beginning to raise other foot; or stops completely between steps; or step length varies over cycles
Path deviation [observe from behind; observe one foot over several strides; observe in relation to line on floor (e.g., tiles) if possible; difficult to assess if patient uses a walker]	Foot follows close to straight line as patient advances	Foot deviates from side to side or toward one direction
Trunk stability (observe from behind; side-to-side motion of trunk may be a normal gait pattern; need to differentiate this from instability)	Trunk does not sway; knees or back are not flexed; arms are not abducted in effort to maintain stability	Any of preceding features present
Walk stance (observe from behind)	Feet should almost touch as one passes other	Feet apart with stepping
Turning while walking	No staggering; turning continuous with walking; steps are continuous while turning	Staggers; stops before initiating turn; or steps are discontinuous

Source: After Tinetti, 1986 (with permission).

205

Table 7-9 Example of a Performance-Based Assessment of Balance*

Maneuver	Normal	Adaptive	Abnormal
Sitting balance	Steady, stable	Holds onto chair to keep upright	Leans, slides down in chair
Arising from chair	Able to arise in a single movement without using arms	Uses arms (on chair or walking aid) to pull or push up and/or moves forward in chair before attempting to arise	Multiple attempts required or unable without human assistance
Immediate standing balance (first 3–5 s)	Steady without holding onto walking aid or other object for support	Steady, but uses walking aid or other object for support	Any sign of unsteadiness (e.g., grabbing objects for support, staggering, more than minimal trunk sway)
Standing balance	Steady, able to stand with feet together without holding object for support	Steady, but cannot put feet together	Any sign of unsteadiness or needs to hold onto an object
Balance with eyes closed (with feet as close together as possible)	Steady without holding onto any object with feet together	Steady with feet apart	Any sign of unsteadiness or holds onto an object
Turning balance (360°)	No grabbing or staggering; no need to hold onto any objects; steps are continuous (turn is a flowing movement)	Steps are discontinuous (patient puts one foot completely on floor before raising other foot)	
Nudge on sternum (patient standing with feet as close together as possible; examiner pushes with light, even pressure over sternum 3 times; reflects ability to withstand displacement)	Steady, able to withstand pressure	Needs to move feet, but able to maintain balance	Begins to fall, or examiner has to help maintain balance

Maneuver	Normal	Adaptive	Abnormal
Neck turning (patient asked to turn head side to side and look up while standing with feet as close together as possible)	Able to turn head at least halfway side to side and be able to bend head back to look at ceiling; no staggering, grabbing, or symptoms of lightheadedness, unsteadiness, or pain	Decreased ability to turn side to side to extend neck, but no staggering, grabbing, or symptoms of lightheadedness, unsteadiness, or pain	Any sign of unsteadiness or symptoms when turning head or extending neck
One leg standing balance	Able to stand on one leg for 5 s without holding object for support		Unable
Back extension (ask patient to lean back as far as possible, without holding onto object if possible)	Good extension without holding object or staggering	Tries to extend, but range of motion is decreased or needs to hold object to attempt extension	Will not attempt or no extension seen or staggers
Reaching up (have patient attempt to remove an object from a shelf high enough to require stretching or standing on toes)	Able to take down object without needing to hold onto other object for support and without becoming unsteady	Able to get object but needs to steady self by holding onto something for support	Unable or unsteady
Bending down (patient is asked to pick up small objects, such as pen, from the floor)	Able to bend down and pick up the object and able to get up easily in single attempt without needing to pull self up with arms	Able to get object and get upright in single attempt but needs to pull self up with arms or hold onto something for support	Unable to bend down or unable to get upright after bending down or takes multiple attempts to upright self
Sitting down	Able to sit down in one smooth movement	Needs to use arms to guide self into chair or not a smooth movement	Falls into chair, misjudges distances (lands off center)

Source: After Tinetti, 1986 (with permission).

ing that are clearly related to symptoms should be treated. Because it is difficult to diagnose aortic stenosis on physical examination, echocardiography should be considered in all patients with suggestive histories and louder than a grade 2 systolic heart murmur. If the history suggests anterior circulation TIA, noninvasive vascular studies should be considered to rule out treatable vascular lesions. CT scans and electroencephalograms should be reserved for those patients in whom there is a high suspicion of an intracranial lesion or seizure disorder.

MANAGEMENT

The basic principles of managing elderly patients with instability problems and a history of falls are outlined in Table 7-10. Assessment and treatment of physical injury should not be overlooked because it may be helpful in preventing recurrent falls.

When specific conditions are identified by history, physical examination, and laboratory studies, they should be treated in order to minimize the risk of subsequent falls, morbidity, and mortality. Examples of treatments for some of the more common conditions are outlined in Table 7-11. This table is meant only as a general outline;

**Table 7-10   Principles of Management
for Elderly Patients with Complaints
of Instability and/or Falls**

Assess and treat physical injury
Treat underlying conditions (Table 7-11)
Provide physical therapy and education
Gait retraining
Muscle strengthening
Aids to ambulation
Properly fitted shoes
Adaptive behaviors
Alter the environment*
Safe and proper-size furniture
Elimination of obstacles (loose rugs, etc.)
Proper lighting
Rails (stairs, bathroom)

*See Appendix for a checklist.

Table 7-11   Examples of Treatment for Underlying Causes of Falls

Condition and Cause	Potential Treatment
Cardiovascular	
Tachyarrhythmias	Antiarrhythmics*
Bradyarrhythmias	Pacemaker*
Aortic stenosis	Valve surgery (for syncope)
Neurological	
Anterior circulation TIA	Aspirin and/or surgery†
Posterior circulation TIA	Aspirin
Cervical spondylosis (with spinal cord compression)	Physical therapy Neck brace Surgery
Parkinson's disease	Antiparkinsonian drugs
Visual impairment	Ophthalmologic evaluation and specific treatment
Seizure disorder	Anticonvulsants
Normal-pressure hydrocephalus	Surgery (shunt)†
Postural hypotension	
Drug-related	Elimination of drug(s)
With venous insufficiency	Support stockings Leg elevation Adaptive behaviors
Autonomic dysfunction or idiopathic	Support stockings Mineralocorticoids Adaptive behaviors
Others	
Foot disorders	Podiatric evaluation and treatment
Gait disorders (miscellaneous)	Properly fitted shoes
Drug overuse (e.g., sedatives, alcohol)	Physical therapy Elimination of drug(s)

*These treatments may be indicated only if the cardiac disturbance is clearly related to symptoms.
†Risk-benefit ratio must be carefully assessed.

most of these topics are discussed in detail in general textbooks of medicine.

Physical therapy and patient education are important aspects of the management of these elderly patients. Gait training, muscle strengthening, the use of assistive devices, and adaptive behaviors (such as rising slowly, using rails or furniture for balance, and techniques of getting up after a fall) are all helpful in preventing subsequent morbidity from instability and falls.

Environmental manipulations can be critical in preventing further falls. The environments of the elderly are often unsafe (Table 7-4), and appropriate interventions can often be instituted to improve safety (Table 7-10).

The Appendix contains an assessment form for patients who fall, as well as a Fall Hazard Checklist.

ACKNOWLEDGMENT

The authors wish to acknowledge Dr. Laurence Rubenstein for his assistance in preparing this chapter.

REFERENCES

Belal A, Glorig A: Dysequilibrium of ageing (presbyastasis). *J Laryngol Otol* 100:1037–1041, 1986.

Buchner DM, Larson EB: Falls and fractures in patients with Alzheimer-type dementia. *JAMA* 257:1492–1495, 1987.

Caird FI, Andrews GR, Kennedy RD: Effect of posture on blood pressure in the elderly. *Br Heart J* 35:527–530, 1973.

Fisher CM: Hydrocephalus as a cause of disturbances of gait in the elderly. *Neurology* 32:1358–1363, 1982.

Gibson TC, Heitzman MR: Diagnostic efficacy of 24-hour electrocardiographic monitoring for syncope. *Am J Cardiol* 53:1013–1017, 1984.

Johnson RH, Smith AC, Spalding JMK, et al: Effect of posture on blood pressure in elderly patients. *Lancet* 1:731–733, 1965.

Kapoor W, Snustad D, Peterson J, et al: Syncope in the elderly. *Am J Med* 80:419–428, 1986.

Lipsitz LA, Nyquist RP, Wei JY, et al: Postprandial reduction in blood pressure in the elderly. *N Engl J Med* 309:81–83, 1983.

Mader SC, Josephson KR, Rubenstein LZ: Low prevalence of postural hypotension among community-dwelling elderly. *JAMA* 258:1511–1514, 1987.

Mathias S, Nayak USL, Isaacs B: Balance in elderly patients: The "get-up and go" test. *Arch Phys Med Rehabil* 67:387–389, 1986.

Ray WA, Griffin MR, Schaffner W, et al: Psychotropic drug use and the risk of hip fracture. *N Engl J Med* 316:363–369, 1987.

Rubenstein LZ, Robbins AS, Schulman BL, et al: Falls and instability in the elderly. *J Am Geriatr Soc* 36:266–278, 1988.

Tinetti ME: Performance-oriented assessment of mobility problems in elderly patients. *J Am Geriatr Soc* 34:119–126, 1986.

Tinetti ME, Ginter SF: Identifying mobility dysfunctions in elderly patients. *JAMA* 259:1190–1193, 1988.

Tinetti ME, Williams FT, Mayewski R: Fall risk index for elderly patients based on number of chronic disabilities. *Am J Med* 80:429–434, 1986.

SUGGESTED READINGS

Branch WT: Approach to syncope. *J Gen Intern Med* 1:49–58, 1986.

Dalziel WB, Kelley FA, Cherkin A: *80 Do's & 58 Don'ts for Your Safety. A Practical Guide for Eldercare.* GRECC, Sepulveda VA Medical Center, 1985, pp 1–16.

Lipsitz LA: Syncope in the elderly. *Ann Intern Med* 99:92–105, 1983.

Nickens H: Intrinsic factors in falling among the elderly. *Arch Intern Med* 145:1089–1093, 1985.

Radebaugh TS, Hadley E, Suzman R (eds): Falls in the elderly. *Clin Geriatr Med* Vol. 1: No. 3, 1985.

Robbins AS, Rubenstein LZ: Postural hypotension in the elderly. *J Am Geriatr Soc* 32:769–774, 1984.

Thomas JE, Schirger A, Fealy RD, et al: Orthostatic hypotension. *Mayo Clin Proc* 56:117–125, 1981.

Chapter 8

Immobility

Immobility is a common pathway by which a host of diseases and problems in the elderly produce further disability. Immobility often cannot be prevented, but many of its adverse effects can be. Improvements in mobility are possible, even in the most immobile elderly patients. Relatively small improvements in mobility can decrease the incidence and severity of complications, improve the well-being of the patient, and make life easier for care givers.

This chapter outlines the common causes and complications of immobility and reviews the principles of management for some of the more common problems associated with immobility in the elderly population.

CAUSES

Many physical, psychological, and environmental factors can cause immobility in the elderly (Table 8-1). The most common causes are musculoskeletal, neurological, and cardiovascular disorders.

Table 8-1   Common Causes of Immobility in the Elderly

Musculoskeletal disorders
   Arthritides
   Osteoporosis
   Fractures (especially hip and femur)
   Podiatric problems
   Other (e.g., Paget's disease)
Neurological disorders
   Stroke
   Parkinson's disease
   Other (cerebellar dysfunction, neuropathies)
Cardiovascular disease
   Congestive heart failure (severe)
   Coronary artery disease (frequent angina)
   Peripheral vascular disease (frequent claudication)
Pulmonary disease
   Chronic obstructive lung disease (severe)
Sensory factors
   Impairment of vision
   Fear (from instability and fear of falling)
Environmental causes
   Forced immobility (in hospitals and nursing homes)
   Inadequate aids for mobility
Other
   Deconditioning (after prolonged bed rest from acute illness)
   Malnutrition
   Severe systemic illness (e.g., widespread malignancy)
   Pain
   Depression
   Drug side effects (e.g., antipsychotic induced rigidity)

Degenerative joint disease (especially that involving the weight-bearing joints), osteoporosis, and hip fractures are probably the most prevalent conditions that predispose to immobility among the elderly. Podiatric problems such as bunions, calluses, and onychomycoses frequently cause pain and reluctance or inability to walk.

The incidence of several neurological disorders that can cause immobility increases with age. About half the individuals who suffer a stroke have residual deficits for which they require assistance; most of these deficits involve immobility. Parkinson's disease, especially in its later stages, causes severe limitations in mobility. Early and active management of these patients can improve their mobility and help to avoid complications.

Severe congestive heart failure, coronary artery disease with frequent angina, peripheral vascular disease with frequent claudication, and severe chronic lung disease can restrict activity and mobility in many elderly patients. Peripheral vascular disease, especially in older diabetics, can cause claudication and limit ambulation and may eventually result in lower extremity amputations, which can restrict mobility further.

Psychological and environmental factors can play an important role in immobility. Decreased mobility (i.e., taking to bed) is a common manifestation of depression. Fear of falling, especially among those with a history of instability problems and previous falls or with impaired vision, can lead to a bed-and-chair existence. Elderly patients with instability problems, impaired vision, and acute illnesses are often inappropriately restricted to bed or chair in acute care hospitals and nursing homes. Lack of mobility aids (e.g., canes, walkers, and appropriately placed railings) also contributes to immobility in acute care hospitals and home settings.

Drug side effects may cause immobility. Sedatives and hypnotics, by causing drowsiness and ataxia, can impair mobility. Antipsychotic drugs (especially the phenothiazinelike agents) have prominent extrapyramidal effects and can cause muscle rigidity and diminished mobility (see Chapter 14).

COMPLICATIONS

Immobility can lead to complications in almost every major organ system (Table 8-2). Prolonged inactivity or bed rest has adverse physical and psychological consequences. Metabolic effects include negative nitrogen and calcium balance, impaired glucose tolerance, and diminished plasma volume, and altered drug pharmacokinetics can result. Immobilized elderly patients often become depressed, are deprived of environmental stimulations, and, in some instances, become delirious and appear demented.

The skin and the musculoskeletal system often bear the brunt of immobility. Pressure sores are all too common. Muscle weakness, atrophy, and contractures can lead to prolonged disability and dys-

Table 8-2   Complications of Immobility

Skin
   Pressure sores
Musculoskeletal
   Muscular deconditioning and atrophy
   Contractures
   Bone loss (osteoporosis)
Cardiovascular
   Deconditioning
   Orthostatic hypotension
   Venous thrombosis, embolism
Pulmonary
   Decreased ventilation
   Atelectasis
   Aspiration pneumonia
Gastrointestinal
   Anorexia
   Constipation
   Fecal impaction, incontinence
Genitourinary
   Urinary infection
   Urinary retention
   Bladder calculi
   Incontinence
Metabolic
   Altered body composition (e.g., decreased plasma volume)
   Negative nitrogen balance
   Impaired glucose tolerance
   Altered drug pharmacokinetics
Psychological
   Sensory deprivation
   Dementia, delirium
   Depression

function. Bone density decreases in immobile patients, predisposing to fractures when the patient is mobilized. Cardiopulmonary complications of immobility are probably the most serious and life-threatening. Prolonged immobility results in cardiovascular deconditioning; the combination of deconditioned cardiovascular reflexes and diminished plasma volume can lead to serious postural hypotension and can impair rehabilitative efforts. Deep venous thrombosis and pulmonary embolism are well-known complications. Immobility, especially bed rest, also impairs pulmonary function. Tidal volume is diminished; atelectasis may occur, and, when combined with the supine position, predisposes to the development of aspiration pneumonia.

Gastrointestinal and genitourinary consequences of immobility are among the most bothersome to the patient and can lead to further complications. Immobility slows down both the gastrointestinal tract and urine flow. This predisposes to constipation, fecal impaction, urinary tract stones and infection, and fecal and urinary incontinence. These latter conditions and their management are discussed in Chapter 6.

ASSESSING IMMOBILE PATIENTS

Several aspects of the history and physical examination are important in the assessment of immobile patients (Table 8-3). Useful historical

Table 8-3 Assessment of Immobile Elderly Patients

History
    Nature and duration of disabilities causing immobility
    Medical conditions contributing to immobility
    Drugs that can affect mobility
    Motivation and other psychological factors
    Environment
Physical examination
    Skin
    Cardiopulmonary status
    Musculoskeletal assessment
        Muscle tone and strength (Table 8-4)
        Joint range of motion
        Foot deformities and lesions
    Neurological deficits
        Focal weakness
        Sensory and perceptual evaluation
Levels of mobility
    Bed mobility
    Ability to transfer (bed to chair)
    Wheelchair mobility
    Standing balance
    Gait (see Chapter 7)

information includes the extent and duration of disabilities causing immobility, the underlying medical conditions that influence mobility, and a review of medications in order to eliminate iatrogenic problems contributing to immobility. Psychological factors such as depression and fear may contribute to immobility and may make recovery difficult. They should, therefore, receive special attention. An assessment of the environment is important in determining measures that may improve the patient's mobility, such as an overhead triangle, bedside commode, railing, and other environmental manipulations.

When examining immobile patients, the skin should be inspected repeatedly to identify early pressure sores. Cardiopulmonary status, especially intravascular volume, and postural changes in blood pressure and pulse are important to the process of treatment. A detailed musculoskeletal examination, including evaluation of muscle tone and strength, testing of joint range of motion, and a search for potentially remediable podiatric problems should be carried out. Standardized and repeated measures of muscle strength (performed by rehabilitation therapists) can be helpful in gauging a patient's progress (Table 8-4). The neurological examination should identify focal weakness as well as sensory and perceptual problems that can impair mobility and frustrate rehabilitative efforts. Hemianopsia, neglect of and inattention to one side of the body (usually the left side is ignored

Table 8-4   Example of a Grading System for Muscle Strength in Immobile Elderly Patients

	Grade	Observed strength
Normal	5	
Good	4	Muscle produces movements against gravity and can overcome some resistance
Fair	3	Muscle produces movements against gravity but cannot overcome any resistance
Poor	2	Muscle produces movements but not against gravity
Trace	1	Muscle tightens but cannot produce movement, even after gravity is eliminated
None	0	Muscle does not contract at all

in patients with nondominant hemisphere lesions), and various apraxias are common after strokes.

Most importantly, the patient's mobility should be assessed and reassessed on an ongoing basis. There are several levels of mobility (Table 8-3) as well as important distinctions within each level. For example, a patient may be bedbound but may be able to sit up without help, or may be able to transfer independently into a wheelchair but may be unable to propel the wheelchair. Rehabilitation therapists are skilled in making these detailed evaluations of mobility and should be involved in the care of immobile patients.

MANAGEMENT OF IMMOBILE ELDERLY PATIENTS

Optimal management of immobile elderly patients requires a thorough assessment, specific diagnoses, and multimodal treatment directed at specific diseases and disabilities. This process most often involves a team of health professionals. Physical and occupational therapists can be especially helpful in the assessment and management of immobility and associated functional disabilities, and they should be consulted as early as possible when confronted with an immobile patient. In many patients mobility cannot be completely restored, and intensive rehabilitative efforts will not be cost-effective. Specific goals must be individualized, and in some patients these goals will involve preventing complications of immobility and adapting the environment to the individual (and vice versa).

It is beyond the scope of this text to detail the management of all conditions associated with immobility in the elderly; important general principles of the management of some of the most common conditions associated with immobility in the elderly will be reviewed. A brief section at the end of the chapter provides an overview of key principles in the rehabilitation of geriatric patients. The Suggested Readings at the end of this chapter provide more detailed discussions of management for these conditions.

Arthritis

Several different rheumatologic disorders occur in the elderly. They can usually be distinguished from each other by clinical features,

Table 8-5 Clinical Aspects of Common Rheumatologic Disorders in the Elderly

Disorder	Osteoarthritis	Rheumatoid arthritis	Polymyalgia rheumatica	Gout	Pseudogout	Carpal tunnel syndrome	Drug-induced disorder
Gradual onset	+++	+++	+++	0	+	+++	+++
Joint swelling or effusion	+++	++++	+	++++	++++	+	++
Joint pain	++++	+++	+	++++	++++	+	+++
Symmetrical involvement	+	+++	+++			++	+++
Muscle pain	+	+	++++	+	+	0	+++
Radiographic abnormalities	++++	+++	0	+	+++	0	0
Synovial fluid crystals	+	+	0	+++	+++		0
Elevated sedimentation rate	+	+++	++++	+	+	+	+++
Anemia	0	++	+++	0	0	0	++
Positive antinuclear antibody	0	+		0	0	0	++++
Positive rheumatoid factor	0	+++	+	0	0	0	+

Note: 0, does not occur; +, occurs occasionally; ++, occurs frequently; +++, almost always occurs; ++++, difficult to make diagnosis without it.
Source: After Reich, 1982.

radiographic abnormalities, synovial fluid analysis, and selected laboratory studies (see Table 8-5).

It is important to make specific diagnoses for these conditions whenever possible because the most appropriate treatment(s) of the primary disorders, as well as associated abnormalities, may differ. For example, polymyalgia rheumatica is a common condition in elderly women; its clinical features are often nonspecific—fatigue, malaise, muscle aches. Because this disorder requires treatment with systemic steroids and is highly associated with temporal arteritis (a disease that can rapidly lead to blindness if appropriate treatment is not instituted), it is essential to make this diagnosis. Elderly patients with fatigue and symmetrical muscle aches (especially in the shoulders) should be tested for sedimentation rate, which will generally be markedly elevated (almost always greater than 40 mm/h) in patients with polymyalgia rheumatica (Chuang et al., 1982). The sedimentation rate does increase in some people with age, but elevations above normal are usually associated with a clinical disorder (Tinetti et al., 1986; Crawford et al., 1987). Any symptoms suggestive of involvement of the temporal artery—headache, recent changes in vision—especially when the sedimentation rate is very high (over 75 mm/h) should prompt consideration of temporal artery biopsy because treatment of temporal arteritis requires higher doses of steroids than does the treatment of polymyalgia alone (Goodman, 1979). Another example of the importance of making a specific diagnosis is the carpal tunnel syndrome. The disorder may be overlooked when symptoms of pain, weakness, and paresthesias in the hand are mistaken for osteoarthritis. Objective weakness, sensory deficit, and atrophy of intrinsic musculature of the hand should prompt consideration of performing nerve conduction studies and surgical therapy to relieve symptoms and prevent progressive disability.

History and physical examination can be helpful in differentiating osteoarthritis from inflammatory arthritides (Table 8-6); however, other procedures are often essential. Osteoarthritis itself may be inflammatory in some instances.

Synovial fluid analysis can be especially helpful in differentiating osteoarthritis from crystal-induced arthritides such as gout and pseudogout (Table 8-5). Because clinical examination alone cannot determine whether an inflamed joint is infected and joint infections

Table 8-6   Clinical Features of Osteoarthritis versus Inflammatory Arthritides

Clinical feature	Osteoarthritis	Inflammatory arthritides
Duration of stiffness	Minutes	Hours
Pain	Usually with activity	Occurs even at rest and at night
Fatigue	Unusual	Common
Swelling	Common, but little synovial reaction	Very common with synovial proliferation and thickening
Erythema and warmth	Unusual	Common

Note: Osteoarthritis may also be inflammatory.

can occur in conjunction with other inflammatory joint diseases, all newly inflamed joints should be tapped, gram-stained, and cultured to rule out infection. Failure to diagnose and treat joint infections can lead to osteomyelitis, joint destruction, and permanent disability.

In addition to making specific diagnoses of rheumatologic disorders whenever possible, careful physical examination can detect treatable nonarticular conditions such as tendonitis and bursitis.

Table 8-7   Treatment Modalities for Musculoskeletal Disorders

Program of exercise and rest
Heat
Other physical modalities (see Table 8-15)
Splints, braces, and aids for ambulation
Drugs
    Salicylates
    Other nonsteroidal inflammatory agents
    Steroids (e.g., for polymyalgia rheumatica)
Local injections (anesthetic and/or steroid)
    Soft tissue ("trigger point")
    Periarticular (tendon, bursa)
    Intraarticular
Surgery (e.g., hip and knee replacements)

Note: Treatment often involves multiple modalities and depends on the diagnosis of specific problems.

Table 8-8 Examples of Anti-Inflammatory Agents Used for Musculoskeletal Disorders in the Elderly

Drug (brand name)	Anti-inflammatory dose, mg	Available dosage forms, mg	Doses per day	Approximate cost* of 100 tablets, $U.S.
Aspirin, coated (Ecotrin)	3000–6000	325, 650	2–4	2.20†
Diflunisal (Dolobid)	500–1500	250, 500	2	62.83
Ibuprofen (Motrin)	1600–3200	300, 400, 600	3–4	7.18†
Indomethacin (Indocin)	75–150	25, 50	2–4	5.68†
Fenoprofen (Nalfon)	2400–3200	300, 600	3–4	36.50
Naproxen (Naprosyn)	500–1000	250, 375	2	54.44
Piroxicam (Feldene)	20	10, 20	1	154.72
Clinoril (Sulindac)	300–400	150, 200	3–4	69.44
Tolmetin (Tolectin)	600–2000	200, 400	3–4	34.89

*Wholesale cost to pharmacist in 1988 for lowest of dosage forms listed.
†Lowest available price for generic preparation.

Dramatic relief from pain and disability from these conditions can be achieved by local treatments such as the injection of steroids.

Osteoarthritis is by far the most common rheumatologic disorder afflicting the elderly. A wide variety of modalities can be used to treat osteoarthritis, as well as other painful musculoskeletal conditions (Table 8-7). Optimal management often involves the use of multiple treatment modalities, and the best combination of treatments will vary from patient to patient.

In general, patients with osteoarthritis and pain from inflammatory musculoskeletal conditions should be treated with an anti-inflammatory agent unless they respond to local measures alone. Table 8-8 lists many of the nonsteroidal anti-inflammatory drugs. Although their side effects are similar (Table 8-9), there is considerable variation in their price. In general, aspirin is the least expensive; enteric-coated preparations can diminish gastrointestinal irritation and still yield adequate absorption. The half-life of aspirin may be prolonged in elderly patients on higher doses; thus, less frequent administration may provide adequate analgesia. Salicylate blood levels can be used to monitor treatment. When compliance is a problem or when aspirin cannot be tolerated or is ineffective, other nonsteroidal drugs can be tried. These drugs can also cause gastrointestinal upset and bleeding and platelet dysfunction, although the incidence of significant bleeding is probably low (Beard et al., 1987). In addi-

Table 8-9 Common Effects and Side Effects of Anti-Inflammatory Agents

Analgesic effects*
Antipyretic effects
Inhibition of platelet function (effects of one dose may last several days)
Gastrointestinal upset†
Gastrointestinal bleeding†
CNS effects (e.g., somnolence, dizziness, confusion)
Sodium retention (not with aspirin)
Asthma (aspirin-sensitive)
Nephrotoxicity (especially with low baseline glomerular filtration rate)
Hepatotoxicity (not with ibuprofen, naproxen, or tolmetin)

*No major differences within dosage ranges, although individual responses to different drugs may vary.

†Gastrointestinal toxicity more common with aspirin (noncoated) and indomethacin.

tion, they can cause sodium retention and impair renal function, especially in patients with already compromised renal function. Although clinoril has been reported to have less effect on renal function, blood urea nitrogen and creatinine should be monitored in elderly patients on all nonsteroidal agents. Combining lower doses of these drugs with acetaminophen can sometimes improve pain relief and minimize side effects. There is no place for systemic steroids in the treatment of osteoarthritis in elderly patients.

Osteoporosis

Osteoporosis is a common disorder in the elderly and frequently leads to complications that result in pain, disability, and immobility. Approximately one-third of women older than 65 have suffered either a vertebral or hip fracture related to osteoporosis; by age 80, close to 30 percent of women will have suffered a hip fracture. Thus, osteoporosis is a major health problem in the elderly population, resulting in substantial morbidity and cost.

Osteoporosis is a generalized bone disorder in which bone mass is diminished but the relative composition (i.e., the ratio of mineral to organic matrix content) is not changed. This is in contrast to osteomalacia, in which the ratio of mineral to matrix is diminished. Aging is associated with a decrease in bone mass. White women lose the greatest proportion of bone mass with increasing age; the bone loss accelerates after the menopause, and as much as 40 percent of bone mass may be lost by age 90.

Two major types of age-related osteoporosis have been defined (Table 8-10). Type I or postmenopausal osteoporosis affects mainly trabecular bone and is related to accelerated bone loss in women during the first two decades after menopause. Type II or senile osteoporosis affects both trabecular and cortical bone and is related to impaired production of 1,25-dihydroxy vitamin D (Riggs and Melton, 1986). Several factors have been associated with increased risk of osteoporosis among women (Table 8-11); many of them (e.g., gastric resection, steroid or anticonvulsant use, immobility) are also risk factors among men.

Because routine radiographs are relatively insensitive in detecting significant bone loss (20 to 30 percent of bone mass must be lost before the radiograph appears abnormal), the prevalence of osteopo-

Table 8-10   Two Basic Types of Age-Related Osteoporosis

	Type I (postmenopausal)	Type II (senile)
Age (years)	51–75	>70
Sex ratio (F:M)	6:1	2:1
Type of bone loss	Mainly trabecular	Trabecular and cortical
Rate of bone loss	Accelerated	Not accelerated
Fracture sites	Vertebrae (crush) and distal radius	Vertebrae (multiple wedge) and hip
Parathyroid function	Decreased	Increased
Calcium absorption	Decreased	Decreased
Metabolism of 25-OH-D to 1,25-dihydroxy vitamin D	Secondary decrease	Primary decrease

Source: After Riggs and Melton, 1986.

rosis in the elderly is probably underestimated. Even with the use of this insensitive measure, close to 30 percent of elderly women and 20 percent of elderly men have osteoporosis. Lateral radiographs of the thoracolumbar vertebrae can show loss of horizontal trabeculation, prominent end plates, and anterior wedging, and radiographs of the

Table 8-11   Factors Associated with an Increased Risk of Osteoporosis among Women*

Postmenopausal (within 20 years after menopause)
White or Asian
Premature menopause
Positive family history
Short stature and small bones
Leanness
Low calcium intake
Inactivity or immobility
Nulliparity
Gastric or small-bowel resection
Long-term glucocorticoid therapy
Long-term use of anticonvulsants
Hyperparathyroidism
Thyrotoxicosis
Smoking
Heavy alcohol use

*Several of these factors also increase risk among men.
Source: After Riggs and Melton, 1986.

upper femur can reveal loss of the trabecular pattern that normally traverses the greater trochanter. Techniques such as computer-assisted tomography and single- or dual-photon absorptiometry are more sensitive than routine radiographs but are expensive and probably unwarranted in nonresearch settings. Many centers are now using the latter techniques to screen for osteoporosis, but data documenting the ability of photon absorptiometry findings to predict risk for specific types of fracture are not yet available. Thus the cost-effectiveness of these techniques as screening tools remains unproven (American College of Physicians, 1987). Patients with a bone mineral density of less than 1 g/cm^3 are at higher risk for all types of fracture. Bone biopsy may be necessary in certain patients to help distinguish osteoporosis from other disorders such as osteomalacia, metastatic carcinoma, and multiple myeloma.

Laboratory studies in uncomplicated osteoporosis should be normal, including serum calcium, phosphorus, magnesium, alkaline phosphatase, and parathyroid and thyroid hormones, although some elderly patients with senile osteoporosis have elevated parathyroid hormone, presumably related to a primary decrease in 1,25-dihydroxy vitamin D levels. Vitamin D blood levels and 24-h urinary calcium excretion (which should be greater than 100 mg/24 h) should be measured if malabsorption is suspected.

Osteoporosis in the elderly is commonly asymptomatic and discovered on routine radiographs. The presenting manifestations most often relate to a fracture of the hip (discussed below), the wrist (Colles' fracture), or the lower thoracic and upper lumbar vertebrae. Vertebral compression fractures can be asymptomatic and cause progressive kyphosis and loss of height. They may also be excruciatingly painful and be precipitated by relatively minor stress such as sitting down quickly. The pain is exacerbated by twisting and increases in intraabdominal pressure (e.g., from coughing, straining to have a bowel movement). The pain can radiate around the thoracic cavity and mimic cardiac pain. Diagnosing a new compression fracture can be difficult, especially when old radiographs are not available. The combination of the new onset of characteristic pain and radiographic evidence of a compression fracture in a compatible location should be treated with bed rest (for as short a period as possible), heat, and muscle relaxants. Posterior wedging of the fracture, fractures above the midthoracic vertebrae, and irregular-appearing vertebral bodies should raise the suspicion of a metastatic malignancy or plasmacytoma.

Several treatments are available for osteoporosis, including exercise, supplemental dietary calcium, vitamin D, fluoride, calcitonin, and estrogen. The most effective treatment for the different types of osteoporosis remains somewhat controversial and is influenced by a number of patient-related factors. Preventive approaches are clearly the most effective—but to be effective in preventing fractures and associated morbidity later in life treatment should be initiated soon after the menopause and continued for 10–20 years. Exercise probably has modest beneficial effects on bone mass (Chow et al., 1987) and has other potential beneficial effects on muscle strength and agility (which may help prevent falls) and cardiovascular status. Thus, prescribing an exercise program suitable to the individual's preferences is certainly reasonable. Calcium supplementation of at least 1000 mg per day is now routinely recommended, but its effectiveness in preventing postmenopausal bone loss without concomitant estrogen treatment has been questioned (Riis et al., 1987). It would still seem reasonable to encourage patients to either eat a high calcium diet or take an inexpensive calcium supplement if hypercalcemia and nephrolithiasis are not present. Routine vitamin D supplementation is generally not recommended unless osteomalacia is present, because it can accelerate bone turnover and calcium loss. Fluoride can increase bone mass, but its effectiveness in preventing vertebral and hip fractures is not established (Riggs et al., 1982). There is also a high incidence of gastrointestinal toxicity from fluoride; therefore, it is not routinely recommended for the prevention or treatment of osteoporosis. Calcitonin can prevent bone resorption and increase bone mineral content and is, therefore, of potential value in preventing osteoporosis. Its use is limited by its high cost because of the necessity for administration by injection. Intranasal preparations are being tested but are not yet available. Thus, calcitonin treatment is generally reserved for high-risk patients with a contraindication to estrogen therapy. A new treatment approach termed *coherence therapy* or ADFR (activate, depress, free, repeat) using potassium phosphate, etidronate, and calcium administered in a specific protocol has been described, but preliminary studies suggest that it is not as effective as calcium replacement alone or hormonal therapy (Pacifici et al., 1988).

Estrogen is clearly the most effective treatment for preventing bone loss and subsequent fractures (Weiss et al., 1980; Ettinger et al., 1985, 1987; Kiel et al., 1987). Although somewhat controversial, the risks of long-term estrogen treatment for endometrial cancer and vascular complications appear to be outweighed by its beneficial effects on bone and coronary heart disease (Wilson et al., 1985; Stampfer et al., 1985; Hillner et al., 1986; Whitehead and Fraser, 1987; Lufkin et al., 1988). In women who are at high risk for osteoporosis (Table 8-11) and who do not have a uterus, the only significant contraindications to estrogen treatment would be a history of breast cancer or recurrent thromboembolic disease. In women who have a uterus, the risk of endometrial cancer is eliminated by cyclical estrogen administration with the addition of a progestational agent (Gambrell, 1987). Progestogen therapy may also increase bone formation (Christiansen et al., 1985) but may also reverse some of the changes in lipid metabolism which may be responsible for the effects of estrogen on coronary heart disease. Cyclical estrogen-progestogen treatment also results in withdrawal bleeding, which some postmenopausal women may find unacceptable. Thus, the exact estrogen treatment regimen to recommend depends on several factors. The equivalent of at least 0.625 mg of conjugated estrogen is necessary for effect on bone; transdermal administration has not been as yet shown to be as effective as oral. If used cyclically, it is usually prescribed for 21 to 25 days, with a progestational agent (e.g., 10 mg of medroxyprogesterone acetate) during the last 10 days of the cycle. Vaginal bleeding outside the pill-free interval should prompt an endometrial biopsy (Judd et al., 1981).

Hip Fracture

Fractures of the hip and femoral neck, especially when associated with osteoporosis, are among the major causes of immobility, disability, and health care expenditures in the elderly (Wylie, 1977). Fear of hip fracture because of a prior fracture or its occurrence in a friend or relative is a common concern that contributes to limitation of mobility in many elderly persons. This fear is realistic: there are over 250,000 hip fractures in the United States every year, with the incidence increasing dramatically with advanced age. In the year after a hip fracture, close to 20 percent of patients will need nursing home care, and between 10 and 20 percent will die. Thus the prevention and the optimal management of hip fractures are critical to the health of our elderly population.

The degree of immobility and disability caused by a hip fracture depends on several factors, including coexisting medical conditions, patient motivation, the nature of the fracture, and the techniques of management. Many elderly patients with hip fracture already have impaired mobility, and there is a high incidence of medical illnesses which require treatment (e.g., infection, heart failure, anemia, dehydration) at the time of hip fracture. Patients with these underlying conditions and those with dementia are at especially high risk for poor functional recovery. The location of the fracture is especially important in determining the most appropriate management and the outcome of treatment (Table 8-12, Figure 8-1). Subcapital fractures (which are inside the joint capsule) disrupt the blood supply to the proximal femoral head, thus resulting in a higher probability of necrosis of the femoral head and nonunion of the fracture. Replacement of the femoral head is often warranted in these cases. Inter- and subtrochanteric fractures generally do not disrupt the blood supply to the femoral head, and open reduction and pinning is usually successful.

In general, it takes 12 weeks for a hip fracture to heal. Newer

Table 8-12   Characteristics of Selected Treatments for Hip Fracture

Type of fracture	Surgical technique	Comments
Displaced subcapital	Femoral head endoprosthesis (e.g., Austin-Moore)	Allows almost immediate ambulation
Non- or minimally displaced subcapital	Closed reduction with multiple pinnings	Protected weight bearing for 8–12 weeks or until fracture heals
Intertrochanteric and low subcapital	Open reduction with compression screw and side plate	Allows early ambulation
Subtrochanteric	Open reduction with Zickel nail and intramedullary rod	Protected weight bearing until fracture heals

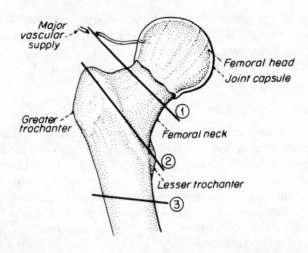

TYPE OF FRACTURE	ANATOMY	IMPLICATIONS
① Subcapital (Intracapsular)	Disrupts blood supply to femoral head	Higher incidence of non-union and necrosis of femoral head
② Intertrochanteric ③ Subtrochanteric	Blood supply to femoral head intact	Lower incidence of non-union and necrosis of femoral head

Figure 8-1 Characteristics of different types of hip fractures.

surgical techniques such as the Austin-Moore prosthesis and the Richard's compression screw allow for almost immediate ambulation in many patients. Like almost all acute conditions in elderly patients, early mobilization is critical to the outcome. When combined with good rehabilitation and patient motivation, early mobilization can minimize disability and immobility from hip fracture. The long-term outcome of elderly patients with hip fracture depends, however, on many other factors besides the type of fracture and patient motivation. Many hip fracture patients have functional disabilities prior to the fracture, active medical conditions at the time of the fracture, and suffer complications while in the acute care hospital (Campion et al., 1987). A recent prospective study of 75 elderly patients with hip fractures revealed a 1-year mortality rate of 29 percent, and only 26 percent of the survivors regained their prefracture functional status (Jette et al., 1987). An intensive rehabilitation program did not appear to improve outcome in this patient population. Thus, even under the best of circumstances hip fracture is a morbid event and a predictor of mortality in the elderly.

Parkinson's Disease

The first step in successful management of Parkinson's disease is to recognize its presence. Although many parkinsonian patients have the classic triad of resting tremor, rigidity, and bradykinesia, many others do not. Early in the disease, the symptoms and signs can be subtle and sometimes unilateral. Many elderly patients, especially in institutions, carry a diagnosis of chronic brain syndrome (or other similar diagnoses) and actually have undiagnosed and treatable forms of parkinsonism. Left untreated, these patients eventually become highly immobile; develop flexion contractures, pressure sores, and malnutrition; and often die of aspiration pneumonia.

Because Parkinson's disease often responds to treatment, especially early in its course, there should be a high index of suspicion for this diagnosis. Patients with Parkinson's disease frequently appear depressed or demented (sometimes both); in fact, many parkinsonian patients become depressed and develop cognitive dysfunction. Experienced neurologists or psychiatrists should be consulted when the diagnosis is in question and when the clinical picture is complicated by dementia and/or depression.

Pharmacological treatment of Parkinson's disease is based on an attempt to increase the ratio of dopamine to acetylcholine in the central nervous system, specifically the nigrostriatal system. Several drugs can be used, sometimes in combination (Table 8-13). Many experts recommend that anticholinergics or amantadine be used initially; others begin with a combination of carbidopa and levodopa. The choice may be based in part on the most prominent clinical manifestations; resting tremor may respond better to anticholinergics, whereas bradykinesia and rigidity may respond better to dopaminergic agents. There remains considerable controversy about whether levodopa should be started at the time of diagnosis, rather than waiting until substantial disability amenable to therapy is present (Duvoisin, 1987). Some authors suggest that early treatment leads to earlier

Table 8-13 Drugs Used to Treat Parkinson's Disease

Drug (brand name)	Usual dosages	Mechanism of action	Potential side effects
Levodopa (Dopar, Larodopa)	2000–5000 mg per day in divided doses	Increases availability of dopamine by providing metabolic precursor	Nausea, vomiting, anorexia Dyskinesias Orthostatic hypotension Behavioral disturbances Vivid dreams and hallucinations
Carbidopa (Lydosyn)	Up to 100 mg per day in divided doses	Decreases peripheral dopamine metabolism	May enhance toxicity of levodopa
Carbidopa/levodopa (Sinemet)	40/400 to 200/2000* mg per day in divided doses	Increases dopamine availability (both above mechanisms)	As above
Amantadine (Symmetrel)	100–300 mg per day†	Increases dopamine release	Delirium and hallucinations Behavioral changes Hypotension Nausea
Bromocriptine (Parlodel)	1–1.5 mg tid or qid (initial); gradually increase to maximum of 100–200 mg in divided doses	Directly activates dopaminergic receptors	Dry mouth Constipation Urinary retention Blurred vision Exacerbation of glaucoma Tachycardia Confusion Behavioral changes
Anticholinergic agents‡ Trihexyphenidyl (Artane, Tremin)	2–20 mg per day in divided doses	Decreases effects of acetylcholine and helps to restore balance between cholinergic and dopaminergic systems	
Benztropine mesylate (Cogentin)	0.5–8 mg per day in divided doses		As above

*Top number represents carbidopa; bottom number, levodopa.
†Eliminated by kidney; dosages should be adjusted when renal function is diminished.
‡Several other anticholinergic agents are available.

233

treatment resistance and fluctuations in response, whereas others suggest that early treatment reduces subsequent morbidity. Whatever approach is used, all the drugs must be used carefully; treatment should begin with small doses, which are gradually increased. Clinical response may take several weeks. Side effects from these drugs are common and often limit pharmacological treatment. Wide variations in response can also occur, including morning akinesia, peak dose dyskinesias, and freezing episodes (sometimes referred to as the "on-off phenomenon"). There is some evidence that these variations may be due in part to dietary amino acids competing with dopamine for transport into the central nervous system (Nutt et al., 1984), but diets containing the recommended daily allowance do not appear to have a significant effect (Juncos et al., 1987). One- to two-week periods off drug therapy, so-called drug holidays, which were frequently recommended in the past, are not beneficial in the vast majority of patients (Mayeux et al., 1985).

Patients who are difficult to manage or who do not respond should be referred to an experienced neurologist. Parkinsonian patients, especially those with more advanced disease, will also benefit from rehabilitation therapy and an ongoing program of exercise and activity in order to maintain strength and functional capabilities and to prevent complications of immobility.

Stroke

In order to prevent disability from immobility and its complications, patients with completed strokes should receive prompt and intensive rehabilitative therapy. In many elderly patients, coexisting medical conditions (e.g., cardiovascular disease) limit the intensity of rehabilitation treatment; however, all patients should be evaluated and managed as actively as possible during the first several weeks after a stroke. Although all stroke patients deserve an assessment and consideration for intensive rehabilitation, the cost-effectiveness of various approaches to stroke rehabilitation is controversial (Johnston and Keith, 1983; Strand et al., 1985). Whether the rehabilitative efforts occur in the acute care hospital, special rehabilitation unit, or nursing home, these efforts should involve a multidisciplinary team, and the basic principles remain the same (see below).

Despite the lack of data from controlled trials, even some of the most severely affected stroke patients can achieve meaningful improvements in functional status by early rehabilitative efforts. Although complete functional recovery occurs in less than half of stroke patients (Silliman et al., 1987), immobility and its attendant complications can almost always be prevented or minimized. Here again, development of realistic goals for individual patients is essential. Intensive efforts directed at functional recovery are probably not appropriate for patients with large or bilateral strokes causing flaccid paralysis or severe perceptual deficits, or for patients with severe underlying medical conditions or dementia. The goals in these latter patients should be to prevent complications and adapt the environment.

The management of elderly patients with cerebrovascular disease is discussed further in Chapter 9. The Suggested Readings section at the end of this chapter lists comprehensive reviews of stroke management.

Pressure Sores

Pressure sores are one of the most common, preventable, and treatable conditions associated with immobility in the elderly. There are four factors that contribute to the development of pressure sores: pressure, shearing forces, friction, and moisture.

As the name implies, pressure sores develop because areas of the body (most often overlying bony prominences) are exposed to prolonged pressure. The amount of pressure necessary to occlude blood supply to the skin (and thus predispose to irreversible tissue damage) is small and is generated in normal sitting and supine positions. Irreversible tissue damage can occur (especially in aging skin) after only 2 h of continuous pressure that exceeds capillary pressure.

Shearing forces (such as those created when the head of a bed is elevated and the torso slides down and transmits pressure to the sacral area) contribute to the stretching and angulation of subcutaneous tissues. Friction, caused by the repeated movement of skin across surfaces such as bed sheets or clothing, increases the shearing force. This can eventually lead to thrombosis of small blood vessels, thus undermining and then destroying skin. Shearing forces and friction are worsened by loose, folded skin, which is common in the elderly because of loss of subcutaneous tissue and/or dehydration.

Moisture from bathing, sweat, urine, and feces compounds the damage. Other risk factors for pressure sores include those that exacerbate oxygen transport (e.g., anemia) or impede healing (e.g., malnutrition). Hospitalized patients with fractures, fecal incontinence, and hypoalbuminemia are at especially high risk (Allman et al., 1986).

Pressure sores can be classified into four grades, depending on their clinical appearance and extent (Table 8-14). It is important to note that the area of damage below the pressure sore is much larger than the sore itself. (This is caused by the manner in which pressure and shearing forces are transmitted to subcutaneous tissues.) Over 90 percent of pressure sores occur in the lower body, mainly in the sacral and coccygeal areas, at the ischial tuberosities, and in the greater trochanter area.

The cornerstone of management of the skin in immobile patients is prevention of pressure sores (Table 8-15). Once a grade I or II pressure sore develops, all preventive measures listed in Table 8-14 should be used to avoid progression of the sore, and intensive local skin care must be instituted. A myriad of techniques have been advocated for local skin care; none have been proved to be more successful than oth-

Table 8-14   Clinical Characteristics of Pressure Sores

Grade I
  Acute inflammatory response limited to epidermis
  Presents as irregular area of erythema, induration, and/or superficial ulceration
  Often over a bony prominence
Grade II
  Extension of acute inflammatory response through full thickness of dermis to the junction of subcutaneous fat
  Appears as a shallow ulcer with more distinct edges
  Early fibrosis and pigment changes occur
Grade III
  Full-thickness skin ulcer extending through subcutaneous fat, limited by deep fascia
  Skin undermined
  Base of ulcer infected, often with necrotic, foul-smelling tissue
Grade IV
  Extension of ulcer through deep fascia, so that bone is visible at base of ulcer
  Osteomyelitis and septic arthritis can be present

Table 8-15 Principles of Skin Care in Immobile Elderly Patients

Preventive
  Identify patients at risk
  Decrease pressure, friction, and skin folding
  Keep skin clean and dry
  Avoid excessive bed rest
  Avoid oversedation
  Provide adequate nutrition and hydration
Grades I and II pressure sores
  Avoid pressure and moisture
  Prevent further injury
  Provide intensive local skin care*
Grade III pressure sores
  Debride necrotic tissue
  Cleanse and dress wound*
  Culture wound†
  Use topical antimicrobials†
Grade IV pressure sores
  Take tissue biopsy for culture
  Use systemic antimicrobials for cellulitis and/or osteomyelitis
  Have surgical consultation to consider surgical repair

*Many techniques are effective (see text).
†Use is controversial (see text).

ers. The most important factor in all these techniques is the attention (and thus the relief from pressure) that the skin gets. Almost any technique that involves removing pressure from the area and regularly cleansing and drying the skin will work.

The management of grades III and IV pressure sores is somewhat more complicated. Debridement of necrotic tissue and frequent irrigation (two to three times daily), cleansing (with peroxide, saline, and/or iodine-containing compounds), and dressing of the wound are essential. Eschars should, in general, be undermined and removed because they can hide large amounts of necrotic and infected tissue. Some of the newer chemical debriding agents can be helpful. The role of wound cultures and antimicrobials in the management of grade III pressure sores is controversial. Topical antimicrobials may be useful, especially when bacterial colony counts are high, but they are generally not recommended. Systemic antimicrobials should not be used because they do not reach sufficient concentrations in the area of the sore, and local therapy will be more effective, unless cellulitis is present. Routine wound cultures are probably not warranted for grade III lesions because they almost always grow several different organisms and do not detect anaerobic bacteria, which are often pathogenic. Once a lesion has progressed to grade IV, systemic antimicrobials are often necessary. Routine and anaerobic cultures of tissue or bone are most helpful in directing antimicrobial therapy. Patients with large pressure sores who become septic should be treated with broad-spectrum antimicrobials which will cover anaerobes, gram negatives, and *Staphylococcus aureus*. In selected instances, consideration of plastic surgery for grade IV lesions is warranted. Air-fluidized beds are being used with increasing frequency for the management of patients with grade III and IV pressure sores, as well as to prevent deep sores in high-risk patients. These beds are expensive, however, and with the exception of one well-controlled study in the acute care hospital setting (Allman et al., 1987), have not been shown to be cost-effective in treating or preventing pressure sores in the elderly population.

REHABILITATION

The goal of rehabilitation is to restore function and prevent further disability. It is, therefore, a core element of geriatric practice, especially for immobile elderly patients, and usually requires a team

Table 8-16   Basic Principles of Rehabilitation in the Elderly

Optimize the treatment of underlying diseases
Prevent secondary disabilities and complications of immobility
Treat primary disabilities
Set realistic, individualized goals
Emphasize functional independence
   Set measurable goals related to functional performance
   Enhance residual functional capacities
   Provide adaptive tools to maximize function
   Adapt the environment to the patient's functional disabilities when feasible
Attend to motivation and other psychological factors of both patients and care
   givers
Utilize a team approach

effort. It is beyond the scope of this text to provide a detailed discussion of rehabilitation in the elderly. Table 8-16 outlines some of the key principles. Careful assessment of a patient's function, the setting of realistic goals, prevention of secondary disabilities and complications of immobility, repeated measures of functional abilities that are relevant to the patient's environment, and adapting the environment to the patients' abilities (and vice versa) are all essential elements of the rehabilitation process.

Physical and occupational therapists can be extremely valuable in assessing, treating, motivating, and monitoring patients whose mobility is impaired. Physical therapists generally attend to the relief of pain, muscle strength and endurance, joint range of motion, and gait. They use a variety of treatment modalities (Table 8-17). Occupational therapists focus on functional abilities, especially as they relate to activities of daily living. They make detailed assessments of mobility and help patients improve or adapt to their abilities to perform basic and instrumental activities of daily living. Even when mobility and function remain impaired, occupational therapists can

Table 8-17   Physical Therapy in the Management of Immobile Elderly Patients

Objectives
  Relieve pain
  Evaluate, maintain, and improve joint range of motion
  Evaluate and improve strength, endurance, motor skills, and coordination
  Evaluate and improve gait and stability
  Assess the need for and teach the use of assistive devices for ambulation
    (wheelchairs, walkers, canes)
Treatment modalities
  Exercise
    Active (isometric and isotonic)
    Passive
  Heat
    Hot packs
    Paraffin
    Diathermy
  Hydrotherapy
  Ultrasound
  Transcutaneous electrical nerve stimulation

make life easier for these patients by performing environmental assessments and recommending modifications and assistive devices that will improve the patient's ability to function independently (Table 8-18).

Although these basic principles of geriatric rehabilitation are essential in providing optimal care for the growing populations of geriatric patients who may need rehabilitation (Findley and Findley, 1987), the cost-effectiveness of various approaches to rehabilitation in the elderly remains controversial. Most of the data on the effectiveness of rehabilitation for the elderly come from studies of geriatric assessment units, where short-term rehabilitation is a major component of the intervention. Most geriatric assessment units described to date have been in either acute care hospitals or ambulatory settings (Rubenstein, 1987), although some have been located in nursing

Table 8-18   Occupational Therapy in the Management of Immobile Elderly Patients

Objectives
   Restore, maintain, and improve ability to function independently
   Evaluate and improve sensory and perceptual motor function
   Evaluate and improve ability to perform activities of daily living (ADL)
   Fabricate and fit splints for upper extremities
   Improve coping and problem-solving skills
   Improve use of leisure time
Modalities
   Assessment of mobility
     Bed mobility
     Transfers
     Wheelchair propulsion
   Assessment of other ADL using actual or simulated environments
     Dressing
     Toileting
     Bathing and personal hygiene
     Cooking and cleaning
Visit home for environmental assessment and recommendations for adaptation
Provide task-oriented activities (e.g., crafts, projects)
Recommend and teach use of assistive devices (e.g., long-handled reachers, special eating and cooking utensils, sock aids)
Recommend and teach use of safety devices (e.g., grab bars and railing, raised toilet seats, shower chairs)

homes (Schuman et al., 1980; Adelman et al., 1987). The effectiveness of such units has been summarized in detail (Rubenstein, 1987). It is clear that targeting rehabilitative efforts to patients who are most likely to benefit is critical to cost-effectiveness. Unfortunately, much more data is needed to accurately predict which geriatric patients will benefit most from specific types of rehabilitative efforts. Until these data are available, geriatricians should work closely with experienced rehabilitation therapists in setting *realistic* and *individualized* goals for their patients. The goals should be compatible with the patients' preferences and socioeconomic environment and should strive toward the maximum functional outcome realistic for that patient. Ongoing assessment of progress, and the prevention of medical and psychological complications are also fundamental to the rehabilitative process.

REFERENCES

Adelman RD, Marron K, Libow LS, et al: A community-oriented geriatric rehabilitation unit in a nursing home. *Gerontologist* 27:143–146, 1987.

Allman RM, Laprade CA, Noel LB, et al: Pressure sores among hospitalized patients. *Ann Intern Med* 105:337–342, 1986.

Allman RM, Walker JM, Hart MK, et al: Air-fluidized beds or conventional therapy for pressure sores: A randomized trial. *Ann Intern Med* 107:641–648, 1987.

Aloia JF, Cohn SH, Ostuni A, et al: Prevention of involutional bone loss by exercise. *Ann Intern Med* 80:356–358, 1978.

American College of Physicians Health and Public Policy Committee: Bone mineral densitometry. *Ann Intern Med* 107:932–936, 1987.

Beard K, Walker AM, Perera DR, et al: Nonsteroidal anti-inflammatory drugs and hospitalization for gastroesophageal bleeding in the elderly. *Arch Intern Med* 147:1621–1623, 1987.

Campion EW, Jette AM, Cleary PD, et al: Hip fracture: A prospective study of hospital course, complications, and costs. *J Gen Intern Med* 2:78–82, 1987.

Chow R, Harrison JE, Notarius C: Effect of two randomised exercise programmes on bone mass of healthy postmenopausal women. *Br Med J* 295:1441–1444, 1987.

Christiansen C, Riis BJ, Nilas L, et al: Uncoupling of bone formation and resorption by combined oestrogen and progestogen therapy in post-menopausal osteoporosis. *Lancet* 2:800–801, October 12, 1985.

Chuang T, Wunder GG, Istrup DM, et al: Polymyalgia rheumatica: A 10-year epidemiologic and clinical study. *Ann Intern Med* 97:672–680, 1982.

Crawford J, Eye-Boland MK, Cohen HJ: Clinical utility of erythrocyte sedimentation rate and plasma protein analysis in the elderly. *Am J Med* 82:239–246, 1987.

Duvoisin R: To treat early or to treat late? *Ann Neurol* 22:2–3, 1987.

Ettinger B, Genant HK, Cann CE: Long-term estrogen replacement therapy prevents bone loss and fractures. *Ann Intern Med* 102:319–324, 1985.

Ettinger B, Genant HK, Cann CE: Postmenopausal bone loss is prevented by treatment with low-dosage estrogen with calcium. *Ann Intern Med* 106:40–45, 1987.

Findley TW, Findley SE: Rehabilitation needs in the 1990s: Effects of an aging population. *Med Care* 25:753–763, 1987.

Frost R: To treat early or to treat late? *Ann Neurol* 22:2–3, 1987.

Gambrell DR: Use of progestogen therapy. *Am J Obstet Gynecol* 156:1304–1312, 1987.

Goodman BW: Temporal arteritis. *Am J Med* 67:389–852, 1979.

Hillner BE, Hollenberg JP, Pauker SG: Postmenopausal estrogens in prevention of osteoporosis—benefit without risk if cardiovascular effects are considered. *Am J Med* 80:1115–1128, 1986.

Jette AM, Harris BA, Cleary PD, et al: Functional recovery after hip fracture. *Arch Phys Med Rehabil* 68:735–740, 1987.

Johnston MV, Keith RA: Cost-benefits of medical rehabilitation: Review and critique. *Arch Phys Med Rehabil* 64:147–154, 1983.

Judd H, Cleary R, Creasman W, et al: Estrogen replacement therapy. *Obstet Gynecol* 58:267–275, 1981.

Juncos JL, Fabbrini G, Mouradian MM, et al: Dietary influences on the antiparkinsonian response to levodopa. *Arch Neurol* 44:1003–1005, 1987.

Kiel DP, Felson DT, Anderson JJ, et al: Hip fracture and the use of estrogens in postmenopausal women: The Framingham Study. *N Engl J Med* 317:1169–1174, 1987.

Lufkin EG, Carpenter PC, Ory SJ, et al: Estrogen replacement therapy: Current recommendations. *Mayo Clin Proc* 63:453–460, 1988.

Mayeux R, Stern Y, Mulvey K, et al: Reappraisal of temporary levodopa withdrawal ("drug holiday") in Parkinson's disease. *N Engl J Med* 313:724–728, 1985.

Nutt JG, Woodward WR, Hammerstad JP, et al: The "on-off" phenomenon in Parkinson's disease. *N Engl J Med* 310:483–488, 1984.

Pacifici R, McMurtry C, Vered I, et al: Coherence therapy does not prevent axial bone loss in osteoporotic women: A preliminary comparative study. *J Clin Endocrinol Metab* 66:747–753, 1988.

Reich ML: Arthritis: Avoiding diagnostic pitfalls. *Geriatrics* 37:46–54, 1982.

Riggs BL, Melton JL: Involutional osteoporosis. *N Engl J Med* 314:1676–1684, 1986.

Riggs BL, Seeman E, Hodgson SF, et al: Effect of the fluoride/calcium regimen on vertebral fractures occurrence in postmenopausal osteoporosis. *N Engl J Med* 306:446–450, 1982.

Riis B, Thomsen K, Christiansen C: Does calcium supplementation prevent postmenopausal bone loss? A double-blind, controlled clinical study. *N Engl J Med* 316:173–177, 1987.

Rubenstein LZ: Geriatric assessment: An overview of its impacts. *Clin Geriatr Med* 3:1–27, 1987.

Schuman JE, Beattie EJ, Steed DA, et al: Rehabilitative and geriatric teaching programs: Clinical efficacy in a skilled nursing facility. *Arch Phys Med Rehabil* 61:310–315, 1980.

Silliman RA, Wagner EH, Fletcher RH: The social and functional consequences of stroke for elderly patients. *Stroke* 18:200–203, 1987.

Stampfer MJ, Willett WC, Colditz GA, et al: A prospective study of postmenopausal estrogen therapy and coronary heart disease. *N Engl J Med* 313:1044–1049, 1985.

Strand T, Asplund K, Eriksson S, et al: A non-intensive stroke unit reduces functional disability and the need for long-term hospitalization. *Stroke* 16:29–34, 1985.

Tinetti ME, Schmidt A, Baum J: Use of the erythrocyte sedimentation rate in chronically ill, elderly patients with a decline in health status. *Am J Med* 80:844–848, 1986.

Weiss NS, Ure CL, Ballard JH, et al: Decreased risk of fractures of the hip and lower forearm with postmenopausal use of estrogen. *N Engl J Med* 303:1195–1198, 1980.

Whitehead MI, Fraser D: Controversies concerning the safety of estrogen replacement therapy. *Am J Obstet Gynecol* 156:1313–1325, 1987.

Wilson PWF, Garrison RJ, Castelli WP: Postmenopausal estrogen use, cigarette smoking, and cardiovascular morbidity in women over 50. *N Engl J Med* 313:1038–1043, 1985.

Wylie CM: Hospitalizations for fractures and bone loss in adults—Why do we regard these phenomena as dull? *Public Health Rep* 92:33–38, 1977.

SUGGESTED READINGS

Immobility, General

Bortz WM: Disuse and aging. *JAMA* 248:1203–1208, 1982.
Kottke FJ: Deterioration of the bedfast patient. *Public Health Rep* 80:437–451, 1965.

Musculoskeletal Disorders

Davis MA: Epidemiology of osteoarthritis. *Clin Geriatr Med* 4:241–256, 1988.
Frymoyer JW: Back pain and sciatica. *N Engl J Med* 318:291–300, 1988.
Gall EP: Analgesic and anti-inflammatory agents, in Conrad KA, Bressler R (eds): *Drug Therapy for the Elderly*. St Louis, Mosby, 1982.
Liang MH, Cullen KE, Poss R: Primary total hip or knee replacement: Evaluation of patients. *Ann Intern Med* 97:735–739, 1982.
Lifschitz ML, Harmon CE: Musculoskeletal problems in the elderly, in Schrier RW (ed): *Clinical Internal Medicine in the Aged*. Philadelphia, Saunders, 1982.
Moskowitz RW: Management of osteoarthritis. *Hosp Pract* 14:75–87, July 1979.
Roth SH: Pharmacologic approaches to musculoskeletal disorders. *Clin Geriatr Med* 4:441–461, 1988.
Simon LS, Mills JA: Nonsteroidal anti-inflammatory drugs. *N Engl J Med* 302:1179–1185; 1237–1243, 1980.
Svara CJ, Hadler NM: Back pain. *Clin Geriatr Med* 4:395–410, 1988.

Osteoporosis

Kaplan FS: Osteoporosis. *Ciba Clin Symp* Vol 35, No 5, 1983.
Raisz LG: Osteoporosis. *J Am Geriatr Soc* 30:127–138, 1982.
Riggs BL, Melton LJ: Involutional osteoporosis. *N Engl J Med* 314:1676–1684, 1986.

Parkinson's Disease

Boshes B: Sinemet and the treatment of parkinsonism. *Ann Intern Med* 94:364–370, 1981.
Duvoisin R: Parkinsonism. *Ciba Clin Symp* Vol 28, No 1, 1976.
Nutt JG: Parkinson's disease: Evaluation and therapeutic strategy. *Hosp Prac* 22:107–136, 1987.
Parkes JD: Adverse effects of antiparkinsonian drugs. *Drugs* 21:341–353, 1981.

Stroke

Browne TR, Poskanzer DC: Treatment of strokes. *N Engl J Med* 28:594–602; 650–657, 1969.

Buonanno F, Toole JF: Management of patients with established ("completed") cerebral infarction. *Stroke* 12:7–16, 1981.

Kelly JF, Winograd CH: A functional approach to stroke management in elderly patients. *J Am Geriatr Soc* 33:48–60, 1985.

Pressure Sores

Agris J, Spira M: Pressure ulcers: Prevention and treatment. *Ciba Clin Symp* Vol 31, No 5, 1979.

Reuler JB, Cooney TG: The pressure sore: Pathophysiology and principles of management. *Ann Intern Med* 94:661–666, 1981.

Shea JD: Pressure sores—classification and management. *Clin Orthop Relat Res* 112:89–100, 1975.

Rehabilitation

Clark GS, Blue B, Bearer JB: Rehabilitation of the elderly amputee. *J Am Geriatr Soc* 31:439–448, 1983.

Liang MH, Partridge A, Eaton H, et al: Rehabilitation management of homebound elderly with locomotor disability. *Clin Geriatr Med* 4:431–440, 1988.

Sinaki M: Postmenopausal spinal osteoporosis. Physical therapy and rehabilitation principles. *Mayo Clin Proc* 57:699–703, 1982.

Steinberg FU: Rehabilitating the older stroke patient: What's possible? *Geriatrics* 41:85–97, 1986.

Vallarino R, Sherman FT: Principles of rehabilitation treatment, in Libow LS, Sherman FT (eds): *The Core of Geriatric Medicine*. St Louis, Mosby, 1981.

Williams TF (ed): *Rehabilitation in the Aging*. New York, Raven Press, 1984.

Chapter 9

Cardiovascular Disorders

In the elderly, heart disease is the leading cause of death worldwide and is the most common cause for hospitalization. Physiological changes of the cardiovascular system in aging may modify the presentation of cardiac disease.

PHYSIOLOGICAL CHANGES

In reviewing data on physiological changes of the cardiovascular system, it is important to recognize the selection criteria of the population studied. Because the prevalence of coronary artery disease may be 50 percent in the eighth and ninth decades, screening for exclusion of occult cardiovascular disease may modify findings.

In a population screened for occult coronary artery disease, there is no change in cardiac output at rest over the third to eighth decade (Table 9-1). There is a slight decrease in heart rate and a compensatory slight increase in stroke volume. This is in contrast to studies in

Table 9-1   Resting Cardiac Function in Patients Aged 30 to 80, Compared with That in 30-Year-Olds

	Unscreened for occult CAD	Screened for occult CAD
Heart rate	−	−
Stroke volume	− −	+
Stroke volume index	− −	0
Cardiac output	− −	0
Cardiac index	− −	0
Peripheral vascular resistance	+ +	0
Peak systolic blood pressure	+ +	+ +
Diastolic pressure	0	0

Note: CAD − coronary artery disease; +, slight increase; + +, increase; −, slight decrease; − −, decrease; 0, no difference.

unscreened individuals, where cardiac output has been shown to fall from the second to the ninth decade.

During maximal exercise, however, other changes are manifest even in the screened population (Table 9-2). Heart rate response to exercise is decreased in the elderly, reflecting a diminished beta-adrenergic responsiveness in aging. Because cardiac output is maintained, the heart affects the Starling curve by increasing cardiac volumes—increasing end-diastolic and end-systolic volumes. With this increase in work load and the work of pumping blood against a higher

Table 9-2   Performance at Maximum Exercise in Sample Screened for CAD, Age 30–80

	Compared with 30-year-olds
Heart rate	− −
End-diastolic volume	+ +
Stroke volume	+ +
Cardiac output	0
End-systolic volume	+ +
Ejection fraction	− −
Total peripheral vascular resistance	0
Systolic blood pressure	0

Note: + +, significant increase; − −, significant decrease; 0, no difference.

blood pressure, cardiac hypertrophy occurs even in the screened elderly population.

HYPERTENSION

Hypertension is the major risk factor for stroke, heart failure, and coronary artery disease in the elderly; all are important contributors to mortality and functional disability. Because hypertension is remediable and its control may reduce the incidence of coronary heart disease and stroke, increased efforts at detection and treatment of high blood pressure are indicated.

Hypertension in the elderly is defined as a systolic blood pressure of 160 mmHg or greater and/or a diastolic blood pressure of 95 mmHg or greater. Systolic hypertension is defined as a pressure of 160 mmHg or greater with a diastolic pressure of less than 95 mmHg. With this definition, 40 to 50 percent of individuals over age 65 are hypertensive.

Diastolic pressure rises with age, but stabilizes after age 60, whereas systolic pressure continues to increase with the incidence rising steeply after age 55 in both sexes but to a greater degree in women.

Despite the high prevalence of hypertension in the elderly, it should not be considered a normal consequence of aging. The Framingham Study has demonstrated that hypertension is the major risk factor for cardiovascular disease in the elderly and that the risk increases with each decade (Kannel, 1976). Once coronary artery disease develops, it tends to be more rapidly fatal among patients with hypertension.

Evaluation

The diagnosis should be made on serial blood pressures. In patients with labile hypertension, blood pressure should be averaged to make the diagnosis because these patients are at no less risk than the stable hypertensive. The history and physical examination should be directed toward assessing the duration, severity, treatment, and complications of the hypertension (Table 9-3). Atherosclerosis may interfere with occlusion of the brachial artery by a blood pressure cuff, leading to erroneously elevated blood pressure determinations, "pseu-

Table 9-3   Initial Evaluation of Hypertension in the Elderly

History:
  Duration
  Severity
  Treatment
  Complications
  Other risk factors
Physical examination:
  Blood pressure, including Osler maneuver
  Weight
  Funduscopic, vascular, and cardiac examination for end-organ damage
  Abdominal bruit
  Neurological examination for focal deficits
Laboratory tests:
  Urinalysis
  Electrolytes
  Creatinine
  Calcium
  Chest x-ray
  Electrocardiogram

dohypertension." Such an effect can be determined by the Osler maneuver. The cuff pressure is raised above systolic blood pressure. If the radial artery remains palpable at this pressure, significant atherosclerosis is probably present and may account for a 10- to 15-mmHg pressure error. Initial laboratory evaluation should include complete urinalysis and measurement of serum electrolytes and creatinine levels. A chest film and electrocardiogram should also be included. An intravenous pyelogram is not indicated in the initial evaluation and should be reserved for the patient resistant to therapy.

Secondary forms of hypertension are uncommon in the elderly but should be considered in resistant patients and in those with diastolic pressures >115 mmHg (Table 9-4). Primary hyperaldosteronism and pheochromocytoma are uncommon in the elderly and are particularly unusual in those past the age of 75. Although also uncommon, renovascular disease should be considered in resistant patients. It is almost always secondary to atherosclerotic occlusive disease in the elderly.

With the use of automated calcium determinations, the fre-

Table 9-4   Secondary Hypertension in the Elderly

Renovascular disease (atherosclerotic)
Hyperparathyroidism (calcium)
Estrogen administration
Renal disease (decreased creatinine clearance)

quency of diagnosis of primary hyperparathyroidism is increasing, particularly in postmenopausal women. Because there is a causal link between this disorder and hypertension, the diagnosis and treatment of hyperparathyroidism may ameliorate the elevated blood pressure.

Estrogen therapy in the postmenopausal woman may be associated with hypertension. Such an association can be assessed by withdrawing estrogen therapy for several months and following the blood pressure response.

Treatment

Although the issue of treatment of hypertension in individuals over the age of 75 remains controversial, it is not an issue in those under age 70 who have diastolic hypertension. The Veterans Administration Cooperative Study (1972), the Hypertension Detection and Follow-Up Program Study (1979), a smaller Australian trial (1980), and more recently the European Working Party on High Blood Pressure in the Elderly (EWPHE) (Amery et al., 1985, 1986) have all demonstrated that treating hypertension decreases morbidity and mortality from coronary artery disease and stroke. Although there has been concern about the hazard of treating individuals with cerebrovascular disease, the evidence suggests that the presence of cerebrovascular disease is an indication for, rather than a contraindication to, hypertensive therapy. Prospective controlled studies have not been performed to assess the benefits and risks of treating isolated systolic hypertension, although the associated cardiovascular risk of systolic hypertension suggests that treatment may be beneficial. The national multicenter Systolic Hypertension in the Elderly Program (SHEP) has been designed to assess the benefits and risks of drug therapy of isolated systolic hypertension in individuals 60 years of age or older.

The EWPHE study did not demonstrate a benefit of drug treatment for individuals over the age of 80 years. However, the number of subjects in this age subgroup was small. Decision on therapy in this age group remains difficult; congestive heart failure from hypertension is an indication for therapy. Although only a small number of patients have been studied, there is a suggestion that cerebral blood flow does not decrease, and may actually increase, in treated hypertensives who respond to therapy. In hypertensives who do not respond, cerebral blood flow decreases with therapy. The therapeutic response in lowering blood pressure might therefore be used to decide which patients should be continued on therapy.

Specific Therapy

Although life-style changes are not easily accomplished, weight reduction and lowering of dietary sodium intake should be attempted. Each of these measures may lower diastolic pressure by 5 to 10 mmHg. Exercise may also be beneficial in lowering blood pressure. Strenuous exercise is not necessary. A modest walking and running program may have a positive effect on blood pressure reduction (Rippe et al., 1988). Other risk factors, such as smoking and diabetes mellitus, should also be modified.

If dietary measures fail to control blood pressure, drug therapy should be considered. Physiological and pathological changes of aging should be considered in individualizing the therapy. Changes in volumes of distribution and hepatic and renal metabolism may alter pharmacokinetics (see Chapter 14). Changes in vessel elasticity and baroreceptor sensitivity may alter responses to posture and drug-induced falls in blood pressure.

Oral diuretics are usually the initial step in therapy (Table 9-5). They are well tolerated, are relatively inexpensive, and can be given once a day; results from the European study indicate that 65 percent of elderly hypertensives can be treated with diuretics as the only medication. The SHEP trial and several other studies have demonstrated that low-dose thiazides (e.g., 12.5 to 25 mg of chlorthalidone) are efficacious in lowering blood pressure while minimizing metabolic side effects (Morledge et al., 1986; Vardan et al., 1987b). Higher doses had a minimal additional effect on blood pressure with a more marked effect on hypokalemia. Postural hypotension is uncommon, but serum potassium should be monitored. Diabetics may have

Table 9-5 Thiazide Diuretics for Antihypertensive Therapy

Advantages	Adverse effects
Well tolerated	Hypokalemia
No CNS side effects	Volume depletion
Relatively inexpensive	Hyponatremia
Infrequent dosing	Hyperglycemia
Good response rate	Hyperuricemia
Orthostatic hypotension uncommon	
Can be used in conjunction with other agents	

increased requirements for insulin or oral hypoglycemic agents. Although short-term trials of thiazide diuretics have demonstrated increases in serum cholesterol, this effect of the drug does not seem to persist at 1 year (Vardan et al., 1987a). Beta-blocking agents may be used as the initial drug, especially when another indication for their use exists, such as coronary heart disease, arrhythmias, or essential tremor. The 1988 Report of the Joint National Committee on Detection, Evaluation, and Treatment of High Blood Pressure has included calcium antagonists and angiotensin-converting enzyme (ACE) inhibitors as potential monotherapy agents for the elderly hypertension patient.

If thiazides alone do not control blood pressure, a second agent is added (Table 9-6), or a thiazide is added if one of the other agents has failed. The choice should be individualized and usually selected from among beta blockers, calcium antagonists, or ACE inhibitors. Where beta blockers would be used for treatment of other disorders in association with hypertension, they would be the drug of choice. These agents are contraindicated in patients with cardiac conduction deficits, overt heart failure, bradyarrhythmias, reactive airways disease, peripheral vascular disease, and insulin-dependent diabetes mellitus.

The advantages of beta blockers might make them the general drug of choice in the second step of therapy, except that they may not be as effective in the elderly as they are in the young. Their mode of action is unknown, but three mechanisms have been proposed: (1) CNS action, (2) decreased cardiac output, and (3) inhibition of renin secretion. Myocardial beta-adrenergic responsiveness decreases with age, and thus the effect of beta blockade on cardiac output may be

Table 9-6   Antihypertensive Medications

Agent	Advantages	Disadvantages
Beta blockers	Useful in associated coronary artery disease or arrhythmias Newer, water-soluble agents have fewer CNS side effects	Contraindicated in cardiac conduction defects, overt heart failure, bradyarrhythmia, reactive airways disease, peripheral vascular disease, and insulin-treated diabetes Propranolol may cause fatigue, somnolence, or depression If cardiac output is decreased, renal blood flow and glomerular filtration rate may fall Must be withdrawn slowly in presence of coronary artery disease
Methyldopa	Increased renal blood flow	Somnolence, depression (may be minimized by low dosage) Orthostatic hypotension
Clonidine	Increased renal perfusion	Somnolence, depression Dry mouth, constipation Rarely withdrawal hypertensive crisis
Reserpine	Inexpensive	Depression (minimized with low dosage)
Prazosin	May be useful in systolic hypertension	Orthostatic hypotension with initial dose
Hydralazine	May be useful in systolic hypertension	Reflex tachycardia, aggravation of angina Lupuslike syndrome at high dosage
Calcium channel blockers	Peripheral vasodilator Coronary blood flow maintained Potency increased with age	Headaches Sodium retention Negative inotropic effect Conduction abnormality
Angiotensin-converting enzyme inhibitors	Preload and afterload reduction Use in CHF	Hyperkalemia Hypotension Decreased renal function

Note: With all these agents, initiation with low dosage and careful titration may minimize side effects.

diminished. Most elderly hypertensives have a low-renin form of hypertension; thus this effect may be less in the aged. However, in those elderly patients without contraindications and who do respond, beta blockers may be the drug of choice.

The newer, more water-soluble beta blockers may be well suited for the geriatric population because they enter the central nervous system less readily and thus have fewer of the CNS side effects such as somnolence and depression, which would be a particular advantage in the elderly. However, if cardiac output is decreased, renal perfusion and glomerular filtration rate may be affected. One concern with beta blockers is the production of bradycardia with reduced cardiac output. One simple test to monitor for this side effect is the patient's response to mild exercise after each dosage increase; a failure to increase pulse by at least 10 beats per minute is an indication to reduce the dosage. If a patient is to be taken off a beta-blocking agent, withdrawal should be done slowly over a period of several days to avoid rebound of original symptoms.

Methyldopa has the disadvantage of CNS side effects, including fatigue, somnolence, and depression. These side effects can be minimized with low dosage levels, and the drug may be quite useful in the elderly if blood pressure control can be achieved at these lower levels. Methyldopa has the advantage of improving renal perfusion. Clonidine may also cause somnolence and depression, but it also increases renal perfusion. The newer clonidine transdermal patch may lessen some of these adverse effects. However, local skin reactions may occur in about 15 percent of users. The once-per-week application of the patch may be an asset in improving compliance.

The major disadvantage of reserpine is the high incidence of depression as a side effect. This can be minimized with low dosages.

The major side effect of prazosin, an alpha blocker, is orthostatic hypotension with initial doses. This makes it difficult to use in the elderly, especially because the orthostasis may be induced each time the drug is stopped and restarted when drug dosages are missed.

Although hydralazine is usually a third-step drug, it may occasionally be used as a second-step drug in the elderly because reflex tachycardia rarely occurs. If used with diuretics alone, it should be initiated in low dosages, which should be increased slowly. It should not be used in the absence of a beta blocker if coronary artery disease is present.

Calcium antagonists are peripheral vasodilators with the advantage of maintaining coronary blood flow. These agents appear to have increased potency with age, possibly as a result of the decreased reflex tachycardia and myocardial contractility in the elderly when compared to younger individuals. Headache, sodium retention, negative inotropic effects—especially in combination with beta-blockers—and conduction abnormalities may limit their use. Dosing several times a day may increase compliance problems. As long-acting agents become available, this may become less of an issue.

ACE inhibitors are both preload and afterload reducers and thus are particularly useful in the face of congestive heart failure. Newer long-acting agents may have an advantage in compliance. Renal function, which may deteriorate on administration of these agents, needs to be monitored carefully. These agents may also induce hyperkalemia and should not be used with a potassium-sparing diuretic. The elderly are also more prone to the hypotensive effects of these drugs.

With the newer, more effective agents, drug-resistant hypertension is unusual. In such cases, drug compliance should be monitored and sodium intake assessed. If such factors are not contributing to drug resistance, secondary causes of hypertension should be considered, especially renovascular disease.

STROKE AND TRANSIENT ISCHEMIC ATTACKS

Although the incidence of stroke is declining, it is still a major medical problem affecting approximately 50,000 individuals in the United States every year. Stroke is clearly a disease of the elderly; about 75 percent of strokes occur in those over age 65. The incidence of stroke rises steeply with age, being 10 times greater in the 75-to-84 age group than in the 55-to-64 age group.

The causes and outcomes of stroke are listed in Table 9-7. In cerebral infarct, thrombosis, usually arteriosclerotic, is the commonest cause, with embolization from an ulcerated plaque or myocardial thrombosis less frequent. Outcomes for survivors are listed in Table 9-8.

Table 9-7   Stroke

Cause	Relative frequency, percent	Mortality rate, percent
Subarachnoid hemorrhage	10	50
Intracerebral hemorrhage	15	80
Cerebral infarction (thrombosis and embolism)	75	40

Source: Robbins, 1978.

Hypertension, diabetes mellitus, and lipid abnormalities are associated with increased risk of cerebrovascular disease; hypertension is the major risk factor. In the Framingham Study (Kannel, 1976), systolic hypertension was associated with a three- to fivefold increased risk for stroke. Hypertension accelerates the formation of atheromatous plaques and damages the integrity of vessel walls, predisposing to thrombotic occlusion and cerebral infarction. Hypertension also promotes growth of microaneurysms in segments of small intracranial arteries. Those lesions are sites of intracranial hemorrhage and lacunar infarcts.

The data associating stroke with transient ischemic attacks are varied. Completed stroke as a sequel of TIA is reported to occur in 12 to 60 percent or more of untreated TIA patients who become asymptomatic; however, some estimates are at 25 percent or less. More TIA patients may die of cardiac disease than of a subsequent stroke (50 percent versus 36 percent, respectively, in a Mayo Clinic 15-year follow-up study) (Robbins, 1978). In retrospective studies of patients

Table 9-8   Outcome for Survivors of Stroke

Outcome	Percent
No dysfunction	10
Mild dysfunction	40
Significant dysfunction	40
Institutional care	10

Source: Robbins, 1978.

with completed stroke, previous TIA is reported to have occurred in 50 to 75 percent.

The keystone to the diagnosis of stroke is a clear history of sudden, acute neurological deficit. When the history is not clear, especially if the deficit could have had a gradual onset, consideration should be given to a mass lesion. In such cases, brain scanning with computerized tomography is indicated. Electroencephalography is only occasionally helpful in the differential diagnosis. Lumbar puncture is indicated in stroke patients if hemorrhage is suspected but not if there is evidence of increased intracranial pressure. An electrocardiogram should be performed routinely in cases of TIA or stroke because it may relate the episode to myocardial infarction or cardiac arrhythmia. Invasive techniques are not usually necessary in stroke patients.

In the elderly, symptoms acceptable as evidence of cerebral ischemia are often misinterpreted. Presenting symptoms for TIA in the carotid and vertebral-basilar systems are given in Table 9-9. When they occur or recur alone without other neurological symptoms, certain symptoms should not be attributed to vascular causes. These include lightheadedness, nonspecific dizziness, vertigo, diplopia, drop attacks, forgetfulness, amnestic attacks, syncope, seizures, episodes of unconsciousness, and drowsy spells (Barnett, 1982).

The decision for surgical intervention in patients with TIA is complex. Doppler studies have allowed noninvasive evaluation of carotid disease, but arteriography is the gold standard in evaluating the feasibility of carotid or subclavian endarterectomy. Because this procedure carries some risk, it is indicated only in patients considered operable. Factors in deciding operability include the clinical profile, expected years of life remaining, collateral disease, possibility of the patient succumbing to another disease, and the risks and benefits of surgery. Age per se is usually not a major consideration; the other factors noted are more important.

Surgical mortality for endarterectomy is under 5 percent in experienced centers. It is 1 to 2 percent in neurologically stable patients without other medical risk, and rises to 10 percent in neurologically unstable patients. Of TIA patients, 70 to 90 percent are asymptomatic or improved after carotid surgery, but 5 to 15 percent become worse or die as a result of surgery. Thus, a 1 to 5 percent risk

Table 9-9   TIA: Presenting Symptoms

Symptom	Carotid	Vertebral-basilar
Paresis	+ + +	+ +
Paresthesia	+ + +	+ + +
Binocular vision	0	+ + +
Vertigo	0	+ + +
Diplopia	0	+ +
Ataxia	0	+ +
Dizziness	0	+ +
Monocular vision	+ +	0
Headache	+	+
Dysphasia	+	0
Dysarthria	+	+
Nausea and vomiting	0	+
Loss of consciousness	0	0
Visual hallucinations	0	0
Tinnitus	0	0
Mental change	0	0
Drop attacks	0	0
Drowsiness	0	0
Lightheadedness	0	0
Hyperacusia	0	0
Weakness (generalized)	0	0
Convulsion	0	0

Note: + + +, most frequent; 0, least frequent.

of operative mortality must be weighted against a 25 to 50 percent risk of developing a stroke (which may result in only partial incapacity).

The alternative to surgery is drug therapy, although the results have not been dramatic. The general trend has been to use aspirin more and anticoagulants less. This is particularly true in the elderly, where the complications of anticoagulants are a greater problem. Persantine alone or in combination with aspirin does not appear to be of benefit.

Stroke Rehabilitation

Factors in the prognosis for rehabilitation of the older stroke patient are presented in Table 9-10. Although the benefit of stroke rehabilitation is controversial, if it is to be of benefit, it should be initiated

Table 9-10   Factors in Prognosis for Rehabilitation

Prognosis for neurological return
Mentation
Motivation
Vigor
Availability and implementation of sound program

early in the course. Generally, most neurological return occurs during the first month after the stroke. By the end of the third month, little, if any, further return can be expected. Not all dysfunctions result in the same level of disability. Motor loss is often the least disabling. Perceptual and/or sensory loss, aphasia, loss of balance, hemicorporal neglect, hemianopsia, and/or cognitive damage may cause more severe and often untreatable disabilities.

In the immediate stage, treatment is directed to avoiding complications such as pressure sores, contractures, phlebitis, pulmonary embolism, aspiration pneumonia, and fecal impaction.

In the next stage of rehabilitation, treatment is directed to reeducating muscles (affected areas) and enhancing remaining capabilities (unaffected areas). Table 9-11 describes measures to be taken during this phase.

When the patient stops making progress after intensive therapy,

Table 9-11   Stroke Rehabilitation

Acute phase:
    Change of patient's position at least every 2 h
    Positioning of patient's joints to prevent contractures
    Positioning of patient to prevent aspiration pneumonia
    Range-of-motion exercises
Later phase:
    Perceptual training
    Muscle reeducation exercises
    Functional activities for affected side
    Ambulation training
    ADL training
    Training in transfer technique

the goal of rehabilitation shifts to finding ways for the patient to cope with the dysfunction. At this stage, the patient is assessed for the need for braces and assistive devices for both ambulation and performance of activities of daily living. With a sound program of rehabilitation, the elderly patient who survives a stroke can return to the community.

CORONARY ARTERY DISEASE

Hypertension is the major risk factor for coronary artery disease in the elderly. Hypercholesterolemia and cigarette smoking become less important risk factors in this age group, although they are still significant when associated with other risk factors.

Angina pectoris has a similar presentation in both the elderly and in younger patients, with familiar pain characteristics and radiation. Treatment includes reducing factors that precipitated anginal attacks and also pharmacological intervention. Smokers should be advised to discontinue smoking; physical and emotional stresses that precipitate pain should be modified.

Pharmacologically, episodes of angina pectoris can be treated with sublingual nitroglycerin, which should be taken in the sitting position to avoid severe orthostatic hypotension. Chronic stable angina is treated with nitrates and beta-adrenergic antagonists. These agents have different mechanisms of action and thus may be used in combination with some benefit. Calcium channel blockers may also be of benefit, but may be limited by orthostatic hypotension.

About 20 percent of patients admitted to a coronary care unit with myocardial infarction are over the age of 70. In this age group, incidence of males and females is about equal. The elderly patient with myocardial infarction may present with symptoms other than chest pain (Table 9-12). Mortality rate from acute myocardial infarction increases with age.

Treatment of the elderly patient with acute myocardial infarction is similar to that of the young patient, with particular attention to avoiding drug toxicity and to beginning early mobilization when possible. Early mobilization may decrease deconditioning, orthostatic hypotension, and thrombophlebitis.

Table 9-12   Presenting Symptoms of Myocardial Infarction

Chest pain
Syncope
Confusion
Dyspnea
Worsening congestive heart failure
Rapid deterioration of health

Indications for coronary artery surgery are controversial, but this surgery can be performed with excellent symptomatic results. Morbidity and mortality, however, are higher than in younger patients. The strongest indication for surgery is angina pectoris refractory to medical management. In patients with left main coronary artery disease, surgery significantly improves survival over medical therapy. Patients with three-vessel disease may also have improved survival. In the elderly, however, improved survival must be considered in the light of the patient's projected survival and the higher operative risk.

VALVULAR HEART DISEASE

Calcific Aortic Stenosis

Pathologically, degenerative calcification of the aortic and mitral valves is common among the elderly; it is found at autopsy in about one-third of individuals over age 75. In most cases, aortic valve calcification is of no clinical significance except as a source of aortic systolic murmur. In some patients, however, calcification is extensive enough to result in aortic stenosis. The frequency of aortic stenosis increases with age, occurring in about 4 to 6 percent of those over age 65 at autopsy. Isolated aortic stenosis is more common among men than women (except over the age of 80, where women predominate). Aortic insufficiency may coexist with calcific aortic stenosis, although regurgitation is usually mild and a regurgitant murmur usually not heard.

The usual clinical presentation of aortic stenosis in the elderly consists of fatigue, syncope, angina pectoris, and congestive heart failure. Because systolic murmurs are a frequent finding in the elderly, differentiation of mitral regurgitation, aortic sclerosis, or aortic stenosis by auscultation is a challenge. The location of the murmur is usually along the lower left sternal border and apex and often does not radiate to the axilla or carotids. It is characteristically a crescendo-decrescendo systolic murmur ending before the second heart sound. Aspects that may help differentiate mitral regurgitation from aortic murmurs are described in Table 9-13.

Differentiation of aortic stenosis from aortic sclerosis may be difficult in the elderly. The typical murmur and pulse of aortic stenosis may be modified in the elderly. Systemic hypertension may shorten the systolic murmur of stenosis, giving it the characteristic of an aortic sclerosis murmur. Loss of vascular elasticity may modify the pulse pressure so that the typical pulse contour of aortic stenosis is absent. Therefore, the physical examination alone is not reliable in diagnosing aortic stenosis in the elderly. Echocardiography may not differentiate aortic stenosis from a nonstenotic calcified valve, and the presence of left ventricular hypertrophy may also not assist in the diagnosis because this may be caused by systemic hypertension. The addition of Doppler flow studies to echocardiography has improved the diagnostic accuracy of noninvasive procedures for aortic stenosis. Left ventricular catheterization remains the most reliable method of assessing aortic stenosis in the elderly, but should be reserved for patients who are symptomatic.

Surgical mortality for valve replacement is higher in elderly individuals, but results have recently improved. Significant coexistent

Table 9-13   Differentiation of Systolic Murmurs

	Post PVC*	Amyl nitrate	Valsalva	Squatting
Aortic sclerosis	↑†	↑	↓	↑
Aortic stenosis	↑	↑↑	↓	↑
Mitral regurgitation	—	↓	↑↑	—
IHSS	↑	↑↑	↑↑	↓↓

*Beat following a premature ventricular contraction.
†Effect of maneuver on intensity of murmur.
Note: PVC = premature ventricular contraction.

coronary artery disease should be treated with bypass surgery at the time of valve replacement. Choice of a valve depends on the size of the patient's aortic valve annulus and ability to tolerate anticoagulation. When anticoagulation is contraindicated, a biological prosthetic valve is preferred. The shorter life span of biological valves should be borne in mind in those between 60 and 70.

Recently several studies have described the benefit of percutaneous transluminal valvuloplasty for elderly patients with aortic stenosis who are high-risk surgical candidates or who refuse surgery (Cribier et al., 1987). Most patients have undergone successful procedures with improvement in symptoms and function and a low mortality rate. The use of this procedure in low-risk surgery patients has yet to be assessed.

Calcified Mitral Annulus

Mitral ring calcification is a disease of the elderly and is most frequently found in patients over 70. It is reported in 9 percent of autopsies in individuals over age 50 and has a striking increase with advancing age, particularly in women, in whom it rises from 3.2 percent below age 70 to 44 percent over age 90.

This lesion often results in mitral insufficiency or conduction abnormalities, and rarely in stenosis. It is an important contributing factor to congestive heart failure in the elderly and is a site for endocarditis. As many as two-thirds of patients with mitral annulus calcification present with an apical systolic murmur of mitral regurgitation. Echocardiography is the best technique for diagnosing mitral annulus calcification. Regurgitation is usually mild to moderate, and surgery is usually indicated only if endocarditis is superimposed. Subacute bacterial endocarditis prophylaxis is recommended. There is a higher incidence of cerebral embolism in this disorder, and thus anticoagulation may be indicated.

Mitral Valve Prolapse

Mucoid degeneration affects mainly the mitral valve. This process allows stretching of the mitral valve leaflet under normal intracardiac pressure, with subsequent prolapse into the left atrium during systole. Although the classic murmur is late systolic, the murmur can occur any time in systole. Mucoid degeneration of the mitral valve has been described in about 1 percent of autopsies on patients over 65. It is associated with mitral insufficiency; left atrial dilatation and regurgitant murmurs are common. Mitral insufficiency caused by this disorder is usually well tolerated and rarely requires surgery. Some patients with this syndrome have abnormal electrocardiograms and chest pain suggestive of coronary artery disease; sudden death has been reported. Death directly from the valve disease is usually related to rupture of the chordae tendineae. Mucoid degeneration also predisposes to infective endocarditis. Subacute bacterial endocarditis prophylaxis is indicated.

Idiopathic Hypertrophic Subaortic Stenosis (IHSS)

In the elderly, IHSS may be misdiagnosed as aortic valve stenosis or mitral regurgitation. Presenting symptoms are similar to those of aortic stenosis or coronary artery disease. The presence of a bisferious arterial pulse in the presence of a systolic ejection murmur and in the absence of an aortic regurgitation murmur should suggest IHSS. The IHSS murmur usually does not radiate to the carotids. Squatting, which increases left ventricular filling, usually decreases the murmur of IHSS. Factors that decrease left ventricular volume (Valsalva maneuver, standing) increase the intensity of the murmur.

Documentation of IHSS is accomplished by echocardiography. Therapy usually relies on beta-adrenergic antagonists. Symptoms may be worsened by cardiac glycosides (which increase myocardial contractility) and diuretics (which create volume depletion). Atrial fibrillation is poorly tolerated and may require cardioversion in the rapidly deteriorating patient. In patients refractory to medical therapy, surgery should be considered after cardiac catheterization to assess severity of outflow obstruction and state of coronary artery flow.

ARRHYTHMIAS

Although the prevalence of arrhythmias increases with age, most elderly patients without clinical heart disease are in normal sinus rhythm. Atrial fibrillation occurs in 5 to 10 percent of asymptomatic ambulatory elderly and more frequently in hospitalized patients. It is usually associated with underlying heart disease; the causes are the same as in younger individuals. Atrial fibrillation does, however, occur more frequently in elderly patients with thyrotoxicosis. Treatment, if indicated to control ventricular response, relies on digoxin. The maintenance dose of digoxin is usually lower in the elderly because of decreased muscular mass and decreased renal clearance.

The incidence of premature ventricular contractions increases with age, and occurs in about 10 percent of electrocardiograms and 30 to 40 percent of Holter monitoring. The decision to treat with antiarrhythmic therapy is difficult except in the immediate post-myocardial infarction period, when it is recommended. Criteria for therapy are the same as in younger patients. The half-life of antiarrhythmic drugs is prolonged in the elderly. Therapy should be initiated at lower doses, and blood levels should be monitored (see Chapter 14).

The sick sinus syndrome is particularly common among elderly patients. Diagnosis is made by Holter monitor. Symptoms, usually related to decreased organ perfusion, are listed in Table 9-14. There is no satisfactory medical therapy. Symptomatic patients may require pacemakers, which do not seem to decrease mortality in this syndrome but can alleviate symptoms. A pacemaker may be indicated in patients with cardiac side effects from drugs used to control tachycardias in the bradycardia-tachycardia syndrome.

CONGESTIVE HEART FAILURE

Although congestive heart failure is prevalent in the elderly, it is often overdiagnosed. Pedal and pretibial edema are not sufficient to

Table 9-14   Manifestations of Sick Sinus Syndrome

Palpitations
Angina pectoris
Congestive heart failure
Dizziness
Syncope
Memory loss
Insomnia

warrant the diagnosis. Venous stasis may produce a similar picture. Care is needed to establish the presence of other signs (e.g., cardiac enlargement, S_3 heart sound, basilar rales, enlarged liver). Determination of ejection fraction by two-dimensional echocardiography may assist in diagnosis.

The use of digitalis preparations must be approached with corresponding caution. Patients once begun on digoxin tend to remain on it long after the indications have ceased. Subtle signs of toxicity may be missed as the drug accumulates in the presence of decreased renal function. Because of decreases in lean body mass and glomerular filtration rate, lower doses of digoxin are generally required in the elderly. Initial maintenance doses should be lower; blood levels should be monitored to avoid toxic levels. Because the therapeutic window is narrowed in the elderly, patients who have been on digoxin therapy for long periods of time after an acute episode of cardiac decompensation not related to arrhythmias should be considered for discontinuation of digoxin. Weight should be monitored closely so that digoxin can be reinstated before congestive symptoms occur. With such evaluation and monitoring, many elderly patients on chronic digoxin therapy for other than antiarrhythmic treatment may not require digoxin therapy. Patients with atrial fibrillation should be kept on digoxin.

ACE inhibitors which have been previously shown to be of benefit in severe congestive failure appear to also be effective in mild to moderate heart failure (The Captopril-Digoxin Multicenter Research Group, 1988). Nitrates also improve symptoms in patients with congestive failure; however, tolerance is a problem with continuous therapy (Abrams, 1988).

REFERENCES

Abrams J: A reappraisal of nitrate therapy. *JAMA* 259:396–401, 1988.

Amery A, Birkenhager W, Brixko P, et al: Mortality and morbidity results from the European Working Party on High Blood Pressure in the Elderly trial. *Lancet* 1:1349–1354, 1985.

Amery A, Birkenhager W, Brixko P, et al: Efficacy of antihypertensive drug treatment according to age, sex, blood pressure, and previous cardiovascular disease in patients over the age of 60. *Lancet* 2:589–592, 1986.

The Australian Therapeutic Trial in Mild Hypertension. *Lancet* 1:1261–1267, 1980.

Barnett HJM: Thrombotic processes in cerebrovascular disease, in Coleman RW et al (eds): *Hemostasis and Thrombosis*. Toronto, Lippincott, 1982.

The Captopril-Digoxin Multicenter Research Group: Comparative effects of therapy with captopril and digoxin in patients with mild to moderate heart failure. *JAMA* 259:539–544, 1988.

Cribier A, Savin T, Berland J, et al: Percutaneous transluminal balloon valvuloplasty of adult aortic stenosis: Report of 92 cases. *J Am Coll Cardiol* 9:381–386, 1987.

Hypertension Detection and Follow-Up Program Cooperative Group: Five-year findings of the hypertension detection and follow-up program. II: Mortality by race, sex, and age. *JAMA* 242:2572–2577, 1979.

1988 Joint National Committee: The 1988 report of the Joint National Committee on Detection, Evaluation, and Treatment of High Blood Pressure. *Arch Intern Med* 148:1023–1038, 1988.

Kannel WB: Some lessons in cardiovascular epidemiology from Framingham. *Am J Cardiol* 37:269–282, 1976.

Morledge JH, Ettinger B, Aranda J, et al: Isolated systolic hypertension in the elderly. A placebo-controlled, dose-response evaluation of chlorthalidone. *J Am Geriatr Soc* 34:199–206, 1986.

Rippe JM, Ward A, Porcari JP, et al: Walking for health and fitness. *JAMA* 259:2720–2724, 1988.

Robbins S: Stroke in the geriatric patient, in Reichel W (ed): *The Geriatric Patient*. New York, HP Publishing, 1978.

Vardan S, Dunsky MH, Hill NE, et al: Effect of one year of thiazide therapy on plasma volume, renin, aldosterone, lipids and urinary metanephrines in systolic hypertension. of elderly patients. *Am J Cardiol* 60:388–390, 1987a.

Vardan S, Mehrotra KG, Mookherjee S, et al: Efficacy and reduced metabolic side effects of a 15-mg chlorthalidone formulation in the treatment of mild hypertension. A multicenter study. *JAMA* 258:484–488, 1987b.

Veterans Administration Cooperative Study Group on Antihypertensive Agents: Effect of treatment on morbidity in hypertension. III: Influence of age, diastolic pressure, and prior cardiovascular disease. *Circulation* 45:991–1004, 1972.

SUGGESTED READINGS

Bloor CM: Valvular disease in the elderly. *J Am Geriatr Soc* 30:466–472, 1982.

Evans JG: "Stroke" predictors, in Sarner M (ed): *Advanced Medicine.* London, Pitman, 1982.

Feinberg LE: Hypertension in the aged, in Schrier RW (ed): *Clinical Internal Medicine in the Aged.* Philadelphia, Saunders, 1982.

Gersh BJ, Kronmal RA, Schaff et al: Comparison of coronary artery bypass surgery and medical therapy in patients 65 years of age or older. *N Engl J Med* 313:217–224, 1985.

Greenspan AM, Kay HR, Berger BC, et al: Incidence of unwarranted implantation of permanent cardiac pacemakers in a larger medical population. *N Engl J Med* 318:158–163, 1988.

Kannel WB: Hypertension and aging, in Finch CE, Schneider EL (eds): *Handbook of the Biology of Aging.* New York, Van Nostrand Reinhold, 1985.

Lakatta EG: Heart and circulation, in Finch CE, Schneider EL (eds): *Handbook of the Biology of Aging.* New York, Van Nostrand Reinhold, 1985.

Lakatta EG, Yin FCP: Myocardial aging: Functional alterations and related cellular mechanisms. *Am J Physiol* 242:H927–H941, 1982.

Lindenfeld J, Groves, BM: Cardiovascular function and disease in the aged, in Schrier RW (ed): *Clinical Internal Medicine in the Aged.* Philadelphia, Saunders, 1982.

Selzer A: Changing aspects of the natural history of valvular aortic stenosis. *N Engl J Med* 317:91–98, 1987.

Stults BM: Digoxin use in the elderly. *J Am Geriatr Soc* 30:158–164, 1982.

Tuck M, Sowers I: Hypertension and aging, in Korenman SG (ed): *Endocrine Aspects of Aging.* New York, Elsevier Biomedical, 1982.

Vallacino R, Sherman FT: Stroke, fractured hip, amputation, pressure sores, and incontinence: Principles of rehabilitation treatment, in Libow LS, Sherman FT (eds): *The Core of Geriatric Medicine.* St Louis, Mosby, 1981.

Winslow CM, Solomon DH, Chassin MR, et al: The appropriateness of carotid endarterectomy. *N Engl J Med* 318:721–727, 1988.

Chapter 10

Decreased Vitality

Among the elderly, decreased vitality is a common complaint; it has a host of underlying causes. This chapter will deal with metabolic factors that may lead to decreased energy in the elderly: endocrine disease, anemia, and nutrition.

ENDOCRINE DISEASE

Carbohydrate Metabolism

Of the elderly population, 50 percent have glucose intolerance with normal fasting blood sugar levels. This abnormality can be demonstrated by oral, intravenous, tolbutamide, or glucocorticoid primed glucose tolerance tests. Although diet, obesity, and lack of exercise may account for some of these findings (Hollenbeck et al., 1984), aging itself is associated with deteriorating glucose tolerance. Most data now suggest a change in peripheral glucose utilization as the major factor in this phenomenon (Fink et al., 1984), although abnormal insulin secretion may also be a contributing factor.

Glucose intolerance, however, should not be diagnosed as diabetes mellitus. The diagnosis of diabetes should be made on the basis of a fasting plasma glucose of 140 mg/dl or greater. This is particularly important in the elderly because the prevalence of glucose intolerance is so high. It follows, therefore, that, for elderly patients, glucose tolerance testing is not indicated in the diagnosis of diabetes mellitus; the fasting plasma glucose is the diagnostic criterion.

The therapeutic goal for most elderly diabetics is the same as that in younger patients: normal fasting plasma glucose without hypoglycemia. However, in those with short life expectancies, the therapeutic goal may be modified to eliminate symptoms associated with hyperglycemia. This can be accomplished by lowering the blood sugar to levels that avoid glycosuria. The use of oral hypoglycemic agents has remained controversial and has become an individual physician-patient choice. These agents are usually effective in lowering fasting blood sugar to 140 mg/dl or below only in patients with pre-therapeutic fasting blood sugars below 200 to 250 mg/dl. In elderly patients with visual problems, arthritis, or memory deficits, where insulin administration by injection may be complicated, oral agents may be the therapy of choice.

Chlorpropamide, however, is not the drug of choice in the elderly because of the known side effect of inappropriate antidiuretic hormone syndrome and associated hyponatremia as well as its prolonged time of action. Shorter-acting agents, such as acetohexamide, tolazamide, glyburide, or glipizide are more appropriate agents for the elderly patient. They can be administered once a day and do not produce the inappropriate antidiuretic hormone syndrome. Although tolbutamide, also, does not produce this syndrome, it is short-acting and requires multiple daily doses, thereby increasing problems in compliance.

Close control of plasma glucose is now in vogue, although its efficacy or feasibility has not been assessed in the aged. Because atherosclerosis is the major complication of diabetes in this age group and because close control has not been shown to affect this complication, the risk of hypoglycemia with close control must be weighed carefully in designing a treatment plan. Counterregulatory hormones, especially catecholamines and glucagon, are important reactants to hypoglycemia, and catecholamine responsiveness is diminished in the elderly. It is important to observe patients closely for hypoglycemic reactions, and their ability to respond to this stress as a management regimen is prescribed.

Because most adult-onset diabetics are obese, weight reduction should be attempted, although only about 10 percent will maintain a prolonged weight loss. Dietary fats should be reduced. Other atherosclerotic risk factors such as smoking and hypertension should be eliminated or treated.

The elderly have an increased incidence of hyperosmolar nonketotic (HNK) coma. Characteristic symptoms and signs help the physician distinguish this syndrome from diabetic ketoacidotic (DKA) coma. Table 10-1 contrasts HNK and DKA. Whereas DKA frequently develops over hours, HNK typically develops over days to weeks. Focal or generalized seizures are common in HNK and unusual in uncomplicated DKA. The fluid deficit is greater in HNK, thus leading to a higher serum sodium and more marked rise in blood urea nitrogen. Therapy in HNK must, therefore, address the volume and hyperosmolar state of the patient. Because these patients may be quite sensitive to insulin, lowering of glucose should be done cautiously. Volume replacement should be initiated with normal saline. This therapy alone may reduce blood glucose levels. If after 1 h of volume repletion blood glucose levels are not reduced, a bolus of 20 units of regular insulin should be administered intravenously. If glucose levels do not respond, an insulin drip may be started. Such an

Table 10-1   Hyperosmolar Nonketotic (HNK) Coma and Diabetic Ketoacidosis (DKA)

	HNK	DKA
Time of development	Days to weeks	Hours
Seizures	Common	Uncommon
Fluid deficit	Marked	Present
Serum sodium	↑↑	↑
Blood urea nitrogen	↑↑	↑

Note: Double arrow signifies a higher increase than for a single arrow. Correction factor for sodium: 100 mg per deciliter of glucose = 1.6 meq per liter of sodium.

approach should allow repletion of volume without lowering serum osmolarity too rapidly.

Thyroid

Although thyroid function is generally normal in aging, the physician should be aware of thyroid-function test norms for this age group (Table 10-2). The majority of data indicate that T_4 levels are normal while T_3 levels may be low in healthy elderly people. Some elderly have normal T_3 levels; it has been suggested that the low T_3 levels reported in several studies are caused by undiagnosed illness and the low-T_3 syndrome described below. Thyroid-stimulating hormone (TSH) levels are also normal while the TSH response to thyroid-releasing hormone (TRH) is decreased in males (Harman et al., 1984) and normal in females. Thus, the TRH test is less valuable in elderly males. Metabolic clearance of thyroid hormones is decreased in aging. With intact feedback loops, normal thyroid function is maintained despite this change. However, with exogenous replacement of thyroid hormone, such regulatory mechanisms are not maintained; thyroid replacement doses in the elderly should be lower to take into account the lower metabolic clearance (Rosenbaum and Barzel, 1982). Laboratory evaluation tests most useful in thyroid disease are summarized in Table 10-3.

Hypothyroidism Hypothyroidism is primarily a disease of those aged 50 to 70. Goiter is rarely seen with hypothyroidism in the elderly except when it is iodide-induced. Diagnosis is usually made by a low free T_4 index, which assesses total T_4 and thyroid-binding proteins, and an elevated TSH. Because T_4 levels may be depressed in

Table 10-2 Thyroid Function in the Normal Elderly

Normal	Decreased
T_4	TSH response to TRH in males
Free T_4	Thyroid hormone production rate
Free T_4 index	Metabolic clearance rate of thyroid hormone
T_3	
TSH	

Table 10-3   Laboratory Evaluation of Thyroid Disease in the Elderly

	Hypothyroidism	Hyperthyroidism
T_4	E	E
Free T_4 index	E	E
TSH	E	E
Free T_4	D	D
T_3	O	D
Radioactive iodine uptake	O	D
TRH test	D (females)	D (females)
	O (Males)	O (Males)
Reverse T_3	D	D
TSH stimulation	D	O
T_3 suppression	O	O

Note: E – test for initial evaluation; D – helpful in confirming diagnosis or in differentiation of difficult cases; O – not helpful in diagnosis or not indicated.

seriously ill patients, diagnosis of hypothyroidism should not be made on the basis of low T_4 levels alone. In seriously ill patients, a circulatory plasma factor interferes with T_4 and T_3 binding to thyroid hormone–binding proteins; this results in a low total T_4 level but maintenance of normal free T_4 and TSH. This factor also interferes with T_3 binding and resin uptake in vitro and thus leads to a low free T_4 index determination. Laboratory characteristics of the low-T_4 syndrome associated with nonthyroidal illness are listed in Table 10-4. Not all free T_4 methods distinguish the low-T_4 syndrome from hypothyroidism;

Table 10-4   Thyroid-Function Tests in Nonthyroidal Illness

	Low-T_4 Syndrome	Low-T_3 Syndrome
T_4	Decreased	Normal
T_4 index	Decreased	Normal
Free T_4	Normal or increased	Normal
T_3	Decreased	Decreased
Reverse T_3	Normal or increased	Normal or increased
TSH	Normal	Normal

physicians should be aware of the type of determination and interpretation used in their laboratory. The T_3 level may be in the normal range in hypothyroidism and thus is not a helpful test. The low T_3 level associated with a host of acute and chronic nonthyroidal illnesses also contributes to the poor specificity of this test in hypothyroidism. About 75 percent of circulating T_3 is derived from peripheral conversion from T_4. The enzymes that convert T_4 to T_3 or reverse T_3 are under metabolic control. During illness, more T_4 is converted to reverse T_3, leading to the characteristic laboratory findings of the low-T_3 syndrome.

The radioactive iodine uptake is also not helpful because normal values are so low that they overlap with hypothyroidism. The TRH stimulation test can be used in females, but decreased responsiveness to TRH in elderly males does not allow this test to distinguish the normal state from pathology states. In males, a TSH stimulation test may help confirm the presence of hypothyroidism.

Hypothyroidism may be accompanied by other laboratory abnormalities. Creatine phosphokinase (CPK) levels, including the MB fraction, may be elevated. A normocytic, normochromic anemia, which responds to thyroid hormone replacement, may be present. There is an increased incidence of pernicious anemia in hypothyroidism, but the microcytic anemia of iron deficiency remains the commonest anemia associated with hypothyroidism.

The symptoms and signs of hypothyroidism may be overlooked when such complaints as fatigue, memory loss, and decreased hearing are ascribed to aging without further investigation. The prevalence of undiagnosed hypothyroidism in healthy elderly people has varied from 0.5 to 2 percent in multiple studies; a general screening program is thus not cost-effective. The prevalence among the elderly who are ill, however, is sufficient to support screening for hypothyroidism in this population, who have already presented themselves for care.

Therapy for hypothyroidism should be started at 0.025 to 0.05 mg of sodium levothyroxine (Synthroid) per day and increased by the same dose at 1- to 3-week intervals. The decreased metabolic clearance rate of thyroid hormone in aging may lead to a lower maintenance dose of T_4. The physician should monitor heart rate response and symptoms of angina, and in the laboratory, the TSH level. When indicated for symptomatic cardiovascular disease, propranolol may be added to the T_4 regimen. In patients with coronary artery disease, therapy can be initiated with triiodothyronine 5 μg per day and increased by 5 μg at weekly intervals to a level of 25 μg per day when the patient is converted to T_4 therapy. Because T_3 has a shorter half-life than T_4, symptoms will remit more rapidly after discontinuance of therapy if the patient develops cardiovascular complications. Propranolol can also be added to the T_3 regimen.

Myxedema Coma Most patients with myxedema coma are over age 60 (Table 10-5). In about 50 percent of the cases the coma is induced in the hospital by treating hypothyroid patients with hypnotics. A neck scar, from previous thyroid surgery, is a clue to the cause of coma. Because patients with this disorder die of respiratory failure, hypercapnia requires prompt attention. These patients should be treated in an intensive care setting, with intubation and respiratory assistance instituted at the first sign of respiratory failure. The CSF protein level is often over 100 mg/dl and should not in itself be used as an indicator of other CNS pathology. Therapy includes a large initial dose (500 μg) of T_4 intravenously. Although studies have not been done to demonstrate the efficacy of glucocorticoids in this syndrome, it is generally recommended that these patients receive 200 mg of hydrocortisone per day in divided doses for the first 1 or 2 days. Patients with concomitant adrenal insufficiency will require continued steroid therapy.

Hyperthyroidism About 20 percent of hyperthyroid patients are elderly; 75 percent have classic signs and symptoms. Ophthalmopathy is infrequent. Although about one-third have no goiter, toxic

Table 10-5 Myxedema Coma

Usually over 60 years old
50 percent induced by hypnotics
Neck scar
Hypothermia
Delayed relaxation of tendon reflex
Respiratory failure and apnea

multinodular goiter is more frequent than in the young. Severe non-thyroidal disease may disguise thyrotoxicosis (apathetic hyperthyroidism). Congestive heart failure, stroke, and infection are common disorders associated with masked hyperthyroidism. There should be a high threshold of suspicion for hyperthyroidism in the elderly. Unexplained heart failure or tachyarrhythmia, recent onset of of a psychiatric disorder, or profound myopathy should raise questions about masked hyperthyroidism. The triad of weight loss, anorexia, and constipation, which may raise the possibility of neoplastic disease, occurs in 15 percent of elderly thyrotoxic patients. Diagnosis is made by T_4, T_3, and radioactive iodine uptake (Table 10-3). The new ultrasensitive TSH assays can differentiate hyperthyroidism from normal. In the absence of acute nonthyroidal disease, this test alone may confirm the clinical diagnosis of hyperthyroidism. In the presence of acute illness, concomitant determination of TSH and T_4 index may be more appropriate. A T_3 suppression test should not be done in the elderly because of the risk of angina or myocardial infarction.

Therapy is usually by radioactive iodine ablation. Often patients are first treated with antithyroid medications to control hyperthyroidism and deplete the thyroid gland of hormone prior to the radioactive iodine treatment. Surgery is reserved for patients with thyroid glands that are causing local obstructive symptoms.

Severe thyrotoxicosis is treated with antithyroid drugs (preferably propylthiouracil because it blocks conversion of T_4 to T_3) to inhibit new hormone synthesis, iodides to block thyroid hormone secretion, and propranolol to decrease the peripheral manifestations of thyroid hormone action. In the elderly with underlying cardiac disease, propranolol therapy may be a problem; thus the cardiovascular response must be closely monitored. In patients allergic to antithyroid medications or where beta blockers are contraindicated, calcium ipodate (Oragrafin), 3 g every 3 days, can be used because it inhibits peripheral conversion of T_4 to T_3.

Goiter and Thyroid Cancer   The prevalence of multinodular goiter increases with age. At autopsy, multinodular goiter is found in 70 percent of females over age 60.

In the evaluation of a thyroid nodule for possible malignancy, several tests are available to assist in the decision for surgery (Table

Table 10-6   Tests for Thyroid Nodule

Thyroid scan
Ultrasound
Needle aspiration
Soft tissue films for psammoma bodies of papillary carcinoma
Thyroid-function tests
Serum calcitonin for medullary carcinoma
Antithyroid antibodies for chronic thyroiditis

10-6). Hyperfunctioning nodules on scan are less likely to be malignant than normo- or hypofunctioning nodules and require therapy only on the basis of overall thyroid function. Fine-needle biopsy is the diagnostic procedure of choice. Cystic lesions should be aspirated. If cytology of the aspirate is not malignant, the nodule need not be resected unless it recurs or enlarges.

Soft tissue x-rays of the neck may assist in the diagnosis of papillary carcinoma of the thyroid if psammoma bodies are demonstrated. Elevated serum calcitonin levels may indicate medullary carcinoma of the thyroid. Anaplastic carcinoma of the thyroid, a rapidly progressive and fatal neoplasm, occurs mostly in females over age 60.

Hyperparathyroidism

One-third of patients with hyperparathyroidism are over age 60. Symptoms are the same in the elderly as in those younger, but may be overlooked. Bone demineralization, weakness, and joint complaints may be ascribed to aging when they may indicate parathyroid disease. In patients with mild elevation of calcium and no symptoms, the surgical risks must be carefully weighed.

Table 10-7 contrasts some of the basic patterns of the common laboratory tests in hyperparathyroidism with those of other metabolic bone diseases common in the elderly.

Vasopressin Secretion

Basal vasopressin levels are unaltered in normal elderly individuals. Infusion of hypertonic saline, however, leads to a greater increase in plasma vasopressin in elderly compared with younger persons (Helderman et al., 1978). In contrast to the response to the hyperosmolar

Table 10-7   Laboratory Findings in Metabolic Bone Disease

Disease	Ca	P	Alk	PTH
Hyperparathyroidism	High	Low/normal	High/normal	High
Osteomalacia	Low/normal	Low	High/normal	High
Hyperthyroidism	High	High	High/normal	Low
Osteoporosis	Normal	Normal	Normal	Normal/high
Paget's disease	Normal/high	Normal/high	High	Normal

Note: Ca = calcium; P = phosphorus; Alk = alkaline phosphatase; PTH = parathyroid hormone.

challenge, volume changes related to the assumption of upright posture are associated with less of a vasopressin response in elderly subjects when compared with the young (Rowe et al., 1982). Both these findings might be explained by impaired baroreceptor input to the supraoptic nucleus. Volume expansion decreases osmoreceptor sensitivity. Hypertonic saline infusion results in volume expansion and thus decreases osmoreceptor sensitivity. If baroreceptor input is impaired in the elderly, volume expansion would lead to a lesser dampening effect and thus the vasopressin response to hyperosmolar stimuli would be increased.

Hyponatremia is a serious and often overlooked problem of the elderly patient. This syndrome is often associated with one of three general causes: (1) decreased renal blood flow with a decreased ability to excrete a water load, (2) diuretic administration leading to water intoxication (this condition is rapidly corrected by discontinuing diuretics), and (3) excess vasopressin secretion. Although a host of pulmonary disorders (e.g., pneumonia, tuberculosis, tumor) and central nervous system disorders (e.g., stroke, meningitis, subdural hematoma) are associated with the inappropriate antidiuretic hormone syndrome in any age group, the elderly seem more prone to this complication. Certain drugs such as chlorpropamide and barbiturates may cause this syndrome more frequently in the elderly.

In addition to treatment directed at correcting the underlying cause, water restriction and hypertonic saline are indicated when the patient is symptomatic or the sodium level is below 120 meq per liter. Dimethylchlorotetracycline therapy may be needed in resistant patients with inappropriate antidiuretic hormone syndrome. This agent induces a partial nephrogenic diabetes insipidus and thus corrects the hyponatremia. Serum creatinine and blood urea nitrogen should be closely monitored.

Ectopic Hormonal Syndromes

Because the incidence of malignancy increases with age, ectopic hormone syndromes are seen more often in the elderly. The ectopic adrenocorticotropic hormone (ACTH) syndrome, seen with oat cell carcinoma of the lung, often presents with hypokalemia. The hyponatremia of the ectopic antidiuretic hormone syndrome is also associated with oat cell carcinoma of the lung. Ectopic parathyroid hormone (PTH) secretion and its associated hypercalcemia has been described with renal cell carcinoma and hepatomas. The hypercalcemia associated with squamous cell carcinoma of the lung appears not to be an ectopic PTH syndrome but a hypercalcemia of another etiology.

Iatrogenic Endocrine Disease

Endocrine disease can also be induced iatrogenically. Two endocrine syndromes related to drug therapy in the elderly are hyperglycemia induced by diuretics (thiazides, furosemide) and hyponatremia induced by chlorpropamide.

ANEMIA

Anemia is common in the elderly, but should not be attributed simply to old age. Increased weakness, fatigue, and a mild anemia should not be dismissed as a manifestation of aging. In healthy elderly individuals, there is generally no change in normal levels of hemoglobin from younger adult values.

Table 10-8   Signs and Symptoms of Anemia

Weakness	Ischemic chest pain
Postural hypotension	Congestive heart failure
Syncope	Exertional dyspnea
Falls	Pallor
Confusion	Tachycardia
Worsened dementia	

Signs and symptoms of anemia may be subtle. Some of these manifestations are listed in Table 10-8. Anemia should be considered in these circumstances. If anemia is present, a diagnostic evaluation is indicated to define the cause. The appearance of the peripheral blood smear along with the history and physical examination should direct the diagnostic evaluation as described below.

Iron Deficiency

Iron deficiency is the most common cause of anemia in the elderly. Laboratory findings include hypochromia, microcytosis, low reticulocyte count, decreased serum iron, increased total iron-binding capacity (TIBC), low transferrin saturation, and absent bone marrow iron stores. A low serum iron and elevated TIBC indicate iron deficiency even in the absence of changes in red cell morphology. Because transferrin is reduced in many diseases, the TIBC may be normal or low in elderly patients with iron deficiency. However, a transferrin saturation of <10 percent would suggest iron deficiency, even in the presence of a low TIBC. A low serum ferritin level is valuable in confirming the diagnosis because serum ferritin levels are below 12 μg per liter in iron-deficiency anemia. Because inflammatory disease can elevate ferritin levels and liver disease can influence ferritin levels in either direction, the diagnosis of iron deficiency on the basis of a ferritin level must be made with a knowledge of the clinical situation.

Once iron deficiency is identified, it should be treated, and the cause of the anemia must be identified and corrected. Poor dietary intake of iron may contribute to iron deficiency in the elderly. A dietary evaluation is important, both for foods that contain iron and for substances such as tea, which inhibit iron absorption. However, even in the presence of poor nutrition, evaluation for a bleeding lesion must be completed.

The stool should be examined for occult blood. Evaluation for a gastrointestinal lesion should be carried out in a patient with unexplained iron deficiency, even if the stool is negative for occult blood. Although gastrointestinal bleeding may be caused by drugs (especially certain analgesics, steroids, and alcohol), a gastrointestinal lesion must be excluded. Diverticulosis is a common cause of bleeding. Vascular ectasia of the cecum and ascending colon is increasingly a recognized cause of bleeding in the elderly.

Replacement of iron should usually be by daily oral administration. The hemoglobin should improve in 10 days and be normal in about 6 weeks. Normal bone marrow iron stores should occur in an additional 4 months. If the anemia does not improve, one should consider noncompliance, continued bleeding, or an incorrect diagnosis. In unreliable patients or when oral iron is not tolerated, parenteral iron replacement with iron dextran is indicated. Tolerance should be monitored with a test dose, and the patient should be closely observed for an acute reaction. Parenteral iron should not be used routinely, but it is an important therapeutic modality in the appropriate patient.

Chronic Disease

The anemia of chronic disease may display many similarities with iron deficiency. In the elderly, this anemia is frequently associated with chronic inflammatory diseases or neoplasia. There is a defect in bone marrow red cell production and a shortening of erythrocyte life span. The finding of hypochromia, low reticulocyte count, and low serum iron may lead to confusion with iron deficiency. When a high TIBC does not confirm the presence of iron deficiency, a ferritin level can differentiate the two anemias. It is low in iron deficiency and high-normal or elevated in the anemia of chronic disease. Treatment is addressed to the underlying chronic illness because there is no specific therapy for this type of anemia.

Sideroblastic Anemia

Sideroblastic anemia should be considered in an elderly patient with hypochromic anemia who does not have iron deficiency or a chronic disease. Serum iron and transferrin saturation are increased. Hence, synthesis is defective, leading to increased iron stores and the diagnostic finding of ringed sideroblasts in the marrow.

In the elderly, sideroblastic anemia is commonly of the acquired type. The idiopathic group is usually refractory; only a few patients have a partial response to pyridoxine, but all should have a trial of pyridoxine. Although the prognosis is fairly good, about 10 percent of patients develop acute myeloblastic leukemia. Secondary sideroblastic anemia may be associated with underlying diseases such as malignancies and chronic inflammatory diseases. Certain drugs and toxins

Table 10-9   Differential Tests in Hypochromic Anemia

Item	Iron deficiency	Chronic disease	Sideroblastic anemia
Serum iron	Low	Low	High
Total iron-binding capacity	Usually increased*	Low	Normal
Transferrin saturation	Low	Low	High
Ferritin	Low	High	Normal
Bone marrow iron	Absent	Adequate	Increased ringed sideroblasts

*May be normal or even low in the elderly.

can induce sideroblastic anemia (e.g., ethanol, lead, isoniazid, chloramphenicol). The drug-induced syndromes are corrected by administering pyridoxine. Tests that will assist in the differential diagnosis of hypochromic anemias are listed in Table 10-9.

Vitamin B_{12} and Folate Deficiency

Both vitamin B_{12} and folate deficiency may occur on a nutritional basis, although folate deficiency is the more common. Elderly people who live alone or are alcoholics are most likely to have poor nutrition. Poor dietary intake of fresh fruits and vegetables may lead to folate deficiency; lack of meat, poultry, fish, eggs, and dairy products may lead to vitamin B_{12} deficiency. Vitamin B_{12} deficiency also occurs with the loss of intrinsic factor (pernicious anemia) and in gastrointestinal disorders associated with malabsorption of vitamin B_{12}.

The laboratory findings are similar in the two deficiencies, and include macrocytosis, hyperchromasia, hypersegmented neutrophils, and megaloblasts in the marrow. Leukopenia and thrombocytopenia may be present, and serum lactic dehydrogenase (LDH) and bilirubin may be increased. The two are differentiated by measuring serum vitamin B_{12} and folate levels. A Schilling test will help confirm the lack of intrinsic factor when that is the cause.

Treatment is with vitamin B_{12} or folic acid, as appropriate. However, because folate will correct the hematologic disorder but not the neurological abnormalities of vitamin B_{12} deficiency, a correct diagnosis is essential before treatment.

NUTRITION

Recently there has been emphasis on perinatal nutrition; in the past, nutrition during growth has been extensively examined, but little has been done in nutrition of adulthood and senescence. A discussion of nutrition and aging is therefore limited by the lack of adequate studies, defined methods, and standards. Although it is generally accepted that intake moderately above recommended allowances is optimal, animal studies demonstrate increased longevity with lower than recommended levels. In establishing nutritional requirements in humans, we must contend with the multiple factors that confound interpretation of available data, e.g., genetic factors, social environment, economic status, selection of food, and weak methods of assessing nutritional status.

Several national surveys have been performed to assess nutrition

Table 10-10 National Surveys of Nutrition in the Elderly

U.S. Department of Agriculture (1972):
  Nutritional intake for men over age 55 was adequate, except for calcium
  Thiamine, riboflavin, and calcium intake was inadequate for women
  Dietary adequacy declined with income
Ten-State Nutrition Survey (1972):
  Groups considered at risk (poor, migrant workers, inner-city groups) were
    studied
  Those over age 60 did not meet standard food consumption; limiting nutrients
    were protein, iron, and vitamin A
  After age 50, skeletal weight decreased with age
  Obesity more prevalent in those with higher income
  Females aged 45–55 had 40–50% prevalence of obesity, decreased to 20
    to 25% in 75–85 age group
  There was no severe malnutrition
Health and Nutrition Examination Survey (1974):
  In those over age 60, above poverty line, 16–18% had intake of less than
    1000 cal per day; below poverty line, 27–36%
  Protein intake was also related to income
  Intake for calcium and vitamins A and C was low

in the elderly (Table 10-10). Taken as a whole, these surveys do not indicate poor nutritional status or marked deficiency among the elderly in the United States and suggest that intake relates more to health and poverty than to age. However, obesity is a significant problem. In a study of 500 elderly individuals admitted to a hospital with long-term illness, 35 percent were found to have significant primary nutritional problems, 15 percent were undernourished, and 20 percent were obese. Of 107 elderly patients admitted to a county hospital, 5 to 10 percent were found to have low vitamin A and vitamin C levels. Of 234 ambulant, well subjects, 5 percent of males and 13 percent of females had a low hematocrit, 8 percent had low vitamin C levels, and 18 to 21 percent had a low thiamine level (6 percent by transketolase assay). Again, these data suggest a low prevalence of nutritional deficiency in the elderly and provide no basis for recommending massive vitamin replacement.

Vitamins, Protein, and Calcium

Table 10-11 summarizes nutritional requirements in the elderly and demonstrates that there is no general increase in vitamin requirements with age. Studies on vitamin metabolism and requirements reveal no correlation between age and vitamin A, B_1, B_2, or C requirement. Vitamin B_6 and vitamin B_{12} requirements also do not increase with age.

Studies on protein requirements are not in agreement. Based on

Table 10-11   Nutritional Requirements in the Elderly

Vitamins	Unchanged in the elderly
Protein	0.5 to >1.0 g/kg/day
Amino acids	Unchanged to increased
Calcium	850–1020 mg/day
Calories	Declines by 12.4 cal/day per year (maturity to senescence)

nitrogen balance studies, estimates of protein requirement varied from 0.5 to more than 1.0 g/kg daily. Data on amino acid requirements are also conflicting: some data show increased requirements with age, and other data show no change.

For calcium, estimated requirements vary from 850 to 1020 mg per day. All these studies exceed the required dietary allowance for calcium of 800 mg per day. Data on the correlation of calcium intake and osteoporosis are conflicting. Although calcium supplementation alone does not seem to reverse postmenopausal osteoporosis, it is an important adjunct to estrogen replacement therapy. It may be necessary to use a calcium supplement to ensure adequate intake.

Nutritional Deficiency and Physiological Impairments

There is little evidence to correlate age-associated nutritional deficiency with clinical findings. In a study on the consequences of vitamin A levels, there was no significant correlation with dark adaptation, epithelial cells excreted, or percent keratinization. In other studies, there was no correlation between vitamin C levels and gingivitis or vitamin B_{12} and lactic acid, lactic dehydrogenase, or hematocrit. Elderly people with limited sun exposure may be at risk of vitamin D deficiency.

The highest prevalence of osteoporosis is among postmenopausal women. In a study using radiographs of the dorsal and lumbar spine, osteoporosis was present in 50 percent of women aged 65 to 70 and increased to 90 percent in women over age 90. In males, the numbers were 15 and 30 percent in the same age groups. Data are conflicting on correlation of dietary calcium intake and osteoporosis. Problems in assessing this correlation include reduced calcium intake in the elderly, altered calcium and phosphorus ratio, decreased protein intake, and acid-base balance.

Reversal of Deficiency by Supplementation

There is no impairment of vitamin or protein absorption in the elderly. Data have demonstrated conclusively that low vitamin levels in the elderly can be reversed by administration of oral supplementation. Because these deficiencies can be corrected by dietary supplementation, they are most likely related to decreased intake.

Caloric Needs

A study of 250 individuals aged 23 to 99 demonstrated an age-associated decline in total caloric intake at the rate of 12.4 cal per day for a year. A yearly decline in basal metabolic rate accounted for 5.23 cal per day, while 7.6 cal per day related to reduction in other requirements, including physical exercise.

Dietary Restriction and Food Additives

Rats, mice, *Drosophila,* and other lower organisms have demonstrated that nutritional deprivation delays maturation and increases life span. The mechanism, however, is not understood. Animals fed isocaloric diets but decreased protein have increased life span. Based on the free radical theory of aging, it has been proposed that reducing agents would prolong life. Although the data are conflicting, some studies have supported this hypothesis.

In certain animal models, caloric restriction has also been shown to decrease incidence and delay onset of disease, including chronic glomerulonephritis, muscular dystrophy, and carcinogenesis. In humans, however, body weight below ideal is not associated with increased life span (discussed below). In animal experiments, nutrition is maintained during caloric variation. This may not be true in humans, and thus may lead to the differing results.

NUTRITIONAL ASSESSMENT

Because people age at different rates, there is a need for age- and sex-specific normative data as indicators of nutritional status. Unfortunately, adequate data are not available. Such data need also to distinguish among community-dwelling, institutionalized, and hospitalized elderly.

Certain parameters are, however, used in assessing nutritional status in the elderly. Some anthropometric variables are probably effective estimators of major aspects of body composition (Table 10-12). They cannot provide a complete description of the nutritional status of an individual and are not highly correlated with biochemical or hematologic indicators of nutritional status.

Although weight is a global measure, it can be obtained easily from adults and is useful in the absence of edema. Weight/stature

Table 10-12 Assessment of Body Composition

Assessment	Component
Weight	Global
Weight / stature	Total fat
Skin fold	Percent fat
Upper arm circumference	Lean body mass

ratio is best correlated with total body fat. Triceps and subscapular skin folds are highly correlated with the percentage of body fat in the elderly. Upper arm circumference is correlated with lean body mass and may be particularly helpful in edematous patients in whom weight is misleading. The effect of the aging process on lean body mass is so great that it remains a poor reflection of nutritional status in the elderly.

Serum albumin is a practical indicator of malnutrition in the elderly. However, liver disease, proteinuria, and protein-losing enteropathies must be excluded. A low serum albumin may be indicative of malnutrition, but a normal or increased serum albumin concentration does not necessarily indicate normality. Thyroxine-binding prealbumin and/or retinol-binding protein are more sensitive indices than are albumin and transferrin. However, the effect of age on these proteins has not been defined.

In animals, dietary deprivation of protein results in anemia. Because anemia is one of the earliest manifestations of protein-calorie malnutrition, its presence should alert the physician to the possibility of malnutrition. Total lymphocyte count may be a very good marker for nutritional problems. An initial evaluation of the immune system may be obtained with a skin test. *Candida* antigen can be uti-

Table 10-13 Critical Questions in Assessing a Patient for Malnutrition

Is there any reason to suspect malnutrition?
If so, of which nutrient(s) and to what extent?
What are the pathophysiological mechanisms (e.g., alteration in nutrient intake, digestion and absorption, metabolism, excretion, or requirements)?
What etiology underlies the pathophysiological mechanism(s)?

Table 10-14   Factors That Place the Elderly at Risk for Malnutrition

Drugs (e.g., reserpine, digoxin, antitumor agents)
Chronic disease (e.g., congestive heart failure, renal insufficiency, chronic
  gastrointestinal disease)
Depression
Dental and periodontal disease
Decreased taste and smell
Low socioeconomic level
Physical weakness
Isolation
Food fads

lized because virtually all people over age 11 have a delayed-type sensitivity.

Although there are presently no clear-cut criteria for the diagnosis of malnutrition in the elderly, some important factors need to be considered in evaluating a given patient, as shown in Table 10-13. Table 10-14 presents some factors that put elderly patients at risk for malnutrition. Individuals with such problems should be considered for evaluation of nutritional status.

Special Considerations

As will be discussed in Chapter 11, sensory loss, especially in taste and smell, may lead to decreased appetite in the elderly and thus predispose to malnutrition. Dentures may cover the roof of the mouth and secondary taste areas, adding to the sensory loss. Poor dentition may also put the patient at risk for malnutrition because the patient will select soft foods often high in sugars or carbohydrates and low in nutrients. Good dental care and especially prevention are thus important factors in nutrition of the elderly patient.

Although the influence of dietary fiber on colonic carcinoma and diverticular disease is controversial, the use of dietary fiber to maintain bowel regularity has significant support, especially in the elderly, where constipation may present a difficult clinical problem. When dietary intake of fiber is low, bran can be used as a supplement, particularly in cereals, breads, or as bran powder. Intake of bran can be adjusted to maintain normal bowel movements.

Although the food industry is slowly responding, most canned foods still contain large amounts of added sodium and sugar. Because some of these are less expensive than fresh or frozen foods, the elderly with limited incomes may use such prepared foods exclusively. When refined carbohydrates or sodium need to be restricted, these patients should be educated about the use of canned products.

Until recently, actuarial tables have been used to support the position that obesity is associated with excess mortality. Recent data from the Framingham Study (Andres, 1981), however, indicate that modest increases in adiposity may even prolong life. However, in the elderly, the Framingham Study demonstrated increasing mortality with increasing relative body weight above ideal weight. Thus, minimally excessive weight may not be as beneficial to the elderly as it is in younger individuals.

INFECTIONS

Although it is proposed that alterations in host defense mechanisms predispose the elderly to certain infections, there is little evidence to support this hypothesis. It may well be that environmental factors, physiological changes in other than the immune system, and specific diseases are the major elements in the increased frequency of certain infections in the elderly (Table 10-15).

Because the elderly more often have acute and chronic illnesses requiring hospitalization and have longer hospital stays, they are at greater risk for nosocomial infections. Such hospitalization puts the elderly at greater risk for gram-negative and *Staphylococcus aureus* infections. Physiological alterations (Chapter 1), such as occur in the lungs, bladder function, and the skin, and glucose homeostasis may also predispose the elderly to infections.

The incidence of malignancies is increased in the elderly. Many of these neoplastic disorders, especially those of the hematologic system, are associated with a higher frequency of infection. Immunosuppression during therapy is also a predisposing factor. The prevalence of diabetes mellitus is higher in the elderly, thus predisposing them to more frequent urinary tract, soft tissue, and bone infections. Prostatic hypertrophy with obstruction predisposes the elderly male to urinary tract infections.

Table 10-15   Factors Predisposing to Infection in the Elderly

More frequent and longer hospital stays:
  Nosocomial infections
    Gram-negative bacilli
    Staphylococcus aureus
Physiological changes:
  Lung
  Bladder
  Skin
  Glucose homeostasis
Chronic disease:
  Malignancy
    Multiple myeloma and leukemia
    Immunosuppression from therapy
  Diabetes mellitus
    Urinary tract infection
    Soft tissue infections
    Osteomyelitis
  Prostatic hypertrophy
    Urinary tract infection
Host defenses:
  Phagocytosis unaltered
  Complement unaltered
  Cellular and humoral immunity diminished

Phagocytic function appears to be unaltered in aging, as is the complement system. Cell-mediated immunity and, to a lesser extent, humoral immunity, is diminished in aging. The role that these changes play in predisposing the elderly to infection has not been well defined.

With the predisposing factors described above, the spectrum of pathogens causing common infections in the elderly is often different than that in younger adults (Table 10-16). The frequency of gram-negative bacilli increases in each category.

Many infections occur more frequently in the elderly and are often associated with a higher morbidity and mortality (Yoshikawa and Norman, 1987). Atypical presentation of infection in some elderly patients may delay diagnosis and treatment. Underreporting of symptoms, impaired communication, coexisting diseases, and

Table 10-16   Pathogens of Common Infections in the Elderly

Infection	Common pathogens in adults	Common pathogens in the elderly
Pneumonia	S. pneumoniae Anaerobic bacteria	S. pneumoniae Anaerobic bacteria H. influenza Gram-negative bacilli
Urinary tract	E. coli	E. coli Proteus sp. Klebsiella sp. Enterobacter sp. Enterococcus
Meningitis	S. pneumoniae N. meningitidis	S. pneumoniae Listeria monocytogenes Gram-negative bacilli
Septic arthritis	N. gonorrheae S. aureus	S. aureus Gram-negative bacilli

altered physiological responses to infection may contribute to altered presentations.

As an example, failure of patients to seek medical evaluation is one factor in the higher morbidity and mortality of appendicitis in the elderly. Difficulties in communication may also alter presentation. Infections not directly involving the central nervous system may cause confusion in the elderly, particularly in individuals with preexisting dementia. The mechanism by which this occurs has not been defined. Acute unexplained functional deterioration should also alert the physician to a potential acute infectious process.

Existing chronic disease may mask an acute infection. Septic arthritis usually occurs in a previously abnormal joint. It may be difficult to clinically distinguish exacerbation of the underlying arthritis from acute infection. Therefore, the physician should not be hesitant to examine synovial fluid in elderly patients with acute exacerbation of joint disease.

Febrile response may be blunted or absent in some elderly individuals with bacterial infections. This may obscure diagnosis and delay therapy. A poor febrile response may also be a negative prognostic factor. Conversely, a febrile response is more likely to indicate a bacterial rather than viral illness in elderly patients, particularly in the old-old.

Antibiotic therapy in the elderly, as in the young, is directed to the specific organism isolated. However, when empirical antimicrobial therapy is initiated, consideration should be given to including a third-generation cephalosporin and/or aminoglycoside because gram-negative infections are more common, regardless of the site. With all antibiotics, but particularly with the aminoglycosides, renal function must be considered and monitored for toxicity. Monitoring of drug blood level and renal function is mandatory with the aminoglycosides.

Although the incidence of tuberculosis is decreasing, it is decreasing more slowly in the elderly and represents a significant cause of pneumonia in the geriatric population. This cohort has lived through a period of higher incidence of tuberculosis, has probably not been treated with isonicotinic acid hydralazide (INH) prophylaxis, and may have predisposing factors (discussed above) such as physiological changes, malnutrition, and underlying disease that may lead to reactivation. Elderly patients are also at increased risk for primary infection. This is particularly the case for elderly patients in long-term-care institutions (Stead, 1981). Tuberculosis screening programs should be implemented in long-term-care facilities because of this increased risk and because of the potential to prevent active disease among patients whose skin test converts to a strongly positive reaction (Stead and To, 1987; Stead et al., 1987) (see Chapter 17). The American Thoracic Society now recommends preventive therapy for certain types of patients regardless of age, including insulin-dependent diabetic patients, those on steroids and other immunosuppressive treatment, patients with end-stage renal disease, and patients who have lost a large amount of weight rapidly (American Thoracic Society, 1986). A useful rule in geriatric care is to suspect tuberculosis when a patient is inexplicably failing.

Several studies have suggested an association of bacteriuria with increased mortality in the elderly (Dontas et al., 1981; Evans et al., 1982; Platt et al., 1982; Sourander and Kasanen, 1972). However, others have not confirmed this finding (Heinamaki et al., 1986; Nicolle et al., 1987a; Nordenstam et al., 1986). Most of these studies did not differentiate between the effect of bacteriuria and age and/or concomitant disease on mortality. When Nordenstam et al. adjusted for age, they concluded that fatal diseases associated with bacteriuria may account for the increase in mortality among elderly patients with bacteriuria.

Several previous studies in elderly hospitalized or institutionalized patients have not revealed antimicrobial therapy for bacteriuria to be effective because of the high rate of recurring infection (Alling et al., 1975; Brocklehurst et al., 1977; Nicolle et al., 1983; Nicolle et al., 1987b). One study in elderly ambulatory nonhospitalized women with asymptomatic bacteriuria demonstrated that short-course antimicrobial therapy is effective in eliminating bacteriuria in most of the women for at least a 6-month period (Boscia et al., 1987b). Survival was not an outcome measure. In fact, no study has assessed the impact of treatment of asymptomatic bacteriuria on survival.

Bacteriuria in elderly persons is common and usually asymptomatic. At present, in the absence of obstructive uropathy, no evidence exists to support the routine use of antimicrobial therapy for asymptomatic bacteriuria in elderly persons (Boscia et al., 1987a). Among bacteriuric patients with urinary incontinence and no other symptoms of urinary tract infection, the bacteriuria should be eradicated as part of the initial assessment of the incontinence (see Chapter 6).

ACKNOWLEDGMENT

The authors wish to thank Dr. T.T. Yoshikawa for his assistance in preparing material for the section on infections in this chapter.

REFERENCES

Alling B, Brandberg A, Seeberg S, et al: Effect of consecutive antibacterial therapy on bacteriuria in hospitalized geriatric patients. *Scand J Infect Dis* 7:201–207, 1975.

American Thoracic Society: Treatment of Tuberculosis and Tuberculosis Infection in Adults and Children. *Am Rev Respir Dis* 134:355–363, 1986.

Andres R: Aging, diabetes and obesity: Standards of normality. *Mt Sinai J Med* 48:489–495, 1981.

Boscia JA, Abrutyn E, Kaye D: Asymptomatic bacteriuria in elderly persons: Treat or do not treat? *Ann Intern Med* 106:764–766, 1987a.

Boscia JA, Kobasa WD, Knight RA, et al: Therapy vs no therapy for bacteriuria in elderly ambulatory nonhospitalized women. *JAMA* 257:1067–1071, 1987b.

Brocklehurst JC, Bee P, Jones D, et al: Bacteriuria in geriatric hospital patients, its correlates and management. *Age Ageing* 6:240–245, 1977.

Dontas AS, Kasviki-Charvati P, Papanayiotou PC, et al: Bacteriuria and survival in old age. *N Engl J Med* 304:939–943, 1981.

Evans DA, Kass EH, Hennekens CH, et al: Bacteriuria and subsequent mortality in women. *Lancet* 1:156–158, 1982.

Fink RI, Kolterman OG, Koa M, et al: The role of the glucose transport system in the post receptor defect in insulin action associated with human aging. *J Clin Endocrinol Metab* 58:721–725, 1984.

Harman SM, Wehmann RE, Blackman MR: Pituitary-thyroid hormone economy in healthy aging men: Basal indices of thyroid function and thyrotropin responses to constant infusions of thyrotropin releasing hormone. *J Clin Endocrinol Metab* 58:320–326, 1984.

Heinamaki P, Haavisto M, Hakulinen T, et al: Mortality in relation to urinary characteristics in the very aged. *Gerontology* 32:167–171, 1986.

Helderman JH, Vestal RE, Rowe JW, et al: The response of arginine vasopressin to intravenous ethanol and hypertonic saline in man: The impact of aging. *J Gerontol* 33:39–47, 1978.

Hollenbeck CB, Haskell W, Rosenthal M, et al: Effect of habitual physical activity on regulation of insulin-stimulated glucose disposal in older males. *J Am Geriatr Soc* 33:273–277, 1984.

Nicolle LE, Bjornson J, Harding GKM, et al: Bacteriuria in elderly institutionalized men. *N Engl J Med* 309:1420–1425, 1983.

Nicolle LE, Henderson E, Bjornson J, et al: The association of bacteriuria with resident characteristics and survival in elderly institutionalized men. *Ann Intern Med* 106:682–686, 1987a.

Nicolle LE, Mayhew WJ, Bryan L: Prospective randomized comparison of therapy and no therapy for asymptomatic bacteriuria in institutionalized elderly women. *Am J Med* 83:27–33, 1987b.

Nordenstam GR, Brandberg CA, Oden AS, et al: Bacteriuria and mortality in an elderly population. *N Engl J Med* 314:1152–1156, 1986.

Platt R, Polk BF, Murdock B, et al: Mortality associated with nosocomial urinary-tract infection. *N Engl J Med* 307:637–642, 1982.

Rosenbaum RL, Barzel US: Levothyroxine replacement dose for primary hypothyroidism decreases with age. *Ann Intern Med* 96:53–55, 1982.

Rowe JW, Minaker KC, Sparrow D, et al: Age-related failure of volume-pressure-mediated vasopressin release. *J Clin Endocrinol Metab* 56:661–664, 1982.

Sourander LB, Kasanen A: A 5-year follow-up of bacteriuria in the aged. *Gerontol Clin* 14:274–281, 1972.

Stead W: Tuberculosis among elderly persons: An outbreak in a nursing home. *Ann Intern Med* 94:606–610, 1981.

Stead WW, To T: The Significance of the Tuberculin Skin Test in Elderly Persons. *Ann Intern Med* 107:837–842, 1987.

U.S. Department of Agriculture: *Food and Nutrient Intake of Individuals in the United States*. USDA Household Food Consumption Survey, 1965–66. Consumer and Food Economics Research Division. Agricultural Research Service, Government Printing Office, 1972.

U.S. Department of Health, Education and Welfare: *Ten-State Nutrition Survey, 1968–70*. HSM 72-8133. Atlanta, Center for Disease Control, 1972.

U.S. Department of Health, Education and Welfare: *Preliminary Findings of the First Health and Nutrition Examination Survey, U.S. 1971–1972: Dietary Intake and Biochemical Findings*. HRA 74-1219. Government Printing Office, 1974.

Yoshikawa TT, Norman DC: *Aging and Clinical Practice: Infectious Diseases. Diagnosis and Management*. New York, Igaku-Shoin, 1987.

SUGGESTED READINGS

Crapo PA: Nutrition in the aged, in Schrier RW (ed): *Clinical Internal Medicine in the Aged*. Philadelphia, Saunders, 1982.

Davis PJ, Davis FB: Hyperthyroidism in patients over the age of 60 years. *Medicine* 53:161–181, 1974.

Eckel RH, Hofeldt FD: Endocrinology and metabolism in the elderly, in Schrier RW (ed): *Clinical Internal Medicine in the Aged*. Philadelphia, Saunders, 1982.

Elahi D, Muller DC, Tzarkoff SP et al: Effect of age and obesity on fasting levels of glucose, insulin, glucagon, and growth hormone. *J Gerontol* 37:385–391, 1982.

Foley CJ, Libow LS, Sherman FT: Clinical aspects of nutrition, in Libow LS, Sherman FT (eds): *The Core of Geriatric Medicine*. St Louis, Mosby, 1981.

Gambert SR: Effect of age on thyroid hormone physiology and function. *J Am Geriatr Soc* 33:360–365, 1985.

Gardner ID: The effect of aging on susceptibility to infection. *Rev Infect Dis* 2:801–810, 1980.

Greenblatt RB (ed): *Geriatric Endocrinology*. New York, Raven Press, 1978.

Gregerman RI, Bierman EL: Aging and hormones, in Williams RH (ed): *Textbook of Endocrinology*. Philadelphia, Saunders, 1981.

Grieco MH: Use of antibiotics in the elderly. *Bull NY Acad Med* 56:197–208, 1980.

Jackson RA, Blix PM, Matthews JA et al: Influence of aging on glucose homeostasis. *J Clin Endocrinol Metab* 55:840–848, 1982.

Korenman SG (ed): *Endocrine Aspects of Aging*. New York, Elsevier, 1982.

Lipschitz DA: An overview of anemia in older patients. *The Older Patient* 2:5–11, 1988.

Moolten SE: Nutrition in the elderly, in Somers AR, Fabian DR (eds): *The Geriatric Imperative: An Introduction to Gerontological and Clinical Geriatrics*. New York, Appleton-Century-Crofts, 1981.

Morley JE, Silver AJ, Fiatarone M, et al: Geriatric grand rounds: Nutrition and the elderly. *J Am Geriatr Soc* 34:823–832, 1986.

Phais JP, Kauffman CA, Bjornson A et al: Host defenses in the aged: Evaluation of components of the inflammatory and immune responses. *J Infect Dis* 138:67–73, 1978.

Reaven GM, Reaven EP: Age, glucose intolerance, and non-insulin-dependent diabetes mellitus. *J Am Geriatr Soc* 33:286–290, 1985.

Report of the Third Ross Roundtable on Medical Issues: *Assessing the Nutritional Status of the Elderly: State of the Art*. Columbus, OH, Ross Laboratories, 1982.

Rockstein M, Sussman ML (eds): *Nutrition, Longevity, and Aging*. New York, Academic Press, 1976.

Rosenthal MJ, Hartnell JM, Morley JE, et al: UCLA geriatric grand rounds: Diabetes in the elderly. *J Am Geriatr Soc* 35:435–447, 1987.

Sawin CT, Castelli WP, Hershman JM, et al: The aging thyroid. Thyroid deficiency in the Framingham Study. *Arch Intern Med* 145:1386–1388, 1985.

Stead WW, To T, Harrison RW, et al: Benefit-risk considerations in preventive treatment for tuberculosis in elderly persons. *Ann Intern Med* 107:843–845, 1987.

Thomas FB, Mazzaferi EL, Skillman TB: Apathetic thyrotoxicosis: A distinctive clinical and laboratory entity. *Ann Intern Med* 72:679–685, 1970.

Vogel JM: Hematologic problems of the aged. *Mt Sinai J Med* 47:150–165, 1980.

Walsh JR: Hematologic disorders in the elderly. *West J Med* 135:445–446, 1981.

Walsh JR, Cassel CK, Madler JJ: Iron deficiency in the elderly: It's often nondietary. *Geriatrics* 36:121–132, 1981.

Yoshikawa TT: Geriatric infectious diseases: An emerging problem. *J Am Geriatr Soc* 31:34–39, 1983.

Yoshikawa TT: Important infections in elderly persons. *West J Med* 135:441–445, 1981.

Chapter 11

Sensory Impairment

Because as many as 75 percent of the elderly have significant visual and auditory dysfunction not reported to their physicians, adequate screening for these problems is important. These disorders may limit functional activity and lead to social isolation and depression. Correction of remediable conditions may improve ability to perform daily activities.

VISION

Physiological and Functional Changes

The visual system undergoes many changes with age (Table 11-1). Decreases in visual acuity in old age may be caused by morphological changes in the choroid, pigment epithelium, and retina, or by decreased function of the rods, cones, and other neural elements. Elderly patients frequently have difficulties turning their eyes up-

Table 11-1   Physiological and Functional Changes of the Eye

Functional change	Physiological change
Visual acuity	Morphological change in choroid, pigment epithelium, or retina
	Decreased function of rods, cones, or other neural elements
Extraocular motion	Difficulty in gazing upward and maintaining convergence
Intraocular pressure	Increased pressure
Refractive power	Increased hyperopia and myopia
	Presbyopia
	Increased lens size
	Nuclear sclerosis (lens)
	Ciliary muscle atrophy
Tear secretion	Decreased tearing
	Decreased lacrimal gland function
	Decreased goblet cell secretion
Corneal function	Loss of endothelial integrity
	Posterior surface pigmentation

ward or sustaining convergence. Intraocular pressure slowly increases with age.

The refractive error may become either more hyperopic or more myopic. In the young, hyperopia may be overcome by the accommodative power of the ciliary muscle on the young lens. However, with age, this latent hyperopia becomes manifest because of loss of accommodative reserve.

Other elderly patients may show an increase in myopia with age, caused by changes within the lens. The crystalline lens increases in size with age as old lens fibers accumulate in the lens nucleus. The nucleus becomes more compact and harder (nuclear sclerosis), increasing the refractive power of the lens and worsening the myopia.

Another definitive refractive change of aging is the development of presbyopia from nuclear sclerosis of the lens and atrophy of the ciliary muscle. As a result, the closest distance at which one can see clearly slowly recedes with age. At approximately age 45, the near point of accommodation is so far that comfortable reading and near work become cumbersome and difficult. Corrective lenses are then needed to enable the patient to move that point closer to the eyes.

Diminished tear secretion in many older patients, especially postmenopausal women, may lead to dryness of the eyes, which can cause irritation and discomfort. This condition may endanger the intactness of the corneal surface. The treatment consists mainly in substitution therapy, with artificial tears instilled at frequent intervals.

The corneal endothelium often undergoes degenerative changes with aging. Because these cells seldom proliferate during adult life, the cell population is decreased. This may leave an irregular surface on the anterior chamber side, where pigments may accumulate. This type of endothelial dystrophy is frequently seen in older patients, and dense pigment accumulation may slightly decrease visual acuity. In some patients, the endothelial dystrophy will spontaneously progress and lead to corneal edema. Such cases require corneal transplants.

Blindness

The prevalence of visual problems and blindness increases with age (Figure 11-1). The most common causes of blindness are cataracts, glaucoma, macular degeneration, and diabetic retinopathy. Screening for these disorders should include testing visual acuity, performing an ophthalmoscopic evaluation, and checking intraocular pressure (Table 11-2).

Senile Cataract   Opacification of the crystalline lens is a frequent complication of aging. In the Framingham Study, the prevalence of cataracts was associated with age and reached 46 percent at ages 75 to 85 (Kini et al., 1978).

The cause of age-related cataracts is unknown, but the opacifications in the lens are associated with the breakdown of the γ-crystalline proteins. Epidemiologic data and basic research suggest that ultraviolet light may be a contributing factor in cataract development (Straatsma et al., 1985). The pathological process may occur in either the cortex or the nucleus of the lens. Cortical cataracts have various stages of development. Early in the process, opacities are in

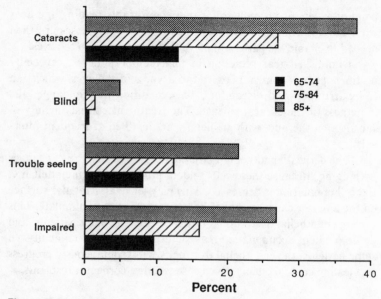

Figure 11-1   Prevalence of vision problems in the elderly, 1984. (*From Havlik, 1986.*)

the periphery and do not decrease visual acuity. At the mature stage, opacifications are more widespread and involve the pupillary area, leading to a slow decrease in visual acuity. In the mature stage, the entire lens becomes opaque. The nuclear cataract does not have these stages of development but is a slowly progressing central opacity, which frequently shows a yellowish discoloration, therefore preventing certain colors from reaching the retina.

Cataract of mild degree may be managed by periodic examination and optimum eyeglasses for an extended period. Ultraviolet

Table 11-2   Ophthalmologic Screening

Visual acuity	Ability to read newspaper-sized print
Lens, fundus	Ophthalmoscopic examination
Intraocular pressure	Tonometry
	Visual fields

lenses may be of benefit. When a cataract progresses to the point where it interferes with activities, cataract surgery is generally indicated. The surgeon may use several methods to remove it, and the decision regarding the best method for each patient should be made by the ophthalmologist.

In intracapsular cataract extractions, the entire cataract and surrounding capsule are removed in a single piece. This removes the entire opacity. In extracapsular cataract extractions, the cataractous lens material and a portion of the capsule are removed. The posterior capsule is left in place to hold an intraocular lens implant.

After cataract removal, the eye has decreased refractive power. Three methods of restoring useful vision are available: eyeglasses, contact lenses, and intraocular lenses (Table 11-3). Approximately 95 percent of those who undergo cataract surgery now receive intraocular lens implants.

Eyeglasses required after surgery are usually thick and heavy. These correct the focus of the eye and permit excellent vision through the central portion. However, they increase the apparent size of the object by about 25 percent, introduce optical distortion, and interfere with peripheral vision. Patients must learn to turn the head instead of the eyes to see clearly to the side. Eyeglasses can be used for patients who have had surgery on both eyes or surgery on one eye and decreased vision in the other. However, eyeglasses cannot usually be used for patients who have had surgery in one eye and have normal vision in the other eye because of the difference in image size.

Contact lenses correct the focus of the eye, permit both central and peripheral vision, and increase apparent object size by 6 percent. However, handling contact lenses is difficult for some individuals, and most lenses must be removed and inserted daily. Extended-wear contact lenses are available, and about 50 to 70 percent of elderly patients are able to wear them after surgery. Contacts are useful in patients who have had cataract surgery in one or both eyes. The lenses correct for distant vision, but eyeglasses are required for reading.

The intraocular lens is surgically placed inside the iris and is expected to remain permanently in place. This lens corrects the focus of the eyes and permits central and peripheral vision; object size is increased by only 1 percent. It is appropriate for patients with cata-

Table 11-3 Methods of Restoring Vision after Cataract Surgery

Eyeglasses
Are thick and heavy
Provide good central vision
Interfere with peripheral vision
Introduce optical distortion
Increase image size by 25%
Cannot be used after surgery on one eye if other eye is normal

Contact lenses
Correct central and peripheral vision
Increase image size by 6%
Are difficult for some patients to handle
Most require daily insertion and removal
About 50–70% can use extended-wear lenses
Can be used after surgery on one or both eyes
Require reading glasses

Intraocular lenses
Correct central and peripheral vision
Increase image size by 1%
Can be used after surgery on one or both eyes
Are useful for aged unable to wear contact lenses
Require bifocal eyeglasses
Introduce added surgical and postsurgical complications

racts in one or both eyes and is particularly useful for patients unable to wear a contact lens. Bifocal eyeglasses are usually required to aid distant or near vision.

Glaucoma The glaucomas are a group of eye disorders characterized by increased intraocular pressure, progressive excavation of the optic nerve head with damage to the nerve fibers, and a specific loss in the visual field. Most cases of primary glaucoma occur in older patients. In the Framingham Study, prevalence of open-angle glaucoma increased with age to 7.2 percent at ages 75 to 85, with men having much higher rates than women (Kini et al., 1978).

Angle-closure glaucoma is an acute and relatively infrequent type of glaucoma, characterized by a sudden painful attack of increased intraocular pressure accompanied by a marked loss in vision. The treatment consists of normalizing the intraocular pressure by the application of miotic eye drops or other medication (such as carbonic anhydrase inhibitors or osmotic agents). The definitive treatment, however, is surgical excision of a peripheral piece of iris or more frequently now by laser iridectomy, ensuring free flow of aqueous humor. Because the disease is usually bilateral, some physicians propose prophylactic iridectomy on the second eye.

Chronic open-angle glaucoma is the more frequent variety of primary glaucoma. It is characterized by an insidious onset, slow progression, and the appearance of typical defects of the visual fields. Early in the disease, intraocular pressure is only moderately elevated, and optic nerve head excavation progresses slowly and sometimes asymmetrically.

While central visual acuity may remain normal for a long time, the defects in the peripheral visual field are characteristic and gradually progressive. Initially there is a paracentral scotoma, which may coalesce. A nasal step of the visual field is another important sign. Finally, the entire field will constrict and eventually involve the visual centers.

The treatment is usually medical, with miotics of various kinds used first. Beta-blocking agents may also be used and have the advantage of not changing the diameter of the pupil. However, caution should be taken because these agents may be systemically absorbed. In severe cases, combination drops may be used with systemic medications such as carbonic anhydrase inhibitors. Surgery or laser therapy is indicated only if disease progresses on maximal medical therapy.

Age-Related Macular Degeneration The macular area of the retina lying at the posterior pole of the globe is the site of highest visual acuity. This area depends entirely on choriocapillaries for nutrition. Any disturbance in the vessel wall of the choroidal capillaries, in the permeability or thickness of Bruch's membrane, or in the retinal pigment epithelium may interfere with exchange of nutrients and oxygen from the choroidal blood to the central retina. Such disturbances occur frequently in older patients. Senile degeneration of the macula is one of the most frequent causes of visual loss in the elderly and is the commonest cause of legal blindness (20/200 or worse). In the Framingham Study, the prevalence was 28 percent at ages 75 to 85, with a higher rate in women than in men (Kini et al., 1978).

Ophthalmoscopic findings vary and do not always parallel loss of vision. In the "dry" form of degeneration, there are areas of depigmentation alternating with zones of hyperpigmentation caused mainly by changes in the retinal pigment epithelium. In another form, the degeneration involves Bruch's membrane, leading to the pigmentation of well-circumscribed, roundish yellow areas.

The second type of degeneration is an exudative or "wet" type. Here there is an elevated focus in the macular area, which at first contains serous fluid but later contains blood derived from blood vessels sprouting from the choroid to the subretinal space. The blood may become organized and form a plaque.

In all these cases, central visual acuity will be markedly affected. These patients will gradually lose the ability to read or see any other details. Most macular degeneration is not treatable; however, laser treatment applied at a specific stage of exudative macular degeneration has been effective in preventing central visual loss in some patients (Folk, 1985). Total blindness does not occur, as patients retain peripheral vision, and therefore are able to perform activities that do not require acute central vision.

Diabetic Retinopathy   In the geriatric population, a significant amount of visual loss is attributed to diabetic retinopathy. The Framingham Study showed an age-associated increase in prevalence up to 7 percent at ages 75 to 85 years (Kini et al., 1978). In the adult-onset diabetic with background changes, the visual loss is usually related to vascular changes in and around the macula. Leakage of serous fluid from vessels surrounding the macula lead to macular edema and deterioration of visual acuity. This may respond to laser photocoagulation. Hemorrhages within the macula may lead to more permanent visual loss. A loss of retinal capillaries may lead to macular ischemia and poor prognosis of visual recovery.

General Factors

Table 11-4 summarizes the general patterns of signs and symptoms associated with common visual problems of the elderly. In addition to the specific treatment discussed above, some simple techniques such as a magnifying glass, large-print reading material, and reduction of glare can help maximize visual function (see Table 11-5).

Health care providers should also be aware of the significant systemic absorption of ophthalmic medications (Anand and Eschmann, 1988). These agents may lead to other organ systems dysfunction and interact with other medications (Table 11-6). The patient's other medical problems and medications should be assessed, and the minimum dose to achieve the desired effect should be used. Patients should also be monitored for systemic toxicity.

HEARING

This section will cover four areas related to hearing problems in the elderly: a review of the major parts of the auditory system, tests used to evaluate the hearing system, effects of aging on hearing performance, and specific pathological disorders affecting the auditory system.

Hearing problems are common in the elderly, especially in a highly industrialized society where noise and age interact to cause hearing loss (Figure 11-2). This loss is usually of the sensorineural type due to damage of the hearing organ, the peripheral nervous system, and/or the central nervous system. These hearing problems are not usually amenable to medical or surgical intervention and thus require hearing aids, aural rehabilitation, and understanding as the major avenues of remediation.

The Auditory System

On a functional basis, the auditory system can be divided into three major parts: peripheral, brainstem, and cortical areas (Table 11-7). Each part of the hearing system has unique functions, which combine to allow hearing and understanding of speech. These functions are listed in Table 11-8.

The main functions of the peripheral auditory system are to

Table 11-4 Signs and Symptoms Associated with Common Visual Problems in the Elderly

Signs and symptoms	Cataract	Open-angle glaucoma	Angle-closure glaucoma	Macular degeneration	Temporal arteritis	Diabetic retinopathy
Pain			X		X	
Red eye			X			
Fixed pupil			X			
Retinal vessel changes					X	X
Retinal exudates				X		X
Optic disk changes		X			X	
Sudden visual loss			X		X	
Loss of peripheral vision		X				
Glare intolerance	X					
Elevated intraocular pressure		X	X			
Loss of visual acuity	X			X		X

Table 11-5 Aids to Maximize Visual Function

Magnifying glass
Soft light, flat paint to avoid glare
Tinted glasses to reduce glare
Night light to assist in adaptation
Large-print newspapers, books, and magazines

Table 11-6 Potential Adverse Effects to Ophthalmic Solutions

Drug	Organ System	Responses
Beta-blockers (e.g., timolol)	Cardiovascular	Bradycardia, hypotension, syncope, palpitation, congestive heart failure
	Respiratory	Bronchospasm
	Neurological	Mental confusion, depression, fatigue, lightheadedness, hallucinations, memory impairment, sexual dysfunction
	Miscellaneous	Hyperkalemia
Adrenergics (e.g., epinephrine, phenylephrine)	Cardiovascular	Extrasystoles, palpitation, hypertension, myocardial infarction
	Miscellaneous	Trembling, paleness, sweating
Cholinergic / anticholinesterases (e.g., pilocarpine, echothiophate)	Respiratory	Bronchospasm
	Gastrointestinal	Salivation, nausea, vomiting, diarrhea, abdominal pain, tenesmus
	Miscellaneous	Lacrimation, sweating
Anticholinergic (e.g., atropine)	Neurological	Ataxia, nystagmus, restlessness, mental confusion, hallucination, violent and aggressive behavior
	Miscellaneous	Insomnia, photophobia, urinary retention

Source: Anand and Eschmann, 1988.

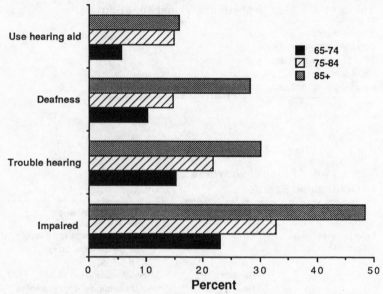

Figure 11-2   Prevalence of hearing problems in the elderly, 1984. (*From Havlik, 1986.*)

change sound into a series of electrical impulses and to transmit those to the brainstem. The major brainstem function is binaural interaction. Binaural interaction allows localization of sound and extraction of a signal from a noisy environment. The cortex brings sound to consciousness and allows interpretation of speech and initiation of appropriate reactions to sound signals.

Assessment

Assessment of hearing function can be divided into three kinds of hearing tests: standard, binaural, and difficult speech. The standard tests are useful for evaluating the peripheral system, binaural tests for evaluating the brainstem, and difficult speech tests for evaluating cortical problems (Table 11-9). Standard tests are performed by presenting pure tones or single words at varying intensity. An audioscope (Welch-Allyn, Inc.) which will deliver pure tones is now available for the office screening of hearing deficits (Lichtenstein et al., 1988).

Table 11-7   Peripheral and Central Auditory Nervous System

A. External ear and peripheral hearing mechanism
   1. Auricle
   2. Tympanic membrane
   3. Ossicular chain
   4. Eustachian tube
   5. Cochlea
      a. Bony labyrinth
      b. Membranous labyrinth
   6. Cochlear nerve
B. Auditory areas in the brainstem
   1. Entrance of the VIIIth cranial nerve
   2. Cochlear nucleus
   3. Superior olivary complex
   4. Lateral lemniscus
   5. Inferior colliculus
   6. Medial geniculate
   7. Auditory radiations (brainstem-to-cortex tract)
C. Auditory areas in the cortex
   1. Temporal lobe
   2. Parietal lobe
   3. Corpus callosum

Table 11-8   Functional Components of the Auditory System

A. Transmission of signals in the periphery
   1. Molecular motion (ear canal)
   2. Mechanical vibration (eardrum and ossicles)
   3. Hydromechanical motion (inner ear)
   4. Electrical impulse (VIIIth nerve)
B. Binaural interaction in the brainstem
   1. Localization and lateralization of sound
   2. Extraction of signals from environmental noise
C. Speech processing in the cortex
   1. Conscious sensation of hearing
   2. Interpretation of speech
   3. Initiation of response to sound

Table 11-9   Assessment of Hearing Function

A.   Standard test measures
   1.   Sensitivity for tones and speech
   2.   Speech discrimination / understanding
   3.   Movement of tympanic membrane
B.   Binaural tests
   1.   Loudness comparison
   2.   Lateralization
   3.   Masking level differences
C.   Difficult speech tests
   1.   Monotic degraded tasks
   2.   Dichotic tasks

Tympanic membrane movement is assessed with a probe. Loudness comparison assesses the individual's ability to balance intensity of sound coming from both ears; lateralization tests the individual's ability to fuse sounds from both ears; and masking level differences assesses the ability to pick out specific sounds from a background of noise. Monotic degraded tasks present difficult sounds such as noise background, filtered sound, and time-compressed speech; dichotic tasks simultaneously present sense and nonsense speech, which the individual is asked to repeat.

Aging Changes

Many changes in the peripheral and central auditory system during aging have effects on the hearing mechanism (Table 11-10). These

Table 11-10   Effects of Aging on the Hearing Mechanism

Atrophy and disappearance of cells in the inner ear
Angiosclerosis in the inner ear
Calcification of membranes in the inner ear
Bioelectric and biomechanical imbalances in the inner ear
Degeneration and loss of ganglion cells and their fibers in the VIIIth cranial nerve
VIIIth nerve canal closure, with destruction of nerve fibers
Atrophy and cell loss at all auditory centers in the brainstem
Reduction of cells in auditory areas of the cortex

changes lead to diminished performance by older subjects (Table 11-11), including the loss of sensitivity and distortion of signals that succeed in passing to higher levels, difficulty in localizing signals and in taking advantage of two-ear listening, difficulty understanding speech under unfavorable listening conditions, and problems with language, especially when aging is compounded by stroke.

Three major factors enhance the progression of hearing loss with advancing age: previous middle-ear disease, vascular disease, and exposure to noise. These factors alone do not, however, account for the hearing loss of old age, called *presbycusis*. Although clinically and pathologically complex, this is a distinct progressive sensorineural hearing loss associated with aging. The deterioration is not limited to the peripheral sensory receptor. Presbycusis affects 60 percent of individuals over age 65 in the United States. However, only a fraction of these have a functional deficit requiring aural rehabilitation.

Sensitivity

Beginning with the third decade of life, there is a deterioration in the hearing threshold. At first, sensitivity at the high frequencies declines gradually. This age-associated loss has been confirmed in populations not exposed to high levels of noise. This gradual impairment is sensorineural and can be tested by pure tone audiometry, which reveals useful information about the physiological condition of hearing but does not disclose some important aspects of deterioration.

Table 11-11   Hearing Performance in the Elderly

A. Peripheral pathology
  1. Hearing loss for pure tones
  2. Hearing loss for speech
  3. Problems understanding speech
B. Brainstem pathology
  1. Problems localizing sounds
  2. Problems in binaural listening
C. Cortical pathology
  1. Problems with difficult speech
  2. Language problems

Speech

Although there is a close relationship between pure tone loss and ability to hear speech, the audiogram does not precisely measure hearing for speech. To assess this auditory function, speech audiometry can be performed by presenting the undistorted test words above threshold intensities in the absence of background noise.

Elderly people with hearing impairment may have difficulty understanding speech under less favorable conditions, such as with background noise, under poor acoustic conditions, or when spoken quickly. This difficulty may be caused in part by the longer time required by higher auditory centers to identify the message. Such hearing loss may require testing of desired signals with the presentation of a competing signal. This will more accurately reflect hearing of speech in social circumstances.

Speech occurring in rooms that cause long reverberations is also much less intelligible to the elderly. Auditory temporal discrimination and auditory reaction time and frequency discrimination also decline with age. Because consonant sounds are of higher frequency and shorter duration, the loss of high-frequency hearing in the elderly may affect these sounds, which encode much of speech information. Lipreading may compensate to some extent for this effect on understanding speech, but other factors of processing information still remain.

Loudness

A common auditory problem of the elderly is abnormal loudness perception. This can occur as hypersensitivity to sounds of high intensity and as manifested by increased "loudness recruitment" in which gradually increasing loudness such as amplified sound is unpleasantly harsh and difficult to tolerate. In the elderly with hearing impairment, this abnormality is manifest when a speaker is asked to speak louder or the output of a hearing aid is increased. This abnormality may result from a sensorineural loss attributable to changes in the hair cells of the inner ear.

Localization

Sound localization contributes to effectiveness of signal detection and helps with discrimination. Loss of directional hearing results in greater hearing difficulty in a noisy environment. Localization is disturbed in the elderly with hearing loss and may be partly caused by the aging brain's deranged processing of interaural intensity differences and time delays. A strongly asymmetrical hearing loss also disturbs localization.

Tinnitus

Tinnitus, an internal noise generated within the hearing system, occurs in many types of hearing disorders at all ages, but is much more frequent in the elderly. Tinnitus, however, is not necessarily associated with hearing loss and may occur in the elderly without hearing impairment. Estimates of prevalence in those aged 65 to 74 are about 11 percent (Fisch, 1978). Treatment is generally unsatisfactory.

Other Hearing Disorders

One of the most easily treatable, but too easily overlooked, causes of hearing loss is cerumen that occludes the external auditory canal (see Table 11-12). Cerumen usually affects low-frequency sounds and complicates existing hearing impairments.

Hearing loss in the geriatric patient may be caused by scarring of the tympanic membrane. In tympanosclerosis, there is calcification of the tympanic membrane that results in stiffening of the drumhead.

Otosclerosis may cause fixation of the ossicular chain and lead to a conduction hearing loss. The bony capsule may also be affected and

Table 11-12 Disorders of Hearing in the Elderly

Cerumen plug
Tympanosclerosis
Otosclerosis
Paget's disease
Ototoxic medications
Sound trauma
CNS lesions
Pseudodeafness (depression)

lead to sensorineural loss. Paget's disease may also lead to both kinds of hearing loss and should be evaluated radiologically and by an alkaline phosphatase determination.

Ototoxic medication is an acquired cause of hearing loss producing cochlear damage. The aminoglycoside antibiotics require special caution. At high doses, ethacrynic acid and furosemide may be ototoxic. High doses of aspirin may cause a reversible hearing impairment. Unfortunately, except for aspirin, removal of the offending drug usually does not reverse the sensorineural loss.

Sound trauma is an environmental factor with neurosensory consequences. Superimposed on the changes of aging, sound trauma can have severe impact on a patient's communicative ability.

Vascular or mass lesions may affect hearing at one of several levels, including the middle and inner ear, auditory nerve, brainstem, and cortical level.

Aural Rehabilitation

Every individual who has communication difficulties caused by a permanent hearing loss should have an ear, nose, and throat evaluation to rule out remediable disease and then an audiological evaluation to assess the roles of amplification and aural rehabilitation. Factors that should be considered during the evaluation for a hearing aid are listed in Table 11-13. In the severely impaired, aural rehabilitation with

---

Table 11-13   Factors in Evaluation for a Hearing Aid

Exclude contraindicating medical or other correctable problem

Greatest satisfaction is achieved with aid if loss is 55–80 dB; there is only partial help if loss is greater than 80 dB

Less satisfaction is achieved when poor discrimination is present

Aid is specifically designed for face-to-face conversation; patient's expectations should be realistic

Aid may need to be combined with lipreading

Loudness perception abnormalities may make aid unacceptable

More severe hearing loss requires aid worn on the body rather than behind-the-ear device

Assess for monaural or binaural aids

Assess for patient's ability to handle aid independently

Assess patient's motivation for using an aid

---

speech reading may be necessary in addition to a hearing aid. Family counseling may also improve utilization and satisfaction with an aid.

Improvements and modifications in design and construction of hearing aids have enabled a greater proportion of the hearing-impaired population to profit from amplification. The old adage that hearing aids will not help people with sensorineural loss is simply not true. The aid can be adjusted to a specific frequency rather than all frequencies, thus decreasing loudness problems, improving discrimination, and making the aid more acceptable. Binaural aids improve sound localization and discrimination.

The hearing aid that is worn on the body provides the greatest amplification but is necessary only for patients with the most severe hearing loss. The controls are large and therefore more easily managed by some elderly persons. However, many elderly people prefer behind-the-ear or in-the-ear devices. The in-the-ear devices are small, cosmetically more acceptable, but more difficult to manipulate.

TASTE

During aging there is a significant loss of lingual papillae and an associated diminution of ability to taste. Salivary secretion also diminishes, thus decreasing solubilization of flavoring agents. Upper dentures may cover secondary taste sites and decrease taste acuity.

Olfactory bulbs also show significant atrophy with old age. Taste and olfactory changes together may account for the lessened interest in food shown by the elderly.

ACKNOWLEDGMENT

The authors wish to thank Dr. Douglas Noffsinger for his assistance in preparing material for the section on hearing in this chapter.

REFERENCES

Anand KB, Eschmann E: Systemic effects of ophthalmic medication in the elderly. *NY State J Med* 88:134–136, 1988.

Fisch L: Special senses: The aging auditory system, in Brocklehurst JC (ed): *Textbook of Geriatric Medicine and Gerontology.* New York, Churchill Livingstone, 1978.

Folk JC: Aging macular degeneration. Clinical features of treatable disease. *Ophthalmology* 92:594–602, 1985.

Havlik RJ: Aging in the eighties, impaired senses for sound and light in persons age 65 years and over. *NCHS Advancedata* No. 125, 1986.

Kini MM, Liebowitz HM, Colton T, et al: Prevalence of senile cataract, diabetic retinopathy, senile macular degeneration, and open-angle glaucoma in the Framingham eye study. *Am J Ophthalmol* 85:28–34, 1978.

Lichtenstein MJ, Bess FH, Logan SA: Validation of screening tools for identifying hearing-impaired elderly in primary care. *JAMA* 259:2875–2878, 1988.

Straatsma BR, Foos RY, Horowitz J, et al: Aging related cataract: Laboratory investigation and clinical management. *Ann Intern Med* 102:82–92, 1985.

SUGGESTED READINGS

Blodi FC: Eye problems of the elderly. *Ophthalmologica* 181:121–128, 1980.

Capino DG, Liebowitz HM: Age-related macular degeneration. *Hosp Pract* 23–42, 1988.

Koopmann CF Jr: Symposium of Geriatric Otolaryngology. *Otolaryngol Clin North Am* 15(2), May 1982.

Kornzweig AL: Visual loss in the elderly, in Reichel W (ed): *The Geriatric Patient*. New York, HP Publishing, 1978.

Liesegang TJ: Cataracts and cataract operations. *Mayo Clin Proc* 59:622–632, 1984.

Mader S: Hearing impairment in elderly persons. *J Am Geriat Soc* 32:548–553, 1984.

Margolis M, Levy B, Sherman FT: Hearing disorders, in Libow LS, Sherman FT (eds): *The Core of Geriatric Medicine*. St Louis, Mosby, 1981.

Roush J (ed): Aging and hearing impairment. *Seminars in Hearing* 6:99–219, 1985.

Ruben RJ: Otolaryngologic problems, in Reichel W (ed): *The Geriatric Patient*. New York, HP Publishing, 1978.

Chapter 12

Disorders of Temperature Regulation

Temperature dysregulation in the elderly demonstrates the narrowing of homeostatic mechanisms that occurs with advancing age. Elderly persons are less able to adjust to extremes of environmental temperatures. Hypo- and hyperthermic states are predominantly disorders of the elderly. Despite underreporting of these disorders, there is evidence that morbidity and mortality increase during particularly hot or cold periods, especially among ill elderly (Hope et al., 1984; Collins et al., 1977; Rango, 1984). Much of this illness is caused by an increased incidence of cardiovascular disorders (myocardial infarct and stroke) or infectious diseases (pneumonia) during these periods.

Studies in the United Kingdom reveal that hypothermia is a common finding among the elderly during the winter, when homes are heated below 70°F.

Table 12-1   Pathophysiology of Temperature Dysregulation

Hyperthermia	Hypothermia
Higher threshold of central temperature to sweating	Diminished sensation to cold
Diminished or absent sweating	Impaired sensation to change in temperature
Impaired warmth perception	Abnormal autonomic vasoconstrictor response to cold
Abnormal peripheral blood flow response to warming	Impaired shiver response
Compromised cardiovascular reserve	Diminished thermogenesis

Table 12-2   Factors Predisposing to Hypothermia

Decreased heat production
  Hypothyroidism
  Hypoglycemia
  Starvation and malnutrition
  Immobility and decreased activity (e.g., stroke, arthritis, parkinsonism)
Increased heat loss
  Decreased subcutaneous fat
  Exposure to cold (immersion)
Thermoregulatory impairment
  Hypothalamic and CNS dysfunction
    Heat trauma
    Hypoxia
    Tumor
    Cerebrovascular disease
  Drug-induced impairment
    Alcohol
    Barbiturates
    Major and minor tranquilizers
    Glutethimide
    Reserpine
    Tricyclic antidepressants
    Salicylates, acetaminophen
    General anesthetics
  Old age
Miscellaneous
  Sepsis
  Cardiovascular disease
  Bronchopneumonia

Table 12-3   Clinical Presentation of Hypothermia

Early signs (32–35°C)	Later signs (28–30°C)	Late signs (<28°C)
Fatigue	Cold skin	Very cold skin
Weakness	Hypopnea	Rigidity
Slowness of gait	Cyanosis	Apnea
Apathy	Bradycardia	No pulse—ventricular
Slurred speech	Atrial and ventricular	fibrillation
Confusion	arrhythmias	Areflexia
Shivering (±)	Hypotension	Unresponsiveness
Cool skin	Semicoma and coma	Fixed pupils
Sensation of cold (±)	Muscular rigidity	
	Generalized edema	
	Slowed reflexes	
	Poorly reactive pupils	
	Polyuria or oliguria	

PATHOPHYSIOLOGY

The basic pathophysiology of hypo- and hyperthermic states in the elderly is represented in Table 12-1. The thermoregulatory center maintains body temperature through control of sweating, vasoconstriction and vasodilation, chemical thermogenesis, and shivering. Impaired temperature perception, diminished sweating (Foster et al., 1976) in hyperthermia, and abnormal vasoconstrictor response in hypothermia are major pathophysiological mechanisms in these disorders.

Table 12-4   Complications of Severe Hypothermia

Arrhythmias
Cardiorespiratory arrest
Bronchopneumonia
Aspiration pneumonia
Pulmonary edema
Pancreatitis
Gastrointestinal bleeding
Acute tubular necrosis
Intravascular thrombosis

Table 12-5   ECG Abnormalities in Hypothermia

Bradycardia
Prolonged PR interval, QRS complex, and QT segment
J wave (Osborn wave)
Atrial fibrillation
PVCs
Ventricular fibrillation
Muscle tremor artifact

HYPOTHERMIA

Hypothermia is defined as a core temperature (rectal, esophageal, tympanic) below 35°C. Essential to the diagnosis is early recognition with a low-recording thermometer. Ordinary thermometers will not serve. The factors predisposing to hypothermia are listed in Table 12-2.

Table 12-3 illustrates the clinical spectrum of hypothermia. Because early signs are nonspecific and subtle, a high index of suspicion must exist to allow an early diagnosis. A history of known or potential exposure is helpful, but elderly patients can become hypothermic at modest temperatures. Frequently the most difficult differential diagnosis in more severe hypothermia is hypothyroidism. A previous history of thyroid disease, a neck scar from previous thyroid surgery, and a delay in the relaxation phase of the deep tendon

Table 12-6   Supportive Therapy for Hypothermia

Use intensive care unit (for temperature below 30°C).
Maintain continuous ECG monitoring.
Use intravenous fluid replacement (assess individually).
Arrhythmias are resistant to cardioversion and drug therapy (drugs given during hypothermia may cause problems when patient is rewarmed).
Treat only severe hyperglycemia.
Use caution when correcting severe acidosis with HCO_3.
If central venous pressure necessary, avoid entrance into the heart.
Follow blood gases to assess respiratory function.
O_2 therapy, suctioning, and endotracheal intubation may be required.
Monitor chest films—pneumonia is common.
In myxedema, treat with levothyroxine 500 μg IV and corticosteroids.

reflexes may assist in diagnosing hypothyroidism. Patients may sometimes be mistaken for dead. Case reports reveal patients who have survived after being discovered without respiration and pulse.

Complications of severe hypothermia are listed in Table 12-4. The most significant early ones are arrhythmias and cardiorespiratory arrests. Later complications involve the pulmonary, gastrointestinal, and renal systems. ECG abnormalities are frequent (Table 12-5). The most specific ECG finding is the J wave (Osborn wave) following the QRS complex. This abnormality disappears as temperature returns to normal.

General supportive therapy for severe hypothermia consists of intensive care management of complicated multisystem dysfunctions (Table 12-6). Every attempt should be made to assess and treat any contributing medical disorder (e.g., hypothyroidism, hypoglycemia). While patients should have continuous ECG monitoring, central lines should be avoided if possible because of myocardial irritability. Because there is delayed metabolism, most drugs have little effect on a severely hypothermic patient, but they may cause problems once the patient is rewarmed. It is preferable to stabilize the patient and immediately undertake specific rewarming techniques (Table 12-7).

Table 12-7   Specific Rewarming Techniques

Passive rewarming
   Removal from environmental exposure
   Insulating material
   Placement in warm environment ($>70°F$)
Active external rewarming
   Immersion in heated water ($42°C$ or $107.6°F$)
   Electric blankets
   Heated objects (water bottle)
Active core rewarming
   Intragastric balloon
   Colonic irrigation
   Mediastinal irrigation via thoracotomy
   Hemodialysis
   Peritoneal dialysis
   Extracorporeal blood rewarming
   Inhalation rewarming
   Cardiopulmonary bypass

Serious arrhythmias, acidosis, and fluid and electrolyte disorders will usually respond to therapy only after rewarming has been accomplished.

Passive rewarming is generally adequate for those with mild hypothermia ($>32°C$). Active external rewarming has been associated with increased morbidity and mortality because cold blood may suddenly be shunted to the core, further decreasing core temperature; and peripheral vasodilatation can precipitate hypovolemic shock by decreasing circulatory blood volume. For more severe hypo-

Table 12-8   Factors Predisposing to Heatstroke

Exogenous heat gain
    High ambient temperature
    Increased risk in
        Extremes of age
        Debilitating illness
        Alcohol ingestion
Increased heat production
    Exercise and exertion
    Infection (febrile state)
    Agitated and tremulous states
    Drugs (amphetamines)
    Hyperthyroidism
Impaired heat dissipation
    Lack of acclimatization
    High ambient temperature
    High humidity
    Obesity
    Heavy clothing
    Cardiovascular disease
    Dehydration
    Extremes of age
    Central nervous system lesions
    Drugs
        Phenothiazines
        Anticholinergics
        Diuretics
        Propranolol
    Sweat gland dysfunction
    Potassium depletion

thermia (<32°C), core rewarming is necessary. Several techniques for core rewarming have been used (Table 12-7), but positive results have been reported only from small, uncontrolled studies. Peritoneal dialysis and inhalation rewarming may be the most practical techniques in most institutions.

Mortality is usually greater than 50 percent for severe hypothermia. It increases with age and is particularly related to underlying disease.

HYPERTHERMIA

Heatstroke is defined as a failure to maintain body temperature and is characterized by a core temperature of >40.6°C (105°F), severe central nervous system dysfunction (psychosis, delirium, coma), and

Table 12-9 Complications of Heatstroke

Myocardial damage
   Congestive heart failure
   Arrhythmias
Renal failure (20–25%)
Cerebral edema
   Seizures
   Diffuse and focal findings
Hepatocellular necrosis
   Jaundice
   Liver failure
Rhabdomyolysis
   Myoglobinuria
Bleeding diathesis
   Disseminated intravascular
     coagulation
Electrolyte disturbances
Acid-base disturbances
   Metabolic acidosis
   Respiratory alkalosis
Infection
   Aspiration pneumonia
   Sepsis
Dehydration and shock

anhidrosis (hot, dry skin). The two groups primarily affected are the elderly who are chronically ill and the young undergoing strenuous exercise. Mortality is as high as 80 percent once this syndrome is manifest.

Table 12-8 illustrates predisposing factors relevant to the elderly. Usually there are multiple factors, but most often there is a prolonged heat wave. Again, the diagnosis requires a high level of suspicion. In view of the poor survival, efforts must be directed toward prevention. Elderly patients should be cautioned about the dangers of hot weather. For those at particularly high risk, temporary relocation to more protected environments should be considered.

Table 12-9 lists some of the more serious complications resulting from heat damage to organ systems. Once the full syndrome has developed for any length of time, the prognosis is very poor. While management at this stage requires intense multisystem care, the key is rapid specific therapy consisting of cooling by ice bath, with vigorous massage, ice massages, and vaporization, to 102°F within the first hour.

Prevention appears to be the most appropriate approach to management of temperature dysregulation in the elderly. Education of older adults to their susceptibility to hypo- and hyperthermia in extremes of environmental temperature, education to appropriate behavior in such conditions, and close monitoring of the most vulnerable elderly should help reduce the morbidity and mortality from these disorders.

ACKNOWLEDGMENT

The authors wish to acknowledge the assistance of Dr. Alan Robbins in preparing this chapter.

REFERENCES

Collins KJ, Dore C, Exton-Smith AN, et al: Accidental hypothermia and impaired temperature homeostasis in the elderly. *Br Med J* 1:353–356, 1977.

Foster KG, Ellis FT, Dore C, et al: Sweat responses in the aged. *Age Ageing* 5:91–101, 1976.

Hope W, Donnel HD Jr, McKinley TW, et al: Illness and death due to environmental heat: Georgia and St Louis, 1983. Leads from the MMWR. *JAMA* 252:20–23, 1984.

Rango N: Exposure related hypothermia mortality in the United States, 1970–79. *Am J Publ Health* 74:1159–1160, 1984.

SUGGESTED READINGS

Avery CE, Pestle RE: Hypothermia and the elderly: Perceptions and behavior. *Gerontologist* 27:523–526, 1987.

Collins KJ, Exton-Smith AN: Thermal homeostasis in old age. *J Am Geriatr Soc* 31:519–524, 1983.

Collins KJ, Exton-Smith AN, James MH, et al: Functional changes in autonomic nervous responses with ageing. *Age Ageing* 9:17–24, 1980.

Hudson LD, Conn RD: Accidental hypothermia: Associated diagnoses and prognosis in a common problem. *JAMA* 227:37–40, 1974.

Khogali M, Weiner JS: Heat stroke: Report on 18 cases. *Lancet* 2:276–278, 1980.

Knochel JP, Dallas MD: Environmental heat illness: An eclectic review. *Arch Intern Med* 133:841–864, 1974.

MacMillan AL, Corbett JL, Johnson RH, et al: Temperature regulation in survivors of accidental hypothermia of the elderly. *Lancet* 2:165–169, 1967.

O'Keeffe K: Accidental hypothermia: A review of 63 cases. *J Am Coll Emerg Phys* 6:491–496, 1977.

Reuler J: Hypothermia: Pathophysiology, clinical settings, and management. *Ann Intern Med* 89:519–527, 1978.

Rosin AJ, Exton-Smith AN: Clinical features of accidental hypothermia with some observations on thyroid function. *Br Med J* 1:16–19, 1964.

Treatment of hypothermia. *Med Lett Drugs Ther* 28:123–124, 1986.

Trevino A, Bazi B, Beller BM, et al: The characteristic electrocardiogram of accidental hypothermia. *Arch Intern Med* 127:470–473, 1971.

Wheeler M: Heat stroke in the elderly: Symposium on geriatric medicine. *Med Clin North Am* 60:1289–1296, 1976.

Wong KC: Physiology and pharmacology of hypothermia. *West J Med* 138:227–232, 1983.

Part Three

General Management
Strategies

Chapter 13

Iatrogenesis

The aging individual is an organism in fine balance with its environment. Like the early stages of life, the latter stage is characterized by an increased sensitivity to the environment. As noted in Chapter 1, aging is typified by a decreased capacity to respond to stress. Whereas a mature adult is likely to adapt to or alter the environment, the aged individual is very affected by changes of setting.

It is hardly surprising then that the elderly patient is vulnerable to the variety of stresses imposed by modern medical care. Table 13-1 lists some of the iatrogenic problems elderly patients may suffer. The elderly patient generally presents with a much narrower therapeutic window than does a younger person. Figure 13-1 portrays in a very conceptual manner this narrowing as the response to therapy decreases and the susceptibility to toxic side effects increases. These changes are attributable to both a change in receptor behavior and an altered chemical environment produced by other simultaneous drugs.

**Table 13-1   Common
Iatrogenic Problems
of the Elderly**

Overzealous labeling
  Dementia
  Incontinence
Bed rest
Polypharmacy
Enforced dependency
Transfer trauma

This narrowing of the therapeutic window is perhaps most easily recognized in the pharmacological treatment of the elderly. In the face of reduced capacity for metabolizing and excreting many drugs, the older patient can develop high blood levels on "normal" dosages. Changes in receptors may alter sensitivity to chemicals in either

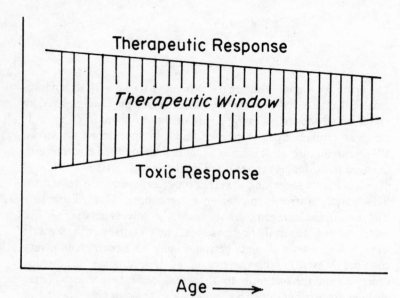

Figure 13-1   Narrowing therapeutic window.

direction. Use of numerous drugs transforms the elderly patient into a living chemistry set. Because of their prevalence and importance, drugs are discussed separately in Chapter 14. Here we will focus attention on some of the more subtle ways in which other types of treatment can adversely affect the elderly.

HOSPITALS

Hospitals are dangerous places for any patient. Most of us are resilient enough to enter an acute care hospital and suffer the vicissitudes of care with the expectation that we will emerge better (certainly in the long run). The calculation of benefits received for risks undertaken needs to be more carefully thought through with older patients. Just a little thought reveals the litany of familiar hazards of hospitalization—from the risk of nosocomial infection to getting the wrong drug to the stress of major surgery or the danger of certain diagnostic procedures. All these are imposed on the general hazards of bed rest discussed in Chapter 8. Table 13-2 offers some examples of potential hazards in the hospital.

The elderly are more likely to experience an untoward event during a hospital stay. In part, this is because elderly patients present with more physical problems, but they are also more vulnerable.

Among 815 consecutive admissions to a hospital's general medical service, an overall rate of 497 iatrogenic events developed, involving 36 percent of patients; 9 percent of the patients had complications classified as major, and in 2 percent the complications contributed to death. Patient characteristics associated with increased risk of iatrogenic complications are listed in Table 13-3. Of these, only the first two, source of admission and condition on admission, remained significant when other factors were controlled (Steel et al., 1981). Because elderly patients are more likely to come from nursing homes and to be in poor condition on admission, they should be considered at high risk for iatrogenic complications.

In a study of patients hospitalized on a general medical service, the incidence of functional symptoms unrelated to diagnosis was over 4 times higher among patients aged 70 and over than among younger patients. As shown in Table 13-4, younger patients were more likely

**Table 13-2   The Hazards
of Hospitalization**

Diagnostic procedures
  Cardiac catheterization
  Arteriography
Therapeutic procedures
  Intravenous therapy
  Urinary catheters
  Nasogastric tube
  Dialysis
  Transfusion
Drugs
  Medication error
  Drug-drug interaction
  Drug reaction
  Side effect
Surgery
  Anesthesia
  Infection
  Metabolic imbalance
  Hypovolemia
Bed rest
  Hypovolemia and hypertension
  Calcium metabolism
  Fecal impaction
  Urine incontinence
  Thromboembolism
Nosocomial infection
Falls

**Table 13-3   Risk Factors
for Iatrogenic Hospital
Event**

Admission from nursing home or other
  hospital
Physician's assessment of overall
  condition on admission
Age
Number of drugs
Length of stay

Table 13-4   Rate of Functional Symptoms and Consequent Intervention in Hospital Admissions of the Young and Old

Functional symptom	Incidence, %		Intervention	Frequency, %	
	Young	Old		Young	Old
Confusion	3.6	29.5	Psychotropic drugs	58.3	13.7
			Restraints	58.3	52.9
Not eating	1.8	15.6	Nasogastric tube	0	29.6
Incontinence	5.5	26.6	Foley catheter	11.1	15.2
Falling	0.9	5.2	None		
At least one symptom	8.8	40.5	Any intervention	37.9	47.1

Source: After Gillick, et al., 1982.

to be treated for symptoms of confusion but older patients were more likely to be treated for problems of not eating and incontinence (Gillick, Serrel, and Gillick, 1982).

The elderly patient's vulnerability extends to a more subtle level. Admission to a hospital means entering an unfamiliar world. Moreover, the patient enters the hospital at a time of great stress. The anxiety of unknown consequences is in addition to the physical stress of the illness.

The hospital presents physical and organizational barriers to which the patient must adapt. Not only the geography but the routines are different. The things we rely on to preserve our sense of identity are among the first things taken away: our clothing, our personal effects. It is hardly surprising, then, that many elderly persons who are able to function in their familiar surroundings become disoriented and often agitated in the hospital. Just as a blind person can move flawlessly in familiar surroundings, an elderly person may have developed a host of adaptive mechanisms to function in his or her home situation, overcoming problems of memory loss and impaired vision. Transferred into the sterile, rigid hospital room, such an individual may decompensate. The syndrome of "sundowning," whereby older patients in the hospital become agitated and disoriented as dusk falls, is likely a function of visual or hearing impairments, diminished sensory stimuli, and resultant disorientation.

The older person accustomed to coping with nocturia may wander at night in the dark to where the bathroom at home ought to be and wet the floor. In the crisis of urinary urgency, the patient may be unable to scale the side rails and make it to the bathroom in time. To label an individual who suffers such environmentally exacerbated accidents as incontinent is to inflict double jeopardy.

We fail to appreciate the dangers of bed rest in the elderly. Bed is actually a very dangerous place for an older person, besides the risk of falling out of bed. Table 13-5 lists some of the potential complications of putting a geriatric patient in bed for a sustained period. In addition to the familiar propensity to thrombosis, confinement to bed may produce other adverse effects in an older patient. Calcium metabolism is impaired; in an osteoporotic individual, such an added burden can be harsh. Cardiovascular function is diminished. There are problems of orthostatic hypotension and general lack of reserve cardiac output when it becomes necessary to ambulate. The threat of pressure sores is ever present.

The hospital breeds dependency. Even with younger patients, hospital personnel are accustomed to performing basic functions for the patient. Use of the bathroom is by prescription only. Bathing is often a supervised event. Patients are transported from one location to another. Although most of us as patients may have enjoyed being indulged for a while, we soon begin to rail against the imposed depen-

**Table 13-5   Potential
Complications
of Bed Rest
in the Elderly**

Pressure sores
Bone resorption
Postural hypotension
Pneumonia
Thrombophlebitis and
   thromboembolism
Urinary incontinence
Constipation and fecal impaction
Contractures

---

dency. In older patients who need to be urged, encouraged, and cajoled into doing as much for themselves as possible, such an atmosphere can be especially debilitating.

Encouraging patients to act independently requires patience and time; unfortunately, both are scarce in the acute care hospital. It is much faster and easier to do a task for a person who performs slowly and uncertainly than to take the time to encourage that person to do that task independently. Moreover, the result of a professionally performed task is usually neater and more in keeping with hospital standards. Thus, well-meaning staff bowing to the pressures for efficiency may be inclined to do things for elderly patients rather than urging the patients to do as much as possible for themselves. This well-intentioned behavior fosters dependency at a time when independent function is crucial.

The hospital is notoriously averse to risk taking. Hospital policies are designed to err on the side of caution. Such behavior can further compromise the independent functioning of older patients. Patients who are not allowed to bathe themselves or who are wheeled rather than walked are likely to become less motivated to use their full capacities. Any fears about their ability are likely to increase.

In the light of the multiple adverse consequences that may be associated with hospitalizing the elderly, we might pause to ask why we have not done more to make hospitals more hospitable for them. Ironically, we have invested great care in minimizing the trauma of hospitalization for children. Creativity in architecture and programs has gone into making pediatric wards as nonthreatening and homelike as possible. Although children are rarely hospitalized and geriatric patients are frequently hospitalized, no similar investment of creativity has been devoted to making the hospital less stressful for the elderly. We know enough about perceptual and functional problems of aging to recognize that even simple architectural modifications can make a hospital stay easier. Use of primary colors, windows at lower heights, better-designed furniture, use of textures and patterns, and better design of rooms can all help the older patient retain maximum functioning capacity.

Special units for managing geriatric patients are beginning to emerge. Staffed by an interdisciplinary team composed of nurses, social worker, physician, and physical or occupational therapist, these units apply techniques of multidimensional functional evaluation to assess the capacity of the geriatric patient. Often taking patients who have completed a course of acute care hospitalization and are otherwise destined for a nursing home, such geriatric assessment units can uncover treatable conditions, provide rehabilitation to improve functional capacity, and develop a plan of care that will allow the elderly patient to remain in the community (Rubenstein, Rhee, and Kane, 1982).

The geriatric assessment units have routinely uncovered three or four new significant problems in patients just discharged from university-staffed acute care medical services. An iatrogenic danger to the elderly patient thus lies in underdiagnosis, especially of mundane but critical conditions involving hearing, vision, and dentition. In addition, even more clinically important problems such as thyroid disease or aortic aneurysms may be overlooked unless a careful examination is performed.

LABELING

Perhaps even more dangerous than the cases of underdiagnosis are those of overdiagnosis. The physician who too readily labels a disoriented patient as senile or demented or who classifies a urinary accident as incontinence may be sealing the fate of that patient unnecessarily. These two diagnoses are strongly associated with an increased likelihood of nursing home admission, and thus should not be made lightly.

Unfortunately, much of the nursing home care in the United States leaves a great deal to be desired. Such institutions are neither homes nor hospitals; they are most assuredly not therapeutic milieus. Physicians admitting patients to nursing homes are responsible for assuring both themselves and their patients on several scores:

1   The patient truly needs care in such a setting and cannot reasonably get such care elsewhere.
2   The institution is capable of providing the needed care.
3   The patient is prepared for a transfer to the nursing home.

Too frequently, hospital discharge to the nursing home compounds the trauma. Discharge planning is often begun too late. There is not sufficient time to find the best facility for the patient's needs nor to allow the patient and the patient's family a sufficient role in making the decision for nursing home placement.

The physician can play an important role in improving the quality of nursing home care as well. As an outside professional who is serving as the patient's advocate, the physician can press for a more stimulating environment, encourage programs designed to foster a homelike atmosphere, and insist that treatment regimens be carried out as ordered. Too many physicians are reluctant to become meaningfully involved in nursing home care. An indifferent physician leaves the vulnerable patient to cope with a most unrehabilitating situation. The lack of stimulation, the constant companionship of disoriented persons, the lack of privacy, and rigid rules would make even the strongest of us cringe. How much more harmful will these forces be on the already compromised reserves of the elderly? In such a situation, the elderly patient manifests the worst features of the institutionalized victim, often adopting the predominant pattern of behavior.

SUMMARY

The elderly patient represents a different risk-benefit ratio from younger patients. Actions well tolerated in others may produce serious consequences in the old. Bed is a dangerous place for the elderly patient; confinement to bed rest should be avoided whenever possible.

The physician must guard against several potential iatrogenic problems with elderly patients. Diagnostic labels implying incurable problems (like dementia and incontinence) should not be used until a careful search for correctable causes has been undertaken. Special attention should be given to the tendency to create dependency through well-intentioned care. By keeping in mind the need to maintain the patient's functioning, the physician can remain sensitive to the effects of the environment to enhance or impede such activity.

REFERENCES

Gillick MR, Serrel NA, Gillick LS: Adverse consequences of hospitalization in the elderly. *Soc Sci Med* 16:1033–1038, 1982.

Rubenstein LZ, Rhee L, Kane RL: The role of geriatric assessment units in caring for the elderly: An analytic review. *J Gerontol* 37:513–521, 1982.

Steel K, Gertman PM, Crescenzi C, Anderson J: Iatrogenic illness on a general medical service at a university hospital. *N Engl J Med* 304:638–642, 1981.

Chapter 14

Drug Therapy

Elderly persons are frequently prescribed multiple drugs in complex dosage schedules. In some instances this is justified because of the presence of multiple chronic medical conditions on which acute illnesses are superimposed. In most instances, however, complex drug regimens are unnecessary, excessively costly, and predispose to non-compliance and adverse drug reactions.

Several important considerations, some pharmacological and others nonpharmacological, influence the safety and effectiveness of drug therapy in the elderly. This chapter focuses on these considerations and attempts to give practical suggestions for prescribing drugs for this population. Drug therapy for specific geriatric conditions is discussed in several other chapters throughout this text.

NONPHARMACOLOGICAL FACTORS INFLUENCING DRUG THERAPY

Discussions of geriatric pharmacology frequently center around age-related changes in drug pharmacokinetics and pharmacodynamics.

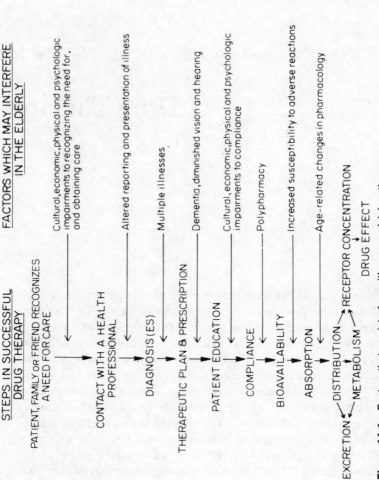

Figure 14-1   Factors that can interfere with successful drug therapy.

Although these changes are sometimes of clinical importance, non-pharmacological factors can play an even greater role in the safety and effectiveness of drug therapy in the elderly population.

Several steps make drug therapy safe and effective (Figure 14-1). Many factors can interfere with this scheme in the elderly, and, as can be seen, most of them come into play before pharmacological considerations arise.

Effective drug therapy can be hampered by inaccurate diagnoses. The elderly tend to underreport symptoms, and when they do complain, their complaints are often vague and multiple. Symptoms of physical diseases frequently overlap with symptoms of psychological illness. To add to this complexity, many diseases present with atypical symptoms. Thus, making the correct diagnoses and prescribing the appropriate drugs are often difficult tasks in elderly patients.

There is a tendency among health care professionals to treat symptoms with drugs rather than to evaluate the symptoms thoroughly. Because elderly patients tend to have multiple problems and complaints and may consult several health care professionals, they often end up with prescriptions for several drugs. All too frequently, neither the patient nor the health care professionals have a clear picture of the total drug regimen. Medication records such as the one shown in Figure 14-2 carried by the patient and maintained as an integral part of the overall medical record may help to eliminate some of the polypharmacy and noncompliance that is all to common in the elderly population.

Compliance plays a central role in the success of drug therapy in all age groups (Figure 14-1). In addition to the tendency for polypharmacy and complex dosage schedules, the elderly face other potential barriers to compliance. The chronic nature of illness in the elderly can play a role in noncompliance. The consequences of these illnesses are often delayed (as opposed to the more dramatic effects of acute illnesses), and chronic illnesses require ongoing prophylactic or suppressive rather than relatively short and time-limited courses of therapy. Compliance tends to be poor for these types of drug regimens. Diminished hearing, impaired vision, and poor short-term memory are relatively common in the elderly population, and all can interfere with patient education and compliance. Problems with transportation can make getting to a pharmacy difficult. Most outpa-

MEDICATION NAME	REASON FOR USE	DESCRIBE OR TAPE MEDICINE HERE	WHEN TO TAKE MEDICINE				SPECIAL NOTES

NAME _____ DOCTOR _____ PHONE: ( ) _____

REMEMBER

BRING THIS CHART TO ALL DOCTOR APPOINTMENTS
INCLUDE ALL THE MEDICATIONS YOU ARE TAKING
DO NOT CHANGE THE WAY YOU TAKE THE MEDICATIONS WITHOUT CALLING THE DOCTOR
DO NOT SHARE MEDICATIONS
IF YOU HAVE ANY QUESTIONS, CALL THE DOCTOR

Figure 14-2 Example of a medication record.

tient prescriptions are not covered by Medicare, thus forcing elderly persons to pay for their drugs from a limited income. Even if the elderly person gets to the pharmacy, can afford the prescription, understands the instructions, and remembers when to take it, the use of childproof bottles and tamper-resistant packaging may hinder compliance in those with arthritic or weak hands.

Several strategies might improve compliance in the elderly (Table 14-1). As few drugs as possible should be prescribed, and the dosage schedule should be as simple as possible. Drugs should be given on the same dosage schedules whenever possible (e.g., twice daily, three times daily), and the administration should correspond to a daily routine in order to enhance the consistency of taking the drugs and compliance. Relatives or other care givers should be instructed in the drug regimen, and they, as well as others (e.g., home health aides and pharmacists), should be enlisted to help the elderly patient comply. Specially designed pill dispensers, dosage calendars, and other innovative techniques can be useful. (At a minimum, prescriptions should instruct the pharmacist not to use the childproof container whenever appropriate.) Elderly patients (as well as their health care professionals) should keep an updated record of the drug regimen (Figure 14-2). Medications should be brought to appointments, especially initial or consultation visits, and health care professionals should regularly inquire about other medications being taken (prescribed by other physicians or purchased over the counter) and review their elderly patients' knowledge of and compliance with the drug regimen.

Table 14-1   Strategies to Improve Compliance in the Elderly

Making drug regimens and instructions as simple as possible
  Use the same dosage schedule whenever feasible (e.g., once or twice per day)
  Time the doses in conjunction with a daily routine
Instruct relatives and care givers on the drug regimen
Enlist others (e.g., home health aides, pharmacists) to help ensure compliance
Make sure the elderly patient can get to a pharmacist (or vice versa), can afford
  the prescriptions, and can open the container
Use aids (such as special pillboxes and drug calendars) whenever appropriate
Keep updated medication records (Figure 14-2)
Review knowledge of, and compliance with, drug regimens regularly

ADVERSE DRUG REACTIONS AND INTERACTIONS

Primum non nocere (first, do no harm), a watchword phrase in the practice of medicine, is nowhere more applicable than when prescribing drugs for the elderly.

Adverse drug reactions are the most common form of iatrogenic illness (see Chapter 13). The incidence of adverse drug reactions in hospitalized patients increases from about 10 percent in those aged 40 to 50 to 25 percent in those older than 80 (Seidel et al., 1966). They account for between 3 and 10 percent of hospital admissions (Caranasos et al. 1974; Williamson and Chopin, 1980) and could result in as much as $3 billion in yearly health care expenditures (U.S. Congress, 1976).

Many drugs commonly prescribed for the elderly produce distressing and sometimes potentially disabling or life-threatening adverse reactions (Table 14-2). Psychotropic drugs and cardiovascular agents are the most common causes of serious adverse reactions in the elderly. In part, this is because of the narrow therapeutic-toxic ratio of many of these drugs. In some instances, age-related changes in pharmacology such as diminished renal excretion and prolonged duration of action predispose to adverse reactions. Some side effects

Table 14-2   Examples of Adverse Drug Reactions

Type of drug	Common adverse reactions
Analgesics	
Anti-inflammatory agents	Gastric irritation
	Chronic blood loss
Narcotic	Constipation
Antimicrobials	
Aminoglycosides	Renal failure
	Hearing loss
Levodopa	Nausea
	Delirium
Anticholinergics	Dry mouth
	Constipation
	Urinary retention
	Delirium

Table 14-2 Examples of Adverse Drug Reactions (*Continued*)

Type of drug	Common adverse reactions
Antiarrhythmics	Diarrhea (quinidine)
	Urinary retention (disopyramide)
Anticoagulants	Bleeding complications
Antihypertensives	Sedation and / or other changes in mental function
	Hypotension
Calcium channel blockers	Decreased myocardial contractility
Diuretics	Dehydration
	Hyponatremia
	Hypokalemia
	Incontinence
Digoxin	Arrhythmias
Hypoglycemic agents	
Insulin	Hypoglycemia
Oral agents	Hyponatremia (chlorpropamide)
Psychotropic agents	
Antidepressants	
Tricyclic drugs	(See Table 5-15)
Lithium	Weakness
	Tremor
	Nausea
	Delirium
Antipsychotics	Sedation
	Hypotension
	Extrapyramidal movement disorders
Sedative and hypnotic agents	Excessive sedation
	Delirium
	Gait disturbances
Others	
Aminophylline	Gastric irritation
	Tachyarrhythmias
Cimetidine	Mental status changes
Terbutaline	Tremor

can have a therapeutic benefit and may be a key factor in drug selection (see below).

Because symptoms can be nonspecific or mimic other illnesses, adverse drug reactions may be ignored or unrecognized. In some instances, another drug is prescribed to treat these symptoms, thus contributing to polypharmacy and increasing the likelihood of an adverse drug interaction. The problem of polypharmacy is exacerbated by elderly people who visit multiple physicians. Medication records kept by the patient (Figure 14-2) as well as in the medical record should help prevent unnecessary polypharmacy when many physicians are involved. Several drugs commonly prescribed for the elderly can interact, with adverse consequences (Medical Letter, 1981) (Table 14-3). The more common types of potential adverse drug interactions in the elderly are drug displacement from protein-

Table 14-3   Examples of Potentially Clinically Important Drug-Drug Interactions

Interaction	Examples	Potential effects
Interference with drug absorption	Antacids interacting with digoxin, INH antipsychotics	Diminished drug effectiveness
Displacement from binding proteins	Warfarin, oral hypoglycemics, aspirin, chloral hydrate, other highly protein-bound drugs (see Table 14-6)	Enhanced effects and increased risk of toxicity
Altered distribution	Digoxin and quinidine	Increased risk of toxicity
Altered metabolism	Cimetidine interacting with propranolol, theophylline, dilantin	Decreased drug clearance, enhanced effects, increased risk of toxicity
Altered excretion	Lithium and diuretics	Increased risk of toxicity and electrolyte imbalance
Pharmacological antagonism	Levodopa and clonidine	Decreased antiparkinsonian effects
Pharmacological synergism	Tricylic antidepressants and antihypertensives	Increased risk of hypotension

binding sites by other highly protein-bound drugs, induction or suppression of the metabolism of other drugs, and additive effects of different drugs on blood pressure and mental function (mood, level of consciousness, etc.). In addition to the potential to interact with other

Table 14-4   Examples of Potentially Clinically Important Drug-Patient Interactions

Drug	Patient factors	Clinical implications
Diuretics	Diabetes	Decreased glucose tolerance
	Poor nutritional status	Increased risk of dehydration and electrolyte imbalance
	Urinary frequency, urgency	Incontinence may result
Beta blockers	Diabetes	Sympathetic response to hypoglycemia masked
	Chronic obstructive lung disease	Increased bronchospasm
	Congestive heart failure	Decreased myocardial contractility
	Peripheral vascular disease	Increased claudication
Narcotic analgesics	Chronic constipation	Worsening symptoms, fecal impaction
Tricyclic antidepressants	Congestive heart failure, angina	Tachycardia, decreased myocardial contractility, postural hypotension exacerbating cardiovascular conditions
Tricyclic antidepressants, antihistamines, and other drugs with anticholinergic effects	Constipation, glaucoma and other visual impairments, prostatic hyperplasia, reflux esophagitis	Worsening of symptoms
Antipsychotics	Parkinsonism	Worsening of immobility
Psychotropics	Dementia	Further impairment of cognitive function

drugs, several drugs can interact adversely with underlying medical conditions in the elderly creating "drug-patient" interactions (Table 14-4).

Health care professionals should have a thorough knowledge of the more common drug side effects, adverse reactions to drugs, and potential drug interactions in the elderly. Careful questioning about side effects should be an important part of reviewing the drug regimen at each visit. Some institutions use computers to detect potential adverse drug interactions and prevent their occurrence. With or without this computer capability, special attention should be given to the potential for a newly prescribed drug to interact with drugs already being taken or with underlying medical or psychological conditions.

AGING AND PHARMACOLOGY

Several age-related biological and physiological changes are relevant to drug pharmacology (Table 14-5). With the exception of changes in renal function, however, the effects of these age-related changes on dosages of specific drugs for individual patients are variable and difficult to predict. In general, an understanding of the physiological status of each patient (taking into account factors such as state of hydration, nutrition, and cardiac output) and how that status affects the pharmacology of a particular drug is more important to clinical efficacy than are age-related changes. Given these caveats, the effects of aging on each pharmacological process are briefly discussed below.

Absorption

Several aging changes occur that could potentially affect drug absorption (Table 14-5). Studies of several drugs, however, have failed to document any clinically meaningful alterations in drug absorption with increasing age. Absorption, therefore, appears to be the pharmacologic parameter least affected by increasing age.

Distribution

In contrast to absorption, clinically meaningful changes in drug distribution can occur with increasing age. Serum albumin, the major drug-binding protein, tends to decline, especially in hospitalized patients. Although the decline is numerically small, it can have a substantial effect on the amount of free drug available for action. This

Table 14-5   Age-Related Changes Relevant to Drug Pharmacology

Pharmacological parameter	Age-related changes
Absorption	Decreases in
	Absorptive surface
	Splanchnic blood flow
	Increased gastric pH
	Altered gastrointestinal motility
Distribution	Decreases in
	Total body water
	Lean body mass
	Serum albumin
	Increased fat
	Altered protein binding
Metabolism	Decreases in
	Liver blood flow
	Enzyme activity
	Enzyme inducibility
Excretion	Decreases in
	Renal blood flow
	Glomerular filtration rate
	Tubular secretory function
Tissue sensitivity	Alterations in
	Receptor number
	Receptor affinity
	Second messenger function
	Cellular and nuclear responses

effect is of particular relevance for highly protein-bound drugs, especially when they are used simultaneously and compete for protein-binding sites (see Table 14-3). Alterations in protein binding itself may occur with increasing age, but the clinical relevance of these changes is not known.

Age-related changes in body composition can prominently affect pharmacology by altering the volume of distribution (Vd). The elimination half-life of a drug varies with the ratio Vd/drug clearance. Thus, even if the rate of clearance of a drug is unchanged with age, changes in Vd can affect the drug half-life and duration of action.

Because total body water and lean body mass decline with increasing age, drugs that distribute in these body compartments (such as most antimicrobial agents, digoxin, lithium, and alcohol) may have a lower Vd and can, therefore, achieve higher concentrations from given amounts of drugs.

On the other hand, drugs that distribute in body fat (such as most of the psychotropic agents) have a large Vd in the elderly. The larger Vd will thus cause a prolongation of the $t_{1/2}$, unless the clearance increases proportionately (which is unlikely to happen with increasing age).

Metabolism

The effects of aging on drug metabolism are complex and difficult to predict. They depend on the precise pathway of drug metabolism in the liver and on several other factors (such as sex and amount of smoking). There is increasing evidence that the first, or preparative, phase of drug metabolism (including oxidations, reductions, and hydrolyses) declines with increasing age, and that the decline is more prominent in men than in women. In contrast, the second phase of drug metabolism (biotransformation, including acetylation and glucuronidation) appears to be less affected by age (Greenblatt et al., 1982). There is also evidence that the ability of environmental factors (most importantly, smoking) to induce drug-metabolizing enzymes declines with age.

Although many studies of drug metabolism in relation to age have been carried out, their results are preliminary and, in many cases, conflicting. Thus, unless liver function is obviously impaired (by intrinsic liver disease, right-sided congestive heart failure, etc.), the effects of aging on the metabolism of specific drugs cannot be predicted at the present time. It is *not* safe to assume, however, that elderly patients with normal liver function tests can metabolize drugs as efficiently as can younger individuals.

Excretion

Unlike metabolism, the effects of aging on renal functions are somewhat more predictable. The tendency for renal function to decline with increasing age can affect the pharmacokinetics of several drugs (and their active metabolites) that are eliminated predominantly by the kidney (Table 14-6). These drugs will be cleared from the body more slowly, their half-lives (and duration of action) will be

Table 14-6 Important Considerations in Prescribing for the Elderly

Drug	Major route of elimination	Other pharmacological considerations	Other considerations
Analgesics			
Nonnarcotic			
Acetaminophen	Hepatic	No substantial age-related change in kinetics	Analgesic effects for noninflammatory condition similar to aspirin and other anti-inflammatory agents
Aspirin	Renal	Highly protein-bound Half-life may be prolonged at higher dosages	Enteric-coated preparations useful Blood levels may be helpful
Nonsteroidal anti-inflammatory agents	Renal (naproxen, ibuprofen) Hepatic (indomethacin)	Highly protein-bound	See Chapter 8
Narcotic	Hepatic	Blood levels may be higher, pain relief longer	Lower doses generally effective for analgesia Constipation a major problem
Antimicrobials			
Antibacterial			
Aminoglycosides (gentamicin, tobramycin, amikacin)	Renal	Half-life prolonged	Nephrotoxicity and ototoxicity are major problems Blood levels important
Cephalosporins	Renal	Half-life prolonged	
Clindamycin	Hepatic		
Erythromycin.	Hepatic		
Penicillins	Renal Hepatic (nafcillin, cloxacillin)	Half-life prolonged Highly protein-bound (nafcillin, cloxacillin, oxacillin)	Carbenicillin in high parenteral doses gives a large sodium load
Sulfonamides	Renal	Highly protein-bound	

353

Table 14-6 Important Considerations in Prescribing for the Elderly (Continued)

Drug	Major route of elimination	Other pharmacological considerations	Other considerations
Tetracyclines	Renal Hepatic (doxycycline)	Half-life prolonged	
Antituberculous			
Ethambutol	Renal		
Isoniazid	Hepatic	Genetic variation in rate of metabolism; no substantial age-related change	Hepatotoxicity increases with age
Rifampin	Hepatic		
Antifungal			
Amphotericin	Nonrenal		Nephrotoxicity a major problem
Antiparkinsonian agents			
Amantadine	Renal		
Bromocriptine	Hepatic		
Carbidopa-levodopa	Hepatic		Cardiovascular toxicity increased in elderly
Trihexyphenidyl	Nonrenal		
Cardiovascular drugs			
Antiarrhythmic			
Disopyramide	Renal, hepatic		Can cause urinary retention
Encainide	Hepatic		
Lidocaine	Hepatic	Volume of distribution increased Half-life prolonged Clearance unchanged	Blood levels helpful

Drug	Elimination	Effect	Comments
Procainamide	Renal	Clearance decreased Steady-state levels higher	Blood levels helpful
Quinidine	Nonrenal	Highly protein-bound Clearance decreased Half-life prolonged	Blood levels helpful
Tocainide	Renal, hepatic		
Verapamil	Hepatic	Clearance decreased Pharmacological effects more pronounced and prolonged	Interacts with and raises digoxin blood levels
Anticoagulant			
Heparin	Nonrenal		
Sulfinpyrazone	Renal	Highly protein-bound	
Warfarin	Hepatic	Sensitivity to effects increased	Bleeding complications increased
Antihypertensives			See Chapter 9 for more detailed discussion of antihypertensive therapy
Atenolol	Renal		
Captopril	Renal		
Clonidine	Renal		
Diltiazem	Hepatic	Clearance decreased	Use carefully with sinus node dysfunction
Enalapril	Renal	Pharmacological effects more pronounced and prolonged	
Hydralazine	Hepatic	Highly protein-bound	
Metoprolol	Hepatic	Blood levels higher	
Methyldopa	Renal		
Nadolol	Renal		
Nifedipine	Hepatic		
Propranolol	Hepatic	Highly protein-bound Blood levels higher Clearance decreased Half-life prolonged Sensitivity to effects decreased	

Table 14-6   Important Considerations in Prescribing for the Elderly (Continued)

Drug	Major route of elimination	Other pharmacological considerations	Other considerations
Prazosin	Hepatic	Highly protein-bound	
Reserpine	Renal		
Diuretics			
Furosemide	Renal	Highly protein-bound	Elderly predisposed to dehydration and electrolyte imbalance
Thiazides	Renal		Potassium supplementation not always necessary
			Glucose intolerance or diabetes may worsen
Triamterene	Hepatic		Many elderly with heart failure and sinus rhythm may not need digoxin (see Chapter 9)
Digoxin	Renal (15–40% nonrenal)	Decreased clearance Half-life prolonged	
Hypoglycemic agents			
Oral			
Acetohexamide	Hepatic, renal	Highly protein-bound (all oral hypoglycemics)	See Chapter 10 for more detailed discussion of hypoglycemic therapy in the elderly
Chlorpropamide	Renal	Long half-life	May cause hypomatremia
Glipizide	Hepatic		
Glyburide	Hepatic		
Tolazamide	Hepatic		
Tolbutamide	Hepatic		

Drug	Elimination	Pharmacokinetics	Comments
Insulin	Hepatic, renal	Renal metabolism may be decreased Sensitivity to effects may be decreased	

Psychotropic drugs

Drug	Elimination	Pharmacokinetics	Comments
Antidepressants (tricyclic, tetracyclic)	Hepatic	Highly protein-bound Blood levels may be higher	See Chapter 5 for more detailed discussion of antidepressant drugs Blood levels important See Tables 14-9, 14-11
Lithium	Renal	Clearance decreased	
Antipsychotics	Hepatic	Highly protein-bound	See Tables 14-10, 14-11
Sedatives and hypnotics			
Benzodiazepines	Hepatic Renal (oxazepam)	Highly protein-bound Diazepam half-life prolonged	
Chloral hydrate	Hepatic	Highly protein-bound	
Diphenhydramine	Hepatic	Highly protein-bound	Anticholinergic side effects may be a problem

Other drugs

Drug	Elimination	Pharmacokinetics	Comments
Aminophylline	Hepatic	Half-life prolonged	Lower doses may give therapeutic blood levels Blood levels helpful
Cimetidine	Renal	Half-life prolonged Steady-state blood levels higher	Can cause mental changes at high doses
Phenytoin	Hepatic	Steady-state blood levels higher Highly protein-bound	Blood levels helpful
Propylthiouracil	Hepatic, renal		
Terbutaline	Hepatic		
Thyroxine	Hepatic	Clearance decreased	Maintenance dose lower Effects can be monitored by TSH blood levels (see Chapter 10)

prolonged, and there will be a tendency to accumulate to higher (and potentially toxic) drug concentrations in the steady state.

Several considerations are important in determining the effects of age on renal function and drug elimination:

1   There is wide interindividual variation in the rate of decline of renal function with increasing age. Thus, although renal function is said to decline by 50 percent between the ages of 20 and 90, this is an *average* decline. A 90-year-old individual may not have a creatinine clearance of only 50 percent of normal. Applying average declines to individual elderly patients could result in over- or underdosing.

2   Muscle mass declines with age; therefore, daily endogenous creatinine production declines. Because of this decline in creatinine production, serum creatinine may be normal at a time when renal function is substantially reduced. Serum creatinine, therefore, does not reflect renal function as accurately in the elderly as it does in younger persons.

3   A number of factors can affect renal clearance of drugs and are often at least as important as age-related changes. State of hydration, cardiac output, and intrinsic renal disease, among other factors, should be considered in addition to age-related changes in renal function.

Several formulas and nomograms have been used to estimate renal function in relation to age. One such formula, validated by direct measurements of creatinine clearance, is shown in Table 14-7. This formula is useful in *initial estimations* of creatinine clearance for the purpose of drug dosing in the elderly. Clinical factors (such as state of hydration and cardiac output), which vary over time, should be considered when determining drug dosages.

When using drugs with narrow therapeutic-toxic ratios, actual

Table 14-7   Renal Function in Relation to Age

$$\text{Creatinine clearance} = \frac{(140 - \text{age}) \times \text{body weight (kg)}}{72 \times \text{serum creatinine level}}$$

Note: Several other factors can influence creatinine clearance (see text). For women, multiply by 0.85.
Source: Cockcroft and Gault, 1976.

measurements of creatinine clearance and drug blood levels (when available) should be utilized.

Tissue Sensitivity

A proportion of the drug (or its active metabolite) will eventually reach its site of action. Age-related changes at this point, i.e., in responsiveness to given drug concentrations (without regard to pharmacokinetic changes), are termed *pharmacodynamic changes*. Elderly persons are often said to be more sensitive to the effects of drugs. For some drugs, this appears to be true. For others, however, sensitivity to drug effects may decrease rather than increase with age. For example, elderly persons seem to be more sensitive to the sedative effects of given blood levels of benzodiazepine drugs (e.g., diazepam) but less sensitive to the effects of drugs that are mediated by beta-adrenergic receptors (e.g., isoproterenol, propranolol). There are several possible explanations for these changes (see Table 14-5). Until further research is done, however, the effects of age-related pharmacodynamic changes on dosages of specific drugs for individual elderly patients remain unknown.

PRESCRIBING FOR THE ELDERLY

General Principles

There is no simple rule for prescribing drugs for the elderly. Certain factors that influence drug pharmacology, such as changes in renal function, are readily quantifiable; thus specific recommendations for prescribing drugs in patients with renal failure can be made (Bennett et al., 1987).

Several considerations make the development of specific recommendations for drug prescribing in the elderly very difficult. These include:

1 Multiple interacting factors influence age-related changes in drug pharmacology.
2 There is wide interindividual variation in the rate of age-related changes in physiological parameters that affect drug pharma-

cology. Thus, precise predictions for individual elderly persons are difficult to make.

3 The clinical status of each patient (including such factors as state of nutrition and hydration, cardiac output, intrinsic renal and liver disease) must be considered in addition to the effects of aging.

4 Research in geriatric pharmacology is just beginning; as more studies are carried out in well-defined groups of elderly subjects, more specific recommendations might be possible.

Adherence to several general principles can make drug therapy in the elderly safer and more effective (Table 14-8). Cardiovascular drugs, which account for a substantial proportion of adverse drug reactions in the elderly, are also discussed in Chapter 9. Because psychotropic drugs are so commonly used and potentially toxic, they are discussed in greater detail below.

Table 14-8 General Recommendations for Prescribing for the Elderly

1. Evaluate elderly patients thoroughly in order to identify all conditions that could (a) benefit from drug treatment; (b) be adversely affected by drug treatment; (c) influence the efficacy of drug treatment
2. Manage medical conditions without drugs as often as possible
3. Know the pharmacology of the drug(s) being prescribed
4. Consider how the clinical status of each patient could influence the pharmacology of the drug(s)
5. Avoid potential adverse drug interactions
6. For drugs or their active metabolites eliminated predominantly by the kidney, use a formula or nomogram to approximate age-related changes in renal function and adjust dosages accordingly
7. If there is a question about drug dosage, start with smaller doses and increase gradually
8. Drug blood concentrations can be helpful in monitoring several potentially toxic drugs used frequently in the elderly
9. Help to ensure compliance by paying attention to impaired intellectual function, diminished hearing, and poor vision when instructing patients and labeling prescriptions (and by using other techniques listed in Table 14-1)
10. Monitor elderly patients frequently for compliance, drug effects, and toxicity

GERIATRIC PSYCHOPHARMACOLOGY

Psychotropic drugs can be broadly categorized as antidepressants (discussed in detail in Chapter 5), antipsychotics (Table 14-9), and sedatives and hypnotics (Table 14-10). These drugs are probably the most misused and overused class of drugs in the geriatric population. Several studies have shown that over half of nursing home residents are prescribed at least one psychotropic drug (Buck, 1988), and frequently these prescriptions are inappropriate (Ray et al., 1980). This is of special concern because of the frequency of adverse reactions to these drugs (see below).

Several considerations can be helpful in preventing the misuse of psychotropic drugs in the elderly:

1 Psychological symptoms (depression, anxiety, agitation, insomnia, paranoia, disruptive behavior), are often caused or exacerbated by medical conditions in elderly patients. A thorough medical evaluation should therefore be done before symptoms are attributed to psychiatric conditions alone and psychotropic drugs are prescribed.

2 Reports of psychiatric symptomatology such as agitation are often presented to physicians by family care givers and nursing home personnel who are inexperienced in the description, interpretation, and differential diagnosis of these symptoms (Cohen-Mansfield and Billig, 1986). "Agitation" or "disruptive behavior" may, in fact, have been a reasonable response to an inappropriate interaction or situation created by the care giver. Psychotropic drugs should, therefore, be prescribed only after the physician is clear as to what the symptoms are and what correctable factors might have precipitated them.

3 Psychological symptoms and signs, like physical symptoms and signs, can be nonspecific in the elderly. Paranoid psychosis, for example, can be the manifestation of an underlying depression. Therefore, appropriate drug treatment often depends on an accurate psychiatric diagnosis. Psychiatrists and psychologists experienced with elderly patients should be consulted when available in order to identify and help target psychotropic drug treatment to the major psychiatric problem(s).

4 Many treatment modalities can either replace or be used in conjunction with psychotropic drugs in managing psychological

Table 14-9 Examples of Antipsychotic Agents

Drug (brand name)	Relative potency	Approximate dosage, mg*	Relative sedation	Potential for side effects	
				Hypotension	Extrapyramidal effects†
Chlorpromazine, (Thorazine, etc.)	1	10–300	Very high	High	Moderate
Thioridazine (Mellaril)	1	10–300	High	Moderate	Low
Thiothixene (Navane)	25	1–5	Low	Low	Very high
Haloperidol (Haldol)	50	0.25–6	Low	Low	Very high

*Per day in three or four divided doses.
†Rigidity, bradykinesia, tremor, akathisia.

Table 14-10 Examples of Sedatives and Hypnotic Agents

Drug (brand name)	Approximate dose equivalent, mg	Relative rapidity of effect after oral administration	Half-life, h	Active metabolites
Benzodiazepines				
Longer-acting				
Diazepam (Valium)	5	Very fast	20–100	Yes
Clorazepate (Tranxene)	7.5	Fast	30–200	Yes
Flurazepam*† (Dalmane)	15	Fast	40–200	Yes
Shorter-acting				
Triazolam* (Halcion)	0.25	Intermediate	2–5	No
Lorazepam (Ativan)	1	Intermediate	10–20	No
Oxazepam (Serax)	15	Slow	5–15	No
Temazepam* (Restoril)	15	Fast	5–15	No
Alprazolam (Xanax)	0.25	Fast	6–20	No
Antihistamines				
Diphenhydramine* (Benadryl, etc.)	25	Fast	4–7	No
Hydroxyzine (Vistaril, Atarax)	10	Very fast	Unknown‡	Unknown
Other				
Chloral hydrate* (Noctec, etc.)	500	Fast	7–10	Yes

*More commonly used as hypnotics.
†When used as a hypnotic in dosages of more than 15 mg, daytime drowsiness, confusion, and ataxia commonly occur in the elderly.
‡Duration of action 4 to 6 h.

symptoms in the elderly. Behavioral modification, environmental manipulation, supportive psychotherapy, group therapy, and other related techniques can be useful in eliminating or diminishing the need for drug treatment.

5 Within each broad category of psychotropic drug, there are considerable differences among individual agents with regard to effects, side effects, and potential interactions with other drugs and medical conditions. Rational prescription of these drugs requires careful consideration of the characteristics of each drug in relation to the individual patient.

6 Because elderly patients are, in general, more sensitive to the effects and side effects of psychotropic drugs, initial doses should be lower, increases should be gradual, and monitoring should be frequent.

7 Careful, ongoing assessment of the response of target symptoms and behaviors to psychotropic drugs is essential. In addition to reports from patients themselves, objective observations by trained and experienced professionals should be continuously evaluated in order to adjust psychotropic drug therapy.

All psychotropic drugs must be used judiciously in the elderly because of their potential side effects. The most common and potentially disabling side effects of psychotropic drugs fall into four general categories: changes in cognitive status (e.g., sedation, delirium, dementia) and extrapyramidal, anticholinergic, and cardiovascular effects. Recent studies have documented that psychotropic drugs can contribute to global cognitive impairment (Larson et al., 1987) and are associated with hip fractures in the elderly population (Ray et al., 1987).

Anticholinergic and cardiovascular side effects are most prominent with the tricyclic antidepressants [see Table 5-12; also Risch et al. (1981)]. Antipsychotic drugs with alpha-adrenergic-blocking properties, including chlorpromazine and thioridazine, also have cardiovascular side effects, most notably hypotension. Extrapyramidal side effects are most common with antipsychotic drugs (Table 14-9). These effects include pseudoparkinsonism (rigidity, bradykinesia, tremor), akathisia (restlessness), and involuntary dystonic movements (such as tardive dyskinesia). These side effects can be severe and cause substantial disability. Rigidity and bradykinesia can lead to immobility and the complications discussed in Chapter 8. Akathisia can make the patient appear more anxious and agitated and lead to the inappropriate prescription of more medication. Tardive dyskinesia can cause permanent disability because of continuous orolingual movements and difficulty with eating.

Although CNS neuropharmacology is very complex and incompletely understood, the basic relationship between the cholinergic and dopaminergic neurotransmitter systems is helpful in understanding the clinical effects (and side effects) of several of the psychotropic drugs. Cholinergic and dopaminergic influences are normally balanced within the central nervous system (Figure 14-3, top). These neurotransmitter relationships have been most intensely studied in the nigrostriatal system. Factors that diminish dopaminergic tone, such as the depletion of dopaminergic neurons in the basal ganglia in Parkinson's disease and phenothiazine-like drugs (which block dopamine receptors), cause a relative increase in cholinergic tone (Figure 14-3, center). Clinically this is manifest by extrapyramidal syndromes. Thus patients treated with haloperidol, thiothixene, chlorpromazine, and other related drugs often develop pseudoparkinsonism (or underlying Parkinson's disease is worsened), akathisia, or tardive dyskinesia. Tardive dyskinesia (repetitive involuntary movements, usually involving the tongue and mouth) is a side effect of long-term treatment with phenothiazine-like drugs and is thought to be related to a "supersensitivity" of dopamine receptors. Although it may respond to increased doses of the phenothiazine (which further blocks dopamine receptors), it has proven unresponsive to most other agents and is often irreversible.

Anticholinergic drugs and dopaminergic agonists (levodopa, bromocriptine, amantadine; see Chapter 8) tip the balance back toward dopamine (Figure 14-3, bottom). Thus anticholinergic drugs are useful in treating both Parkinson's disease and extrapyramidal movement disorders in which there is a relative lack of dopamine. Clinically, dopamine excess can manifest itself by movement disorders (such as choreiform movements) and hallucinations (Figure 14-3, bottom).

Gamma-aminobutyric acid (GABA) is a central neurotransmitter with a negative influence on the dopamine system (Figure 14-3, top). Patients with Huntington's chorea are deficient in GABA, which results in a relative dopamine excess (Figure 14-3, bottom). Benzodiazepine drugs have, among other effects, a net positive effect

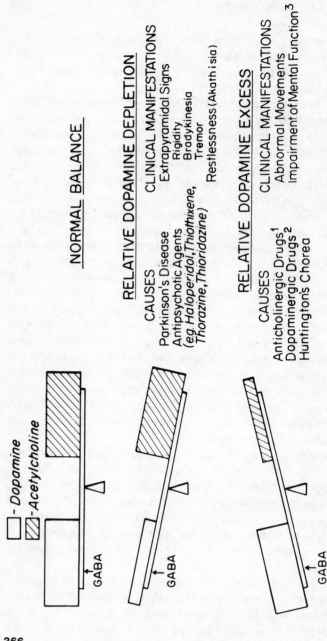

Figure 14-3 Diagrammatic representation of neurotransmitter balance in the nigrostriatal system: (1) e.g., tricyclic antidepressants, certain antiparkinsonian agents, decongestants, and bladder relaxants; (2) e.g., levodopa, bromocriptine, and amantadine; (3) anticholinergic drugs can cause confusion or psychoses; dopaminergic drugs can cause hallucinations and psychoses at higher doses.

on the GABA system and thus are sometimes helpful in the management of movement disorders resulting from excess dopamine.

The preceding discussion, as well as Figure 14-3, is greatly oversimplified, and the complexity of central neurotransmitter relationships should be emphasized. From a clinical perspective, however, these concepts are helpful in understanding the effects and side effects of several psychotropic drugs.

Optimal efficacy of psychotropic drugs requires consideration of characteristics of the drugs in relation to several clinical factors in each patient (Table 14-11). For example, depressed elderly patients with psychomotor retardation may do better with a less sedating antidepressant, whereas those with psychomotor agitation may do better with a more sedating antidepressant (see Chapter 5).

Antipsychotic drugs such as haloperidol (Haldol) and thiothixene (Navane) (Table 14-9) are among the most commonly misused psychotropic drugs. Given the potentially severe and disabling side effects of these drugs, they should be used as infrequently as possible. Unfortunately, there is a tendency to treat agitated elderly patients with an antipsychotic drug without first seeking an underlying cause for the agitation. When an elderly patient becomes agitated (or agitation rapidly worsens), an acute physical illness should be excluded or treated if found. If the agitated patient is depressed, a sedating antidepressant is probably more appropriate than an antipsychotic or a sedative (which might worsen the depression).

In general, the antipsychotic agents should be reserved for treatment of psychoses (i.e., paranoid states, delusions, and hallucinations). Although they are sedating, they are generally less so than adequate dosages of sedatives and are certainly less safe. Much of their "sedative" effect may, in fact, be caused by their pseudoparkinsonian side effects. (Patients become rigid and immobile and appear sedated.) In addition, some patients develop akathisia (restlessness, the jitters) and can appear even more agitated, which, in turn, sometimes leads to an increase in dosage. Identifying the akathisia and switching to a sedative drug is more appropriate. Increasing the antipsychotic dose in these instances is incorrect. There are occasional situations with severely demented elderly patients in which agitation is profound or behavior is excessively disruptive and sedatives are inappropriate or ineffective. Antipsychotics may be helpful in these cases.

Table 14-11 Clinical Considerations in Prescribing Psychotropic Drugs

Clinical indicator	Mose useful types	Comments
Depression with psychomotor retardation	Less sedating antidepressant (e.g., desipramine, nortriptyline)	In choosing antidepressants for the elderly, other considerations are important: anticholinergic effects, potential cardiovascular effects, and potential interactions with antihypertensives (see Chapter 5)
Depression with psychomotor agitation	More sedating antidepressant (e.g., doxepin, trazodone)	
Agitation without psychosis	Short-acting sedative (e.g., alprazolam, oxazepam, lorazepam, hydroxyzine)	Should generally be used on prn basis Nonpharmacological interventions may be more appropriate Can worsen depression
Psychoses without prominent agitation (e.g., delusions and hallucinations in patients with depression or dementia)	Less sedating antipsychotic (e.g., haloperidol, thiothixene)	Extrapyramidal effects may be prominent
Severe agitation poorly controlled by a sedative	More sedating antipsychotic (e.g., thioridazine)	Stronger antipsychotics (haloperidol, thiothixene) sometimes needed Extrapyramidal effects may be prominent Akathisia can make patient appear more agitated
Insomnia	Chloral hydrate Temazepam, triazolam	Underlying cause(s) should be sought Nonpharmacological interventions often helpful (see Chapter 5)

Nonpharmacologic measures (such as individual or group psychotherapy, behavior modification, and activity programs) can be effective in elderly patients with agitation or excessive anxiety; however, these measures are often unavailable, impractical, inappropriate, or unsuccessful. Patients with severe impairment of cognitive function can be especially difficult to manage with nonpharmacological measures alone, particularly when their agitation is interfering with their care (or the care of others around them). Thus, drug treatment of agitation is necessary in some elderly patients. In general, this is best accomplished by using a short-acting sedative such as alprazolam, oxazepam, or lorazepam or (Table 14-10). If antipsychotic drugs are prescribed, initial doses should be very low (e.g., 0.5 mg of haloperidol or 10 mg of thioridazine).

Insomnia, like agitation, can be the manifestation of depression or physical illness. It is a very common complaint in elderly patients and is discussed in greater detail in Chapter 5. Again, nonpharmacological measures (such as increasing activity during the day, prescribing a glass of warm milk or even a small drink of wine or whiskey) are sometimes helpful. When a drug is needed, chloral hydrate or small doses of a benzodiazepine (e.g., temazepam, triazolam) are often effective (Table 14-10). The long-term effects of chronic hypnotic use in the elderly are unknown, but rebound insomnia can become a problem in patients who use hypnotics regularly and then discontinue them. Whatever the indication, it is extremely important that after a psychotropic drug is prescribed, the patient is closely monitored for the effects of the drug on the target symptoms and side effects, and that the drug regimen be adjusted accordingly.

REFERENCES

Bennett WM, Aronoff GR, Golper TA, et al: *Drug Prescribing in Renal Failure: Dosing Guidelines for Adults.* Philadelphia: American College of Physicians, 1987.

Buck JA: Psychotropic Drug Practice in Nursing Homes. *J Am Geriatr Soc* 36:409–418, 1988.

Caranasos GJ, Stewart RB, Cluff LE: Drug-induced illness leading to hospitalization. *JAMA* 288:713–717, 1974.

Cockcroft DW, Gault MH: Predictions of creatinine clearance from serum creatinine. *Nephron* 16:31–41, 1976.

Cohen-Mansfield J, Billig N: Agitated behaviors in the elderly. *J Am Geriatr Soc* 34:711–721, 1986.

Greenblatt DJ, Sellers EM, Shader RI: Drug therapy: Drug disposition in old age. *N Engl J Med* 306:1081–1088, 1982.

Larson EB, Kukull WA, Buchner D, et al: Adverse drug reactions associated with global cognitive impairment in elderly persons. *Ann Intern Med* 107:169–173, 1987.

Medical Letter on Drugs and Therapeutics: Adverse Drug Interactions, Vol 23, No 5, March 6, 1981.

Ray WA, Federspeil CF, Schaffner W: A study of antipsychotic drug use in nursing homes: Epidemiologic evidence suggesting misuse. *Am J Public Health* 70:485–491, 1980.

Ray WA, Griffin MR, Schaffner W, et al: Psychotropic drug use and the risk of hip fracture. *N Engl J Med* 316:363–369, 1987.

Risch SC, Groom GP, Janowsky DS: Interfaces of psychopharmacology and cardiology: Parts I and II. *J Clin Psychol* 42:23–34; 47–59, 1981.

Seidel LG, Thornton GF, Smith JW, et al: Studies on the epidemiology of adverse drug reactions. III: Reactions in patients on a general medical service. *Bull Johns Hopkins Hosp* 119:299–315, 1966.

U.S. Congress. Subcommittee on Aging and Subcommittee on Long Term Care: *Drugs in Nursing Home: Misuse, High Cost, and Kickbacks.* U.S. Government Printing Office, 1976.

Williamson J, Chopin JM: Adverse reactions to prescribed drugs in the elderly: A multicentre investigation. *Age Ageing* 9:73–80, 1980.

SUGGESTED READINGS

Balant-Gorgia AE, Balant L: Antipsychotic drugs: Clinical pharmacokinetics of potential candidates for plasma concentration monitoring. *Clin Pharmacokinet* 13:65–90, 1987.

Conrad KA, Bressler R (eds): *Drug Therapy for the Elderly.* St Louis, Mosby, 1982.

Dement WC: Rational basis for the use of sleeping pills. Pharmacology 27(suppl 2):3–38, 1983/*Internatl Pharmacopsychiatr* 17(supp 2):3–38, 1982.

Foley KM: The Treatment of Cancer Pain. *N Engl J Med* 313(2):84–95, 1985.

Greenblatt DJ, Shader RI, Abernathy DR: Current status of the benzodiazepines. *N Engl J Med* 309:354–358; 410–416, 1983.

Kaye D: Prophylaxis for infective endocarditis: An update. *Ann Intern Med* 104:419–423, 1986.

Lamy PD: *Prescribing for the Elderly*. Littleton, MA, PSG Publishing, 1980.

Nolan L, O'Malley K: Prescribing for the elderly: Part II. Prescribing patterns: Differences due to age. *J Am Geriatr Soc* 36:245–254, 1988.

Ouslander JG: Drug therapy in the elderly. *Ann Intern Med* 95:711–722, 1981.

Plein JB, Plein EM: Aging and drug therapy. *Ann Rev Gerontol Geriatr* 2:211–254, 1981.

Richelson E: Psychotropics and the elderly: Interactions to watch for. *Geriatrics* 39:30–42, 1984.

Roe DA: Diet-drug interactions and incompatibilities, in Hathcock JN, Coon DJ (eds): *Nutrition and Drug Interrelations*. New York, Academic, 1978.

Rossenbaum JF: The drug treatment of anxiety. *N Engl J Med* 306:401–404, 1982.

Sackett DL: Rules of evidence and clinical recommendations on the use of antithrombotic agents. *Arch Intern Med* 146:464–472, 1986.

Salzman C: *Clinical Geriatric Psychopharmacology*. New York, McGraw-Hill, 1984.

Schwartz JB, Abernethy DR: Cardiac drugs: Adjusting their use in aging patients. *Geriatrics* 42:31–38, 1987.

Thompson TL, Moran MG, Nies AS: Psychotropic drug use in the elderly: Parts 1 and 2. *N Engl J Med* 308:134–138; 194–199, 1983.

Chapter 15

Developing Clinical Expectations

Attitudes about the elderly tend to carry over into their care. Elderly patients are in danger of being dismissed as hopeless or not worth the effort. The physician faced with the question of how much time and resources to spend in searching for a diagnosis will want to consider the probability of benefit for the investment. In some cases, older patients are better investments than younger ones. This apparent paradox occurs in the case of some preventive strategies when high risk of susceptibility and the discounted benefits of future health favor the elderly. But it also arises in situations where small increments of change can yield dramatic differences.

Perhaps the most striking example of the latter is found in the case of nursing home patients. Very modest changes in their routine, such as introducing a pet, giving them a plant to tend, or increasing their sense of control over their environment, can produce dramatic improvement in mood and morale (Kane and Kane, 1987).

The narrowed therapeutic window discussed in Chapter 13

argues for more stringent monitoring of the effects of therapeutic interventions. Not only must the actual dosage be ascertained (the amount taken as opposed to the amount prescribed), it must be related to specific changes in performance, either behavioral, physical, or chemical. The management requires careful titration, which, in turn, suggests the need for a careful record that relates dose and effects.

A flowchart is ideally suited to this task. The data selected should represent those parameters that are both significant and most likely to be affected. Because the changes are likely to be subtle, it is often helpful to establish treatment goals with time frames for achieving them. Both the health care team and the patient can then agree on expectations and follow progress toward the goal. It is important that the goals be achievable. Small successes are very important and reinforcing. Thus the units of measurement should be capable of detecting small but meaningful changes.

In many instances, small gains can, in fact, make an enormous difference. The stroke patient, for example, who regains the use of hand muscles greatly improves the ability to function. Being able to change position in bed may be the difference between getting pressure sores and not. Regaining a method of communication, whether by speech or some other means, can restore social contact.

By introducing gradual, small steps, a functional task may appear more achievable. We have all had some experience in getting a bedfast patient to resume a more active role. For an older person who has been at bed rest for a long period, this task requires overcoming both physiological and psychological problems. Small steps will often ease the transition and provide an opportunity to monitor the effects at each stage to minimize risk.

A BENCHMARK APPROACH

We noted earlier in this book that change over time was a hallmark of aging. The basic paradigm consists of gradual decline until a clinical threshold is reached. Medical care for the elderly can respond to this paradigm by altering its approach to take greater cognizance of the pattern. Rather than relying on a fixed plan of periodic contacts determined by the calendar, the physician would do better to use the patient's change over time as a barometer to indicate when intervention is required.

Such an approach requires us to make a prognosis: a prediction of the expected course for the patient. As long as the patient stays on course, minimal intervention is needed beyond simply monitoring progress. The emphasis shifts from routine examination to specific monitoring for predetermined evidence of deviation from the expected course. The earliest sign of such deviation becomes the signal for reevaluation.

The heart of such a system is the set of prognoses and the criteria for predicted progress. The latter are termed *benchmarks*. Ideally each physician would evaluate each patient as a unique combination of problems and potential. However, the costs involved may prove prohibitive in view of time pressures. An alternative is to use a previously conceived set of basic benchmarks geared to the common problems of geriatrics. The generation of a problem list then leads to the implementation of the appropriate benchmarks. These can be modified to fit the more specific characteristics of a given patient. A great advantage of this approach lies in its capacity to enhance delegation. The benchmarks provide a structure to guide ongoing information gathering. They target the pertinent information and can even offer general guidelines about what steps to take when the observed results deviate from those expected. (These actions are usually couched in terms of varying stages of urgency for seeking help.) The benchmark system does not preclude gathering additional data or recognizing the development of a new problem.

One setting ideally suited to such an approach is the nursing home. Because the system guides the collection of information and relates each item to one or more specific problems, it has an educational role as well as a clinical one. Nursing home staff who may feel isolated from the infrequently seen physician now have a more effective means of communication. They know what information is being sought and why. They have a format for recording that data, which offers desired information.

The benchmark system was, in fact, developed for use in the nursing home and has been used effectively in that setting (Woolley et al., 1974). Because the general level of literacy among the nursing home aides was quite low, the system was specifically designed to require minimal narrative by using symbols in a flowchart format.

Table 15-1 presents a sample set of benchmark criteria for hip fracture. The two scales referred to—independence and behavior—

Table 15-1 Example of Benchmark Instructions: Hip Fracture

Observation	Frequency	Benchmark	Action
1. Independence scale score	Every 2 weeks	Decreased score or no change in 6 weeks after therapy is begun	Inform physician
2. Behavioral scale score	Every 2 weeks	Decreased score or no change in 6 weeks after therapy is begun	Inform physician
3. Soreness in either calf (use: R = right soreness, L = left soreness)	Daily; check by pushing foot up with knee extended	Present	Place patient on bed rest Notify physician
4. Temperature (°F)	prn increased hip pain, calf pain, malaise	Above 100° orally for 8–16 h	Notify physician Take temperature every 4–8 h if elevated
5. Contracture or stiff joint, especially foot drop, hip flexion, knee flexion, hip abducted or turned out (+ or −)	Daily	Present	Continue to position properly and give ROM* to tolerance; inform physician; chart location of contracture
6. Distance walked at one time (in yards)	Daily	Decrease over 3 days or no improvement in 1 week after therapy is begun	Inform physician
7. Pain in hip (+ for pain)	prn	No relief by medication after 24 h of administration	Notify physician

*ROM—range of motion.
Note: The charting of this information is demonstrated in Figure 15-1.
Source: Pepper et al., 1972.

were specially developed for the project but could be replaced by measures of activities of daily living and a standardized mood scale such as that for depression. Other clinicians may choose to add, delete, or modify items to fit their pattern of practice. Figure 15-1 offers a hypothetical chart for recording data pertinent to this problem. Specific narrative notes are made only when an event warrants them. The flowchart format readily shows when a change in pattern occurs and intervention is indicated.[1]

Such a system does not easily fit into the current system of regulations for physician attendance to nursing home patients. The present rules are designed to achieve at least a minimal frequency of contact with these patients (usually once a month). Unfortunately, the result is too often superficial attention to the patient's chart. The doctor's signature is the ticket to continued coverage under Medicaid. Particularly when the same system discourages frequent visits, the care of nursing home patients is neglected.

Nursing home care has never attracted a great deal of physician enthusiasm. But this need not continue to be the case. If we can implement a new form of record keeping that provides better information to staff and demands better performance from them, we should see an improvement in morale and hence a more attractive atmosphere in which to practice. It is also worth noting here that the benchmark system was originally developed for use with a nurse practitioner as the person giving primary care, under supervision of physicians. Nurse practitioners have proved themselves very effective in such care roles for nursing home patients, but they are currently precluded from functioning in that capacity by restrictions imposed by the Medicare Part B regulations, which refuse payment if the nurse practitioner is not supervised on site by a physician.

COMPUTERIZED RECORDS

The next major step in long-term care will come with the introduction of computer-driven information systems. Approaches like the benchmark system are readily suitable for computerization. Because long-term care depends so heavily on poorly educated personnel for so much of its core services, the availability of an information support

---

[1]A complete copy of the system is available from the authors.

DATE	8/12	8/13	8/14	8/15	8/16	8/17	8/18	8/19	8/20	8/21	8/22	8/23	8/24	8/25	8/27
Hip Fracture															
1. Independence Scale Score	20														
2. Behavior Scale Score								40							
3. Soreness in either calf (-, R or L	-	-	-	-	-	-	-	*R	R						
4. Contracture (+ or -)	-	+C	+	+	+*	+	+	+	-	-	-	-	-	-	-
5. Distance Walked (yds.)	10	10	11	12	13	14	15	15	C	N					
6. Temperature (°F) prn								101 F	F						

Figure 15-1 Hypothetical example of benchmark chart. The data charted correspond to those outlined in Table 15-1. C = See nurse's notes in chart, as some information about this observation was charted here on this date. F = See form appropriate for charting this observation (I&O, diabetic record, TPR graphic, etc.). * = Physician informed concerning this observation on this day. N = Not determined (*From Pepper et al., 1972.*)

system, which can provide feedback and direction, is especially appropriate.

An automated information system offers other benefits. It can eliminate redundancy by entering information only once. It can structure the way information is collected and organize the way it is displayed. For example, it is easy to incorporate into the structured assessment of persons admitted to long-term care items addressing personal preferences for items such as food, mealtimes, activities, and bedtime. By presenting these issues as part of the routine assessment, the message is subtly given that such considerations are part of routine care and not special issues.

The computer allows data to be fed back in reorganized formats. For example, it is a simple matter to convert functional scores to graphs and to plot the changes in patients or groups of patients over time. Again, much of the value is seen in reorienting thinking, from a custodial mentality to one which anticipates change. It is not a big step to go to the next increment to add information about treatments to look for relationships between what was done and what happened. Again the effort is directed toward changing perceptions about older persons, especially those in long-term care. For too long, long-term care has worked in a negative spiral—a self-fulfilling prophecy which expected patients to deteriorate discouraged both care providers and patients. Such an attitude is hardly likely to attract the best and the brightest in any of the health professions. It would be bad enough if true, but ironically, as noted earlier in this chapter, nursing home patients are among the most responsive to almost any form of intervention. Any information system that can reinforce a prospective view of long-term care, especially one that can display patient progress, represents an important adjunct to such care.

PREVENTION

The physician's concern about a patient's future and the value of that future is reflected in the patient's actions with regard to preventive activities. Enthusiasm for prevention is based on a small set of beliefs:

1 The efficacy of the intervention in preventing disease or dysfunction in the future. This includes an estimate of the likelihood of the patient's following the preventive regimen.

2 The value of the health gained. In the case of older patients, this includes concerns about the likelihood of other problems reducing the benefit.

3 The cost of the preventive activity. This includes both the direct cost and the indirect costs, such as anxiety, restricted life-style, and false-positive results.

Chapter 13 deals with the area in which prevention is most germane: iatrogenic disease. Here some of the major issues and strategies surrounding more conventional preventive activities are discussed. The major thesis here, as with much covered elsewhere in this volume, is that age alone should not be a predominant factor in choosing an approach to a patient. A number of preventive strategies deserve serious consideration in light of their immediate and future benefits for many elderly patients.

Preventive activities can be divided into three types: (1) primary prevention, where some specific action is taken to render the patient more resistant or the environment less harmful; (2) secondary prevention, or screening and early detection for asymptomatic disease or early disease; and (3) tertiary prevention, or efforts to improve care to avoid later complications. Table 15-2 offers examples of activities in each category. Not all the items indicated in Table 15-2 are supported by clear research findings. In some cases, such as seat belts, exercise, and social support, they are based on prudent judgment.

Table 15-2   Preventive Strategies for the Elderly

Primary	Secondary	Tertiary
Immunization	Pap smear	Assessment
Influenza	Breast exam	Foot care
Pneumococcal	? self-exam	Dental care
Tetanus	Mammography	Toileting efforts
Blood pressure	Fecal blood	
Smoking	Hypothyroidism	
Exercise	Depression	
Obesity	Vision	
Social support	Hearing	
Environment	Oral	
Seat belts	Tuberculosis	

In addressing prevention in the elderly, it is important to bear in mind the goals pursued. The World Health Organization (1980) has provided a useful continuum, which progresses from disease to impairment to disability to handicap. Preventive efforts for the elderly can be productively targeted at several points along this spectrum. Efforts can seek to prevent disease, but they can also be designed to minimize its consequences, by reducing the progression to disability. This is, in essence, the heart of geriatrics.

Grimley Evans (1984) has identified several ways in which preventive efforts on behalf of the elderly are special, beyond the emphasis on function. The narrowing of the therapeutic window, discussed in Chapter 13, means that older persons may be susceptible to the side effects of prevention as well as treatment. Some risk factors that strongly predict the onset of disease may not be appropriate for modification in older persons. Perhaps the condition has already become well established and is resistant to change, or the factor may have already exerted its influence at an earlier stage of life.

Clearly, primary prevention is the most desirable. If a brief encounter can confer some form of long-lasting protection at minimal risk, such a strategy will be actively pursued. Unfortunately, the number of activities that are both safe and effective is small. More often, we must rely on the other two strategies, each of which comes at a cost. Screening for one or another condition is useful where the disease process can be detected in advance of the condition's clinical appearance, but this may be excessively costly if the number of treatable cases detected is low. Screening is usually judged on the criteria of sensitivity and specificity. The former refers to the proportion of actual cases correctly identified and the latter to the accuracy of labeling of noncases (normal individuals). Alas, the two factors are usually linked so that an improvement in one comes at the cost of a decrement in the other. The decision about where to set them relative to each other depends on the expected prevalence of the problem and the consequences of a false-positive and a false-negative finding with respect to a given clinical condition. For example, the U.S. Preventive Services Task Force was skeptical about the usefulness of breast self-examination in elderly women (O'Malley and Fletcher, 1987). Moreover, physicians tend to be less enthusiastic about treating older patients with breast cancer (Greenfield et al., 1987).

At the same time, some areas are well served by increased clinical attention. Greater physician sensitivity to identifying depression in older persons can detect an often remediable condition. Detection of mental problems is greatly enhanced by structured screening data (German et al., 1987). Awareness of the likelihood of alcoholism can lead to recognition of a problem that can be corrected. There is more controversy about the desirability of increasing the recognition of cognitive deficiency. Although standardized testing can detect cases that might otherwise be masked by older persons who have skillfully compensated for their loss, it is not immediately clear that there is great benefit in such early uncovering. Indeed, the discussion of labeling in Chapter 13 addresses the problems created by such an act.

Routine screening for geriatric populations tends to uncover problems that are already known. Among a group of elderly persons coming for a health screening, 95 percent had at least one positive finding. About 55 percent were referred to a physician for further evaluation and 15 percent were treated for the finding (Rubenstein et al., 1986). Routine annual laboratory testing of nursing home residents has received mixed reviews. A recent study suggests that a modest panel, including a complete blood count, electrolytes, renal and thyroid function tests, and a urinalysis, may be useful (Levinstein et al., 1987).

Behavior change represents at once the most promising and the most frustrating of the three strategies. While some may argue that "you can't teach an old dog new tricks," or that engrained habit patterns are hard to break, there is no evidence to support such pessimism. Quite to the contrary, anecdotal data about elderly people taking up exercise programs and changing their dietary habits provide reason for more optimism. The critical issue here is the degree to which such changes will sufficiently modify risk factors to justify the disturbance.

In general, moderation seems safest. For example, data from the Alameda County study suggest that no smoking, modest physical activity, moderate weight, and regular meals are associated with lower mortality risks among the elderly (Kaplan et al., 1987). Although our data are scant, the answer will likely vary with the topic addressed. For some behaviors, there is little doubt of benefit. Exercise, for example, will clearly benefit the individual. Although its role in osteoporosis prevention remains controversial (Block et al., 1987), exercise is generally recommended as a safe approach, with more possible benefits than risks (Rodysill, 1987). Figure 15-2 shows that less than a third of older persons report regular exercise, to say nothing of vigorous activity. Although evidence suggests that very active exercise is necessary to reduce risk of cardiovascular accidents, even modest amounts of exercise will improve strength, keep joints more limber, promote a sense of well-being, and improve sleep.

There are epidemiologic data to suggest that even among quite elderly persons cessation of smoking will reduce mortality to levels of nonsmokers in a sufficiently short time to justify actively encouraging quitting (Jaijich et al., 1984). Figure 15-3 traces the change in smoking rates among the elderly from 1979 to 1985. The prevalence of current smokers has increased among older males but decreased among younger males and the youngest females. These changes likely reflect difference in cohorts as well as changes in behavior. In each

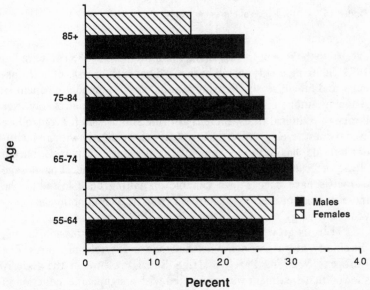

Figure 15-2   Community elderly reporting regular exercise, 1984. (*From LaCroix, 1987.*)

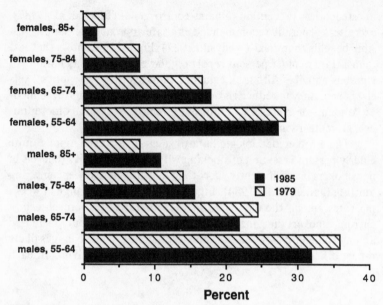

Figure 15-3   Prevalence of current smokers. (*From Havlik, 1987.*)

age group the rate of former smokers was higher in 1985 compared to 1979. Smoking cessation will have rapid benefits for risks of both vascular and lung disease. Wearing seat belts is of immediate benefit in reducing automobile fatalities. Despite the recent controversy over large-scale clinical trials, there is growing enthusiasm for controlling even modest levels of hypertension. Increased calcium, with and without fluoride, has been recommended to prevent osteoporosis, but no clearly efficacious regimen has yet been established. Low-dosage estrogens have been shown capable of halting bone loss, but the increased risk of uterine cancer has thwarted their adoption as a preventive strategy.

There is growing enthusiasm for treating hypertension among the elderly, at least for combined diastolic and systolic pressures. The European Working Party on High Blood Pressure in the Elderly showed that treatment was associated with a significant reduction in cardiac mortality, a nonsignificant reduction in cerebrovascular mortality, but no reduction in overall mortality (Amery et al., 1985).

Studies on the value of controlling pure systolic hypertension in the elderly are currently under way.

It is important to distinguish carefully between the value of uncovering elevated blood pressure and the need to control it over a sustained period. Most older persons with hypertension are aware of it; the challenge is to maintain them in a safe range without producing significant side effects. Hypertension is very common among the elderly. Figure 15-4 shows the range in prevalence of definite hypertension (systolic pressure greater than 160 mmHg, diastolic pressure greater than 90, or currently taking antihypertensives) among different groups. Black females have the highest rates, but even among white males the rate approaches 40 percent.

The effects of dietary changes are less certain. Weight loss for

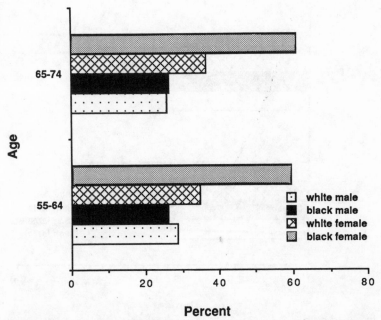

Figure 15-4 Prevalence of definite hypertension, 1976–1980. (*Note: Definite hypertension* is defined as a systolic blood pressure of 160 or more, a diastolic pressure of 90 or more, or taking antihypertensive medications.) (*From Havlik, 1987.*)

obese persons makes sense in terms of reducing cardiovascular load and in the management of adult-onset diabetes and hypertension, but hard data suggest that the benefit may be oversold, certainly for the former. The efficacy of changing diet, especially to reduce the amount of fat consumed, has not yet been clearly established.

Figure 15-5 shows that as much as 60 percent of black females are overweight (body mass index greater than 27.8 kg/m^2 for men and 27.3 for women). Cholesterol has been shown to be a risk factor for heart disease for general populations but has not been specifically tested in the elderly. As shown in Figure 15-6, females are at particular risk for this problem. Over 30 percent of white females have high-risk cholesterol levels (greater than 268 mg/dl).

In areas such as weight, cholesterol, and even blood pressure, the

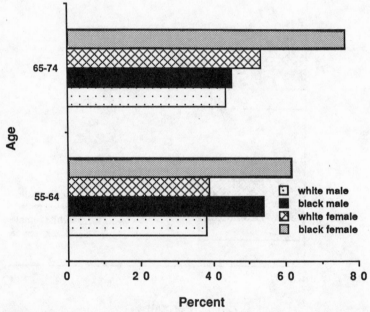

Figure 15-5   Prevalence of overweight, 1976-1980. [*Note: Overweight* is defined as body mass index above 27 kg/m^2 (85th percentile of age group 20-29).] (*From Havlik, 1987.*)

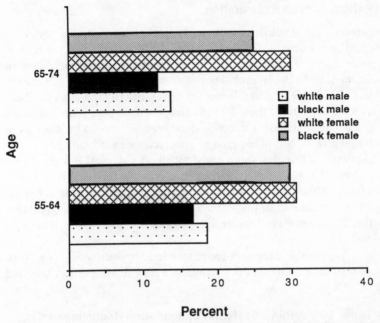

Figure 15-6   Prevalence of high-risk serum cholesterol, 1976–1980. (*Note: High risk* is defined as greater than 268 mg/dl.) (*From Havlik, 1987.*)

clinician must weigh the benefits of intervention against the costs. There is a compelling argument that overzealous activity in the name of prevention may cost more in quality of life than it gains in quality years. Some have suggested that the survivor effect should be taken more seriously. Persons who survive to old age may have demonstrated a biologic ability that deserves more respect. At the very least, any determination to change life-style at this stage in life should be made by the patient after suitable counseling.

One area of behavior with great theoretic promise but little immediate practical application is social support. There is some evidence to suggest that those older persons with strong social support systems, or at least perceived support, are at less risk for adverse events (Zuckerman et al., 1984), but it is not yet clear how one can build such a support system for those without one naturally.

Periodic Health Examination

A simple list of activities that can be incorporated into the routine of practice is offered in Table 15-3. The list is derived from the recommendations of the Canadian Task Force on the Periodic Health Examination (1979), probably the most thorough review of the subject. The procedures and frequency are essentially the same for those aged 65 to 74 as for those 75 and older; the difference is limited to the frequency of assessing functional activity—it should be done more frequently in the older group. The recommended procedures are generally in line with those urged by others (Medical Practice Committee, 1981). One main exception surrounds the pursuit of breast cancer. Although the Canadians recommend neither clinical examination nor mammography after age 59, many authorities suggest that this is an important preventive practice for the elderly female as well.

Three other areas not recommended are worthy of serious consideration. Pneumococcal vaccines are now in widespread use, and

Table 15-3   Periodic Health Examination Recommendations

	Frequency	
	Age 65–74	Age 75+
Tetanus / diphtheria immunization	Every 10 years	Every 10 years
Influenza immunization	Annually	Annually
Hearing: history and clinical testing	Periodically	Periodically
Blood pressure measurement	Every 2 years	Every 2 years
Oral examination: dental caries, periodontal disease, oral cancer	Annually	Annually
Test for occult blood in stool	Annually	Annually
Assessment of physical, psychological, and social functioning	Every 2 years	Annually
Hypothyroidism	Every 2 years	Every 2 years
Skin cancer	Periodically	Periodically
Pap smear	Every 5 years	Every 5 years
Special tests (based on clinical judgment of risk)		
Tuberculin skin test		
Cytology of urine		

Source: After Canadian Task Force on the Periodic Health Examination, 1979.

many consider them to be useful in the care of elderly persons at risk, especially those in institutions, but there remains an active controversy about their cost-effectiveness (Simberkoff et al., 1986; Forrester et al., 1987; Sims et al., 1988). Tuberculosis remains a problem among the elderly, especially those in institutions. Special care must be taken in interpreting a lack of reaction to tuberculin skin tests in elderly persons because of the risk of anergy (Stead, 1987; Stead et al., 1987).

Another area of concern pertains to foot care. Although there are no formal studies to confirm the effects, clinical experience strongly suggests the benefits of podiatry in improving the ambulation of many elderly patients. Not only diabetics should receive attention to their feet, each elderly person should be carefully asked about foot pain and discomfort and checked for bunions and corns. Appropriate treatment can do a great deal to keep such patients ambulatory and stable. Screening for glaucoma—by tonometry and visual fields—is inexpensive and easy. The Canadian panel expressed concern about false-positive results, but the importance of vision in the overall functioning of the elderly patient argues strongly for attention to this area. Community screening with applanation equipment may be another approach that avoids some of the errors of manual tonometry. In a similar vein, the potential for improving function by replacing cataracts with implanted lenses mandates greater attention to visual problems, as well as concern about the excess use of surgery (Applegate, 1987).

Three factors should be borne in mind regarding the Canadian Task Force recommendations:

1 They are intended to be done as part of regular primary care. No special visits for prevention are implied. Particularly in our current system, where Medicare Part B does not pay for preventive services, it is important to appreciate that much can be done in prevention without special visits for that purpose.

2 The procedures cover all three areas of preventive action noted in Table 15-2.

3 Most, if not all, of the procedures can be performed by an appropriately trained nonphysician.

Recommendations for preventive activities in the nursing home setting are discussed in greater detail in Chapter 17.

Prevention of Disability

Although discussions of prevention tend to focus on the prevention of disease, the context of geriatrics—with its emphasis on functioning—urges a broader approach. In the care of the elderly, equal attention must be paid to seeking means to keep the elderly patient as active as possible. While there may be little that can be done to prevent the occurrence of a disease in an elderly person, much can be done to minimize the impact of that disease. Impairments cannot be allowed to become disabilities.

A major component of the efforts to avoid this transition are contained in geriatric assessment programs. The general approaches of such programs are reviewed in Chapter 3. It is important to note that these programs have been very varied in their composition. Table 3-1 in Chapter 3 summarizes the major randomized controlled trials using different approaches to assessment.

A promising line of work has been begun by Williams (1987). In addition to relying more on demonstrated performance than simply on patient report, he has used the time required to complete the task as part of the measure. This additional component provides a way to achieve more variability and may lead to better prediction. It offers a means to detect more subtle change.

Substantial sections of this book deal with various aspects of rehabilitation. One of the most subtle, but nonetheless important, aspects of this approach to prevention—the prevention of inactivity and despair—is the physician's attitude. For the patient, a gain in function or an ability to deal with a chronic problem is essential. It is surely no mean feat. Such behavior should be encouraged and rewarded. Indifference may be enough to discourage the patient from trying.

Enthusiasm is necessary but not sufficient. Attention should be directed toward practical steps. Occupational therapists can be very helpful here in assessing the patient's environment to suggest modifications (see Chapter 8, especially Table 8-18). The Appendix offers a simple environmental assessment form useful in uncovering hazards.

Other programs can be mobilized in the patient's behalf. Self-help groups are available in many communities to offer support with chronic illness, including stress management and drugless pain control techniques. Social activity can play an essential role in maintaining function. Pets have proved to be very effective in improving morale and maintaining function.

Special efforts may be necessary to deal with members of the patient's family. Their concern over dangers of accidents may lead them to become overprotective and thus exaggerate the condition of dependency.

TERMINAL CARE

The physician's concern with the patient's functioning continues throughout the course of the chronic disease. Elderly patients will die. In many cases, death is not a reflection of medical failure. The approach to the dying patient will often raise difficult dilemmas. No simple answers suffice. Perhaps the best advice is not to take on the whole burden. Too often the dying patient is treated as an object. Ignored and isolated, the patient may be discussed in the third person.

Physicians must come to terms with death if they are to treat elderly patients. Often the patients are more comfortable with the subject than are their physicians. Fleeing from the dying patient is inexcusable. Enough has been written on this subject by Kubler-Ross (1969) and others (Duff and Hollingshead, 1968) to make that point clear. Dying patients need their doctors. At a very basic level, everything should be done to keep the patient as comfortable as possible. One simple step is to identify the pattern of discomforting symptoms and arrange the dosage schedule of palliatives to prevent, rather than respond to, the symptoms (Foley, 1985).

Patients need an opportunity to talk about their death. Not everyone will take advantage of that chance, but a surprising number will respond to a genuine offer made without time pressure. Such discussions are not conducted on the run. Often several invitations accompanied by appropriate behavior (i.e., sitting down at the bedside) are necessary.

Some physicians are unable to confront this aspect of practice. For them, the challenge is to recognize their own behavior and get appropriate help. Such help is available at various levels: help for the physician and for the patient. Groups and therapy are readily available to assist doctors to deal with their feelings. Patients of doctors who fear death need the help of other care givers. Often other professionals—nurses, social workers—who are working with these patients already can play the lead role in helping them work through their feelings. But the active intervention of another care giver is not justification to ignore the patient.

The rise of the hospice movement has created a growing cadre of persons and settings to help with the dying patient. The lessons coming from this experience suggest that much can be done to facilitate this stage of life (Saunders, 1978; Fennell, 1980; Zimmerman, 1984), although the formal studies done to evaluate hospice care do not show dramatic benefits (Greer et al., 1986; Kane et al., 1984). Patients should be encouraged to be as active as possible and as interactive as they wish. Even more than in other aspects of care, the physician must be prepared to listen carefully to the patient and to share the decision making about how and when to do things.

SUMMARY

Physicians caring for the elderly patients need to think in prospective terms. They will enjoy their practices more if they can learn to set reasonable goals for patients, to record progress toward these goals, and to use the failure to achieve progress as an important clinical sign of the need for reevaluation. Prospective medicine should also carry over into prevention. Many useful steps can be taken to improve and protect the health of elderly patients.

REFERENCES

Amery A, Birkenhager W, Brixko P, et al: Mortality and morbidity results from the European Working Party on high blood pressure in the elderly trial. *Lancet* 1:1349–1354, 1985.

Applegate WB, Miller ST, Elam JT, et al: Impact of cataract surgery with lens implantation on vision and physical function in elderly patients. *JAMA* 257:1064–1066, 1987.

Block JE, Smith R, Black D, et al: Does exercise prevent osteoporosis? *JAMA* 257:3115–3117, 1987.

Canadian Task Force on the Periodic Health Examination: Periodic health examination. *Can Med J* 121:1193–1254, 1979.

Duff RS, Hollingshead AB: *Sickness and Society.* New York, Harper & Row, 1968.

Evans JG: Prevention of age-associated loss of autonomy: Epidemiological approaches. *J Chron Diseases* 37:353–363, 1984.

Fennell FB: The need for hospice. *N Engl J Med* 303:158–161, 1980.

Foley KM: The treatment of cancer pain. *N Engl J Med* 313:84–95, 1985.

Forrester HL, Jahnigen DW, LaForce FM: Inefficacy of pneumococcal vaccine in a high-risk population. *Am J Med* 83:425–430, 1987.

German PS, Shapiro S, Skiner EA, et al: Detection and management of mental health problems of older patients by primary care providers. *JAMA* 257:489–493, 1987.

Greenfield S, Blanco DM, Elashoff RM, et al: Patterns of care related to age of breast cancer patients. *JAMA* 257:2766–2770, 1987.

Greer DS, Mor V, Morris JN, et al: An alternative in terminal care. Results of the National Hospice Study, *J Chron Diseases* 39:9–26, 1986.

Havlik RJ: Determinants of health—cardiovascular risk factors, in Havlik RJ, Liu MG, Kovar MG, et al. (eds) *Health Statistics on Older Persons, United States, 1986.* Vital and Health statistics, Series 3, No. 25. DHHS Pub. No. (PHS)87-1409. Public Health Service, Washington, DC, US Government Printing Office, June, 1987.

Jaijich CL, Ostfeld AM, Freeman DH: Smoking and coronary heart disease mortality in the elderly. *JAMA* 252:2831–2834, 1984.

Kane RA, Kane RL: *Long-Term Care: Principles, Programs and Policies.* New York, Springer, 1987.

Kane RL, Kane RA, Arnold SB: Prevention and the elderly: Risk factors. *Health Services Research* 19(Part II):945–1006, 1985.

Kane RL, Wales J, Berstein L, et al: A randomised controlled trial of hospice care. *Lancet* i:890–894, 1984.

Kaplan GA, Seeman TE, Cohen RD, et al: Mortality among the elderly in the Alameda County study: Behavioral and demographic risk factors. *Am J Pub Health* 77:307–312, 1987.

Kubler-Ross E: *On Death and Dying.* New York, Macmillan, 1969.

LaCroix AZ: Determinants of health—exercise and activities of daily living, in Havlik RJ, Liu MG, Kovar MG, et al. (eds) *Health Statistics on Older Persons, United States, 1986.* Vital and Health statistics, Series 3, No. 25. DHHS Pub. No. (PHS)87-1409. Public Health Service, Washington, DC, US Government Printing Office, June, 1987.

Levinstein MR, Ouslander JG, Rubenstein LZ, et al: Yield of routine annual laboratory tests in a skilled nursing home population. *JAMA* 258:1909–1915, 1987.

Medical Practice Committee: Periodic health examination: A guide for designing individualized preventive health care in the asymptomatic patient. *Ann Intern Med* 95:729–732, 1981.

O'Malley MS, Fletcher SW: Screening for breast cancer with breast self-examination: A critical review. *JAMA* 257:2197–2203, 1987.

Pepper GA, Jorgensen LB, Kane RL, et al: *Problem-Oriented Process: Nurse's Manual.* Salt Lake City, University of Utah, 1972.

Rodysill KJ: Postmenopausal osteoporosis—intervention and prophylaxis: A review. *J Chron Diseases* 40:743–760, 1987.

Rowe JW, Kahn RL: Human aging: Usual and successful. *Science* 237:143–149, 1987.

Rubenstein LZ, Josephson KR, Nichol-Seamons M, et al: Comprehensive health screening of well elderly adults: An analysis of a community program. *J Gerontol* 41:342–352, 1986.

Saunders C: Hospice care. *Am J Med* 65:726–728, 1978.

Simberkoff MS, Cross AP, Al-Ibrahim M, et al: Efficacy of pneumococcal vaccine in high-risk patients. *N Engl J Med* 315:1318–1327, 1986.

Sims RV, Steinmann WC, McConville JH, et al: The clinical effectiveness of pneumococcal vaccine in the elderly. *Ann Intern Med* 108:653–657, 1988.

Stead WW, To T: The significance of the tuberculin skin test in elderly persons. *Ann Intern Med* 107:837–842, 1987.

Stead WW, To T, Harrison RW, et al: Benefit-risk considerations in preventive treatment for tuberculosis in elderly persons. *Ann Intern Med* 107:843–845, 1987.

Stultz BM: Preventive health care and the elderly. *West J Med* 41:832–845, 1984.

Williams ME: Identifying the older person likely to require long-term care services. *J Am Geriatr Soc* 33:761–766, 1987.

Woolley FR, Warnick R, Kane RL, et al: *Problem-Oriented Nursing.* New York, Springer, 1974.

World Health Organization: *International Classification of Impairment, Disabilities and Handicaps: A Manual of Classification Relating to the Consequences of Diseases.* Geneva, World Health Organization, 1980.

Zimmerman JM: *Hospice.* Baltimore, Urban & Schwartzenberg, 1984.

Zuckerman DM, Kasl SV, Ostfeld AM: Psychosocial predictors of mortality among the elderly poor: The role of religion, well-being and social contacts. *Am J Epidemiol* 119:410–423, 1984.

SUGGESTED READINGS

Breslow L, Somers AR: The lifetime health-monitoring program: A practical approach to preventive medicine. *N Engl J Med* 296:601–608, 1977.

Hamilton M, Reid H (eds): *A Hospice Handbook: A New Way to Care for the Dying.* Grand Rapids, Eerdmans, 1980.

Kane RL, Kane RA: *Values and Long-Term Care.* Lexington, MA, Heath, 1982.

Patriarcia PA, Arden NH, Koplan JP, et al: Prevention and control of type A influenza infections in nursing homes. *Ann Intern Med* 107:732–740, 1987.

Willems JS, Sanders CR, Riddiough MA, et al: Cost effectiveness of vaccination against pneumococcal pneumonia. *N Engl J Med* 303:533–559, 1980.

World Health Organization: *Preventing Disability in the Elderly.* Copenhagen, Regional Office for Europe, 1982.

Chapter 16

Long-Term-Care Resources

A proportion of elderly patients will require substantial long-term care. There is no uniform definition for long-term care, but the following description of the term highlights the important aspects:

> A range of services that addresses the health, personal care, and social needs of individuals who lack some capacity for self-care. Services may be continuous or intermittent but are delivered for sustained periods to individuals who have a demonstrated need, usually measured by some index of functional incapacity.

This statement emphasizes the common thread of most discussions of long-term care: the dependence of an individual on the services of another for a substantial period. The definition is carefully unspecific about who provides those services or what they are. Long-term care is certainly not the exclusive purview of the medical profession; in fact, most of the long-term care in this country is not provided by professionals at all but by a host of individuals loosely referred to as *informal support*. These persons may be family, friends, or neighbors.

The best estimates suggest that about 15 percent of the elderly population need the help of another person to manage their daily lives. As shown in Figure 16-1, this rate increases with age, from about 7 percent at age 65 to 40 percent after age 85. Far fewer older persons suffer from significant limitations of activity such as being confined to bed. Recall that for each person in a nursing home today, there are between one and three equally disabled persons living in the community. Thus, first instincts are not always best. Physicians have been trained to respond to the dependent elderly person by thinking of admission to a nursing home. Nursing home placement should be the *last* resort, not the first. Table 16-1 offers a wider array of treatment choices for various types of patients. The physician, in conjunction with other health professionals (especially social workers and nurses), can do a great deal to steer patients and their families toward these

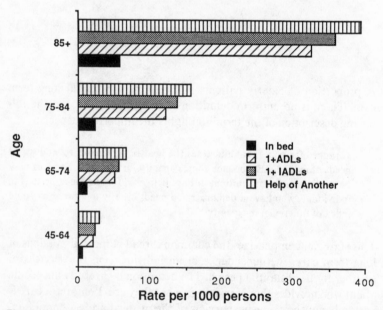

Figure 16-1 Measures of functional dependency among community elderly, 1979–1980. (*From Feller, 1986.*)

Table 16-1 Relationship between Target Groups and Possible Alternatives

Target group now in nursing home	Community alternatives		Institutional backup requirement
	Intermediate	Long-range	
Terminally ill	Home health Home hospice Homemaking Counseling	Narcotic law reform	Possibly a hospice
Those who might benefit from rehabilitation	Home health Day hospital		Rehabilitation hospital
Those requiring skilled nursing care	Home health Day hospital Meals on wheels Homemaking	Personal-care attendant policy	Possibility of acute care hospital service when needed
Those who are mentally ill	Halfway house Day hospital Sheltered workshops Day care	Bereavement counseling Identification of high-risk groups	Possible need for acute care hospital service
Those with social needs and minimal health problems—the frail, the very old	Sheltered housing Day care Social programming Senior centers Primary health care	Preretirement counseling Reeducation Changed income transfer programs Employment programs	Old-age home
The completely disorientated—ambulatory but needing constant supervision	Foster care		Possibility that better services can be provided through institutions

resources. Although the physician is not likely to become actively involved in specific placement decisions, the physician's suggestions and opinions about what should be considered can play a pivotal role. Moreover, the physician's medical certification of need is essential for establishing eligibility for long-term-care services under several reimbursement programs.

In many instances, the family (and often nonrelatives) are the first line of support. A study in Cleveland (U.S. Comptroller General 1977, 1979) indicates that family and friends provide almost 80 percent of the care received by dependent elderly persons living in the community. The ideal program would keep older people at home, relying on family as the first line of support, and bolstering their efforts with more formal assistance to provide professional services and occasional respite care.

Why then does our system rely so heavily on the nursing home? Several reasons can be offered. First, nursing homes are available; there are more nursing home beds than acute care hospital beds in this country. Nonetheless, there is usually a waiting list to get in, especially into a relatively good home. Second, nursing home care is cheap; it is under $60 a day in most states, when a hospital day costs at least $500 and even a good hotel room costs at least $80. Finally, and related to the first two points, the programs to cover long-term-care services have become a complex maze of eligibility and regulations, which has not encouraged anyone to develop innovative alternatives.

It is not altogether true to say that there have been no efforts to develop alternatives. For a period there was great effort expended trying to find less expensive ways of caring for clients in the community. The upshot of these efforts was the recognition that community care is preferable in many cases but not always cheaper. One of the major difficulties in controlling the cost of this care is the potential for widespread use. Because there are a large number of dependent elderly living in the community, a dependency-based eligibility system will include many people who would not opt for a nursing home. This need to control entry has stimulated great interest in case management. The continuing need to improve community care has led to some recent innovations, including new waiver programs that allow use of nursing home funds for community care if the total long-term-care budget is kept constant. As a result, there has been uneven development of community programs in different parts of the country.

At the same time, there is concern that a preoccupation with a search for alternatives to nursing homes may distract efforts from the sorely needed work to improve the quality of nursing home care. Even in the best situation, a substantial number of older persons will continue to need such care. One scenario for the future holds that the form of nursing homes will change. Many of the residents currently cared for in nursing homes will be treated in more flexible situations that emphasize living arrangements with nursing and other services brought to the residents on a more individualized basis. Those patients needing more intensive care will be treated in more medically oriented facilities.

LONG-TERM-CARE PROGRAMS

The physician caring for elderly patients must have at least a working acquaintance with the major programs that support long-term care. We are accustomed to thinking about care of the elderly in association with Medicare. In fact, at least three parts (called *Titles*) of the Social Security Act provide important benefits for the elderly (Table 16-2): Title XVIII (Medicare), Title XIX (Medicaid), and Social Services Block Grants (formerly Title XX). Medicare was designed to address health care, particularly acute care hospital services. It deals with long-term care only to the extent that long-term care can supplant more expensive hospital care. The major funding for long-term care thus falls to Medicaid.

This distinction is a very important one. Whereas Medicare is an insurance-type program to which persons are entitled after contributing a certain amount, Medicaid is a welfare program, eligibility for which depends on a combination of need and poverty. Thus, in order to become eligible for Medicaid, a person must not only prove illness but also exhaustion of personal resources—hardly a situation conducive to restoring autonomy. Figure 16-2 contrasts the funding for health services for the elderly with that for nursing homes to emphasize the difference in source of payment for acute and long-term care.

In 1984, the per capita expenditure for personal health services of older persons was just over $4200: $1900 went to hospitals; $880 went to nursing homes; about $870 went to physicians; and about $550 went for other care such as home care, drugs, tests, and equipment. As seen in Figure 16-2, the pattern of coverage is quite different for the various services covered. Most obvious is that Medicare

Table 16-2 Summary of Major Federal Programs for the Elderly

Program	Eligible population	Services covered	Deductibles and copayments
Medicare (Title XVIII of the Social Security Act)			
Part A: Hospital insurance	All persons eligible for Social Security and others with chronic disabilities such as end-stage renal disease plus voluntary enrollees 65+	Per benefit period, "reasonable cost" for 90 days of hospital care plus 60 lifetime reservation days; 150 days of skilled nursing facility (SNF); home health visits (see text) including 80 hours/year of respite care; hospice care*	Full coverage for hospital care after a deductible of about 1 day and for SNF days 21–29
Part B: Supplemental medical insurance	All those covered under Part A who elect coverage; participants pay a monthly premium	80% of "reasonable cost" for physicians' services; supplies and services related to physician services; outpatient; physical, and speech therapy; diagnostic tests and radiographs; mammogram; surgical dressings; prosthetics; ambulance. 50%, rising to 80% of drug cost after a limit (deductible)	Deductible and 20% copayment. (No copay after a limit reached)
Medicaid (Title XIX of the Social Security Act)	Persons receiving Supplemental Security Income (SSI) (such as welfare) or receiving SSI and state supplement or meeting lower eligibility standards used for medical assistance criteria in 1972 or eligible for SSI or were in institutions and eligible for Medicaid in 1973; medically needy who do not qualify for SSI but have high medical expenses are eligible for Medicaid in some states; eligibility criteria vary from state to state	*Mandatory services for categorically needy:* Inpatient hospital services; outpatient services; SNF; limited home health care; laboratory tests and radiographs; family planning; early and periodic screening, diagnosis, and treatment for children through age 20	None, once patient spends down to eligibility level

402

Program	Eligibility	Services	Payment
Medicaid (cont'd)		*Optional services vary from state to state:* Dental care; therapies; drugs; intermediate care facilities; extended home health care; private duty nurse; eyeglasses; prostheses; personal-care services; medical transportation and home health care services. (states can limit the amount and duration of services)	Fees are charged to those with incomes greater than 80% of state's median income
Social Services Block Grant (Title XX of the Social Security Act)	All recipients of Aid to Families with Dependent Children (AFDC) and SSI; optionally, those earning up to 115% of state median income and residents of specific geographic areas	Day care; substitute care; protective services; family counseling; home-based services; employment, education and training; health-related services; information and referral; transportation; day services; family planning; legal services; home-delivered and congregate meals	
Title III of the Older Americans Act	All persons 60 years and older; low-income, minority, and isolated older persons are special targets	Homemaker; home-delivered meals; home health aides; transportation; legal services; counseling; information and referral plus 19 others. (50% of funds must go to those listed)	Some payment may be requested

*Hospice care was added as a Medicare benefit in 1982; 365 days per year when patient certified as terminal.

Note: Information applies as of July 1988.

403

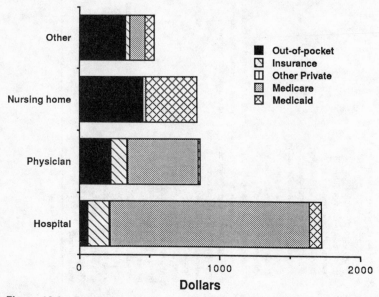

Figure 16-2 Per capita health care expenditures for the elderly, 1984. (*From Waldo and Lazenby, 1984.*)

is a major source of hospital and physician care but is almost absent from nursing home care, whereas just the reverse applies to Medicaid.

Eligibility for Medicare differs for each of its two major parts. Part A (hospital services insurance) is available to all who are eligible for Social Security, usually by virtue of paying the Social Security tax for a sufficient number of quarters. Part B (medical services insurance) is offered for a monthly premium, paid by the individual. Almost everyone over age 65 is covered by Part A. (Federal, state, and local government employees are exceptions; until recently they were not covered by Social Security and have their own pension and medical programs.)

The introduction of prospective payment for hospitals under Medicare has created a new set of problems. Hospitals are now paid a fixed amount per admission according to the Diagnosis-Related Group (DRG) the patient is assigned to on the basis of the admitting diagnosis. The rates for DRGs are, in turn, based on expected lengths of stay and intensity of care for each condition. The incentives in such an approach run almost directly contrary to most of the goals of geriatrics. Whereas geriatrics addresses the functional result of multiple interacting problems, DRGs encourage concentration on a single problem. Extra time required to make an appropriate discharge plan is discouraged. Use of ancillary personnel, such as social workers, is similarly discouraged.

Moreover, the two payment systems now in effect create much confusion. Hospitals are now paid a fixed amount per case, but the patients continue to pay under a system of deductibles. If there was ever a rationale for the copayments under Part A as a way of discouraging unnecessary stays, it has certainly disappeared with the introduction of DRGs. The concerns now focus on the potential adverse consequences of "quicker and sicker" discharges. Not surprisingly, there is a general perception of greater demands on the services for those just discharged from the hospital, especially home health care and nursing home care. The latter has become more a postacute care service than just a long-term-care one. Ironically, this was the role of the nursing home originally designed in the plan for Medicare and the reason for brief coverage after hospitalization.

The recent passage of catastrophic coverage legislation provides new benefits for the elderly. This new universal insurance component for Medicare would eliminate the limitations on hospital days and copayments for hospital care. The only out-of-pocket cost for hospital care is a deductible roughly the equivalent of the first day. This new plan increases potentially covered nursing home days to 150 per year. Home health care is increased to up to 38 days of care per illness for seven days per week; in addition, respite care of 80 hours a year is available. It also provides coverage for ambulatory drugs after a deductible. The precise mechanism to set limits for drug benefits follows a complicated formula designed to control overall drug costs from year to year. For the first time, a preventive service, mammograms, is specifically covered.

A slightly smaller proportion of the elderly population uses Part B; it is a good buy, and Social Security payments were increased to allow people to purchase it. Some elderly persons have also purchased so-called Medi-Gap insurance; unfortunately, most of this insurance covers only the gaps up to the ceilings established by Medicare (i.e., it pays deductibles and coinsurance, but not the difference between billed charges and allowable charges). Medi-Gap policies will essentially disappear with the passage of the Catastrophic Health Care Act of 1988.

Medicare coverage is important but not sufficient for three basic reasons:

1 To control utilization, it mandates deductible and copayment charges for both Parts A and B.

2 To control costs, it sets fees by a complicated formula based, for physicians, on the concept of usual, customary, and reasonable fees; this system essentially means that physicians are paid less than they would usually bill for the service (some opt to bill the patient directly for the difference).

3 The program does not cover several services essential to patient functioning, such as drugs, eyeglasses, hearing aids, and preventive services. Medicare specifically excludes services designed to provide "custodial care"—the very services often most critical to long-term care.

As a result of these three factors, a substantial amount of the medical bill is left to the individual. In 1984, 33 percent of health care costs for the elderly ($1380 per elderly person) came from private sources (Figure 16-3).

Medicaid, in contrast, is a welfare program designed to serve the poor. It is a state-run program to which the federal government contributes (50 to 78 percent of the costs, depending on the state). In some states, persons can be covered as medically indigent even if their income is above the poverty level, if their medical expenses would impoverish them. As a welfare program, Medicaid has no deductibles or coinsurance (although current proposals call for modest charges to discourage excess use). It is, however, a welfare program cast in the medical model.

It is important to appreciate that the shape of the Medicaid expenditures is determined largely by the gaps in Medicare. Medicaid serves primarily two distinct groups: mothers and young children under Aid to Families of Dependent Children and the elderly eligible for Old Age Assistance. The former use some hospital care around birth and for the small group of severely ill children. A large portion

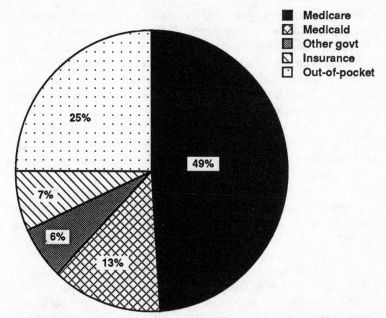

■ Medicare
☒ Medicaid
▨ Other govt
◩ Insurance
▢ Out-of-pocket

Figure 16-3 Source of the elderly's personal health care expenditures, 1984.
(*From Waldo and Lazenby, 1984.*)

of the Medicaid dollar goes to those things needed by the elderly but not covered by Medicare, namely, drugs, nursing home care, and custodial home care.

Because it is the major source of nursing home payments, physicians are often placed in the difficult position of being asked to certify a patient's physical limitations in order to gain the patient admittance to a nursing home for primarily social reasons (i.e., lack of social supports necessary to remain in the community).

Medicaid is the major public payer for nursing home care. Medicaid is thus important in shaping nursing home policies. It pays about half of the nursing costs but covers almost 70 percent of the residents. The discrepancy is explained by the policies that require residents to expend their own resources first. Thus Social Security payments, private pensions, and the like are used as primary sources of payment, and Medicaid picks up the remainder. However, it does not directly pay for most physician care in the nursing home. For elderly persons already covered by Medicaid, the welfare program will pay the Medicare Part B premium and thus reinsure through available federal funds. Medicaid would then pay the deductibles and copayments and those services not covered under Medicare.

The third part of the Social Security legislation pertinent to the elderly is Title XX, now administered as Social Services Block Grants. This is also a welfare program targeted especially to those on categorical welfare programs like Aid to Families with Dependent Children and, more germane, Supplemental Security Income. The latter is a federal program, which, as the name implies, supplements Social Security benefits to provide a minimum income. Title XX funds are administered through state and local agencies, which have a substantial amount of flexibility in how they wish to allocate the available money across a variety of stipulated services. The state also has the option of broadening the eligibility criteria to include those just above the poverty line.

The other major relevant federal program is Title III of the Older Americans Act. This program is available to all persons over age 60, regardless of income. The single largest component goes to support nutrition through congregate meal programs where elderly persons can get a subsidized hot meal, but a wide variety of services are covered as well. Some duplicate or supplement those covered under Social Security programs; others are unique.

Table 16-2 summarizes these four programs and their current scope. It is important to appreciate that this summary attempts to condense and simplify a very complex and ever-changing set of rules and regulations. Physicians should be familiar with the broad scope and limitations of these programs but will have to rely on others, especially social workers, to be familiar with the operating details.

THE NURSING HOME

There is an unfortunate tendency to think of the nursing home as a miniature hospital; it is not. Nursing homes are smaller and less well staffed than hospitals. Whereas a hospital has a ratio of over three staff for each bed, the nursing home has only about a sixth of that number, and most of those staff are aides. Nursing homes are usually divided into at least two categories: skilled care and intermediate care. The distinction is based primarily on the amount of nursing care available. Nursing homes are certified as being capable of caring for patients with different needs based on these levels. In turn, patients are certified as needing a given level of care, but the criteria are vague, and much is left to professional judgment.

This distinction is scheduled to be phased out, as new regulations call for a merger of skilled and intermediate care. The distinction between nursing home care and that provided in purely residential facilities with little or no nursing component will be retained.

As shown in Figure 16-4, most of the nursing home beds, but not the homes, are currently classified as skilled. The residential facilities, by contrast, are smaller but more numerous.

Admission to a nursing home is very much a function of age. Figure 16-5 shows the sharp rise in the rate of nursing home use after age 85. Because this portion of the population is growing rapidly, there is great fear of being inundated with nursing home users.

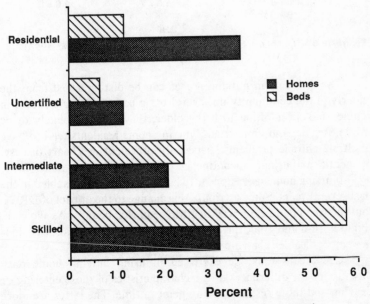

Figure 16-4   Long-term-care inventory, 1986. (*From Sirrocco, 1988.*)

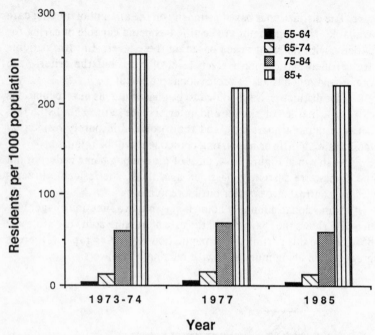

Figure 16-5   Rate of nursing home use. (*From Hing and Sekscenski, 1987.*)

The residents in nursing homes can be distinguished from the elderly in the community on several basic parameters. As shown in Table 16-3, in addition to being older, they are more likely to be white, female, and unmarried. Nursing home residents tend to have multiple chronic problems. Especially prevalent are heart disease, dementia, and urinary incontinence.

Nursing home users appear to have become more disabled in the last several years. Some attribute this change to the impact of DRGs, but the trend had begun well in advance of that change. As shown in Figures 16-6 and 16-7, the contemporary nursing home user is older and more disabled than a decade ago.

Great care must be exercised in using nursing home data because of the differences in the characteristics of those entering or leaving and those resident at any point in time. The latter are more likely to have chronic problems such as dementia, whereas the former

Table 16-3 Comparison of Nursing Home Residents and the Noninstitutionalized Population Age 65 and Over, 1984–1985

	Nursing home residents, %*	Noninstitutionalized population, %†
Age		
65–74 years	16.1	61.7
75–84	38.7	30.7
85+	45.2	7.6
Sex		
Male	25.4	40.8
Female	74.6	59.2
Race		
White (including Hispanics)	93.1	90.6
Black and other	6.9	9.4
Marital status		
Married	12.1	54.7
Widowed	69.3	34.1
Divorced or separated	4.5	6.3
Never married	14.2	4.4

*Source: Hing, 1987.
†Source: Kovar, 1986.

will have problems that are either rehabilitatable or fatal (e.g., hip fracture and cancer). This distinction makes it tricky to talk about nursing home patients and may explain the often contradictory data presented.

For example, it is true that nursing home stays are not nearly as long as one might believe. The commonly cited statistic indicates that about half of those admitted are discharged within 3 months. But this number is deceptive. As shown in Figure 16-8, the length of stay for those discharged alive is much shorter than for those who die in the nursing home. However, many of those discharged alive go not to the community but to hospitals, where they recycle back to the nursing home. Figure 2-21 (Chapter 2) traces the outcomes of a group of nursing home patients followed for two years after their discharge. The dominant pattern suggests that most of the survivors end up back in the nursing home.

The nursing home has not been an attractive place for physicians

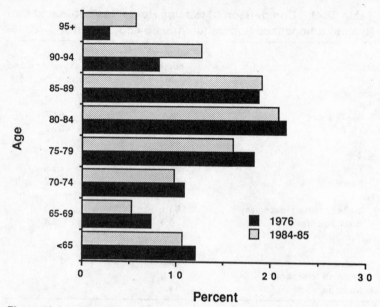

Figure 16-6 Age of persons discharged from nursing homes, 1976 and 1984–1985. (*From Sekscenski, 1987.*)

to practice. The basic environment and the lack of professional staff have daunted many. It is important to recognize that conditions are changing. Nursing homes are upgrading facilities and, under pressure from regulatory agencies, are upgrading staff. The physician can play a critical role in setting the tone for the care of patients in the nursing home. Physicians' expectations of professional performance and their advocacy of their patients' needs can be very influential in shaping staff behavior.

Some physicians have elected to concentrate their work in one or two nursing homes, just as they do with hospitals. This practice increases efficiency and permits more impact on the staff. In some cases, the physician serves as medical director and can thereby become more actively involved in setting policies to improve care. Much can be done to make nursing homes more effective. Some nursing homes have already instituted improved recordkeeping systems, even using computers. These systems provide more usable informa-

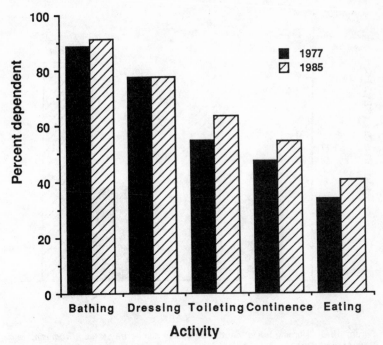

Figure 16-7   Change in nursing home dependence level from 1977 to 1985. (*From Hing, 1987.*)

tion in tabular, or flowsheet, format and have been designed so that even nurses' aides with very limited education can enter useful data. Problem-oriented records, to which nurses and social workers contribute, are especially appropriate in this setting (Woolley et al., 1974).

A study by the Institute of Medicine (1986) pointed to the need for reforms. They made an important distinction between quality assessment and quality assurance. Too often most of the energy goes into measuring the deficiencies and little is devoted to doing something about them. Sometimes the fear of closing a facility in the face of heavy utilization leads to inaction, or even worse, to pouring additional money into an inadequate facility in the hopes of making it better. The rewards are thus perverted.

Regulations intended to upgrade care can also constrain care.

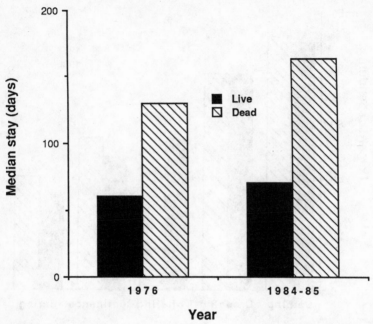

Figure 16-8   Nursing home length of stay, by discharge status. (*From Hing and Sekscenski, 1987.*)

Rather than insisting that all patients be seen on a fixed schedule, more flexibility is needed to adjust care to the patient's condition. New types of personnel can be effectively used to deliver primary care to nursing home patients. Nurse practitioners and physician assistants have been shown to deliver high-quality care in this setting (Kane et al., 1976; Master et al., 1980). Medicare regulations covering Part B were altered to allow greater use of physician assistants, but nurse practitioners elected not to be covered at that time because of their unwillingness to work under the supervision of a physician. Similarly, clinical pharmacists have proved very helpful in simplifying drug regimens and avoiding potential drug interactions. The physician's role in nursing home care is discussed in greater detail in Chapter 17.

HOME CARE

As already noted, we have developed in this country a backward system of long-term care, which focuses on the nursing home. We tend to speak of the nursing home and alternatives to it, when we should begin with the premise that elderly people belong at home and want to be cared for at home. Institutional care will be needed in some cases, when the strain on care givers is too great, but it should not be the resource of first resort. Our system has not evolved that way, and the resources available for home care are meager, but not so underdeveloped as to be ignored. Even today, most communities have at least some home care services, and more are likely to develop.

Home care involves at least two basic types of care: home health services and homemaking and chore services. As shown in Table 16-4, different programs provide one or both types. Most elderly people treated at home require homemaking more than home health services. Sometimes the differences between the two are purely arbitrary. If we consider that the homemaker replaces or supplements a family member, many of the tasks involved are extensions of home nursing (for example, supervising medication or giving baths). The definitions have emerged arbitrarily, often to fit the regulations governing a particular program. The physician will usually find that the home health agency is familiar with these regulations and how to deal with them.

The major problem at present is getting services. Although Medicare has broadened its home health benefit (in contrast to homemaking) to include unlimited home health visits without a prior hospital stay of at least 3 days, the criteria for eligibility for these services severely restricts their use. To get home health services for a patient, a physician must certify that the patient is homebound and that intermittent skilled care is likely to produce a benefit in a reasonable time. Thus, a large number of dependent elderly who need continuing home nursing but are "custodial" are ineligible unless the physician misrepresents their situation. *Skilled service* is defined as a skilled service offered by a nurse, a physical therapist, or a speech therapist. If one of these establishing services is present, the patient may also receive the skilled services of an occupational therapist or medical social worker, and/or the services of a home health aide, if

Table 16-4 Home Care Provided under Various Federal Programs

	Medicare	Medicaid	Title XX
Eligibility criteria	Must be homebound; need skilled care; need and expect benefit in a reasonable period; need certification by physician	State can use homebound criterion; not limited to skilled care; need certification by physician	Vary from state to state
Payment to provider	Reasonable costs	Varies with state	Three modes of payment possible: (1) direct provision by government agency; (2) contract with private agency; (3) independent provider
Services covered	Home health services, skilled nursing, physical or speech therapy as primary services; secondary services (social worker and home health aide) available *only* if primary service is provided; position of occupational therapy in service hierarchy ambiguous*	Limited home-health care mandatory; expanded home care optional; personal care in home optional	Wide variety of home services allowed, including home health aide, homemaker, chore worker, meal services

*Occupational therapy was authorized as a primary service beginning in July 1981; but, as of October 1981, it has become an "extended" secondary service, which may continue if needed after primary services are discontinued.

required by the plan. All reimbursed services must be given by a certified home health agency. (To be certified, the agency needs to offer
nursing plus at least one of the five other services.)

Medicaid funds can be used to provide home health care to persons eligible for nursing home care. Until recently, Medicaid funds
have not been widely used for home care. In fact, until 1980, one state
(New York) accounted for almost 95 percent of the Medicaid moneys
spent on home health care. Home care under Medicaid must have a
physician's authorization, but the patient need not be homebound,
and the care need not be "skilled." All agencies delivering home care
under Medicaid must meet Medicare certification standards, but, if
no organized home health agencies exist in a region, a registered
nurse may be reimbursed for the services. In practice, states have
often modeled their Medicaid home care benefits after the medically
oriented Medicare benefit and thus restricted its use.

Under Medicaid, the nursing care is a required component of
home health services, and the state has the option to provide physical,
occupational, and speech therapy; medical social services; and personal-care services. Medicaid allows homemaking assistance on a
more generous basis than does Medicare. Personal-care services must
be prescribed by a physician and supervised by a registered nurse.
These services may not be delivered by persons related to the patient.
Recent changes in legislation have broadened the permissible use of
Medicaid moneys to support a wide variety of long-term-care services
in an effort to reduce nursing home costs. A number of states have
applied for waivers to develop this broader package of services.

The bulk of support for homemaking services, however, continues to rest with Title III and Title XX. Title XX provides at least
four methods of payment: local public agencies can provide the service directly; they can contract with agency providers (perhaps using
competitive bidding); they can purchase services from agencies at
negotiated prices; or they can permit the recipient to enter into agreement with independent providers, who do not work for an agency. It is
possible to have all these arrangements operating in the same community. This provision for independent vendors has prompted controversy because maintaining standards is difficult in the absence of any
supervisory system or institutional responsibility. Under Title XX, an
employment category known as *chore worker* has emerged; although

performing functions similar to the home health aide and the home-maker, chore workers do not need to be tightly supervised and cannot be reimbursed under Medicare or Medicaid.

Persons eligible for cash assistance from the state and other persons with low incomes and unmet service needs are eligible for Title XX as long as 50 percent of a state's annual federal allotment is expended on those receiving cash assistance. Fees are charged to those whose family income exceeds 80 percent of the state's median income for a family of four.

Home services are one of four priority items under Title III of the Older Americans Act. This source is important because means testing (whereby eligibility is set by income) is prohibited for programs under the Older Americans Act, making it possible to target a group that cannot afford private care but are ineligible for Title XX or Medicaid. Generally speaking, the Area Agency on Aging (AAA) subcontracts for home care services rather than providing them directly. The usual pattern is that Administration on Aging dollars permit existing agencies to develop or expand a home care component. Services vary from area to area but can include personal care, homemaker service, chore service, and service for heavier jobs (e.g., minor home repairs or renovations, insect eradication, gardening, and painting). The provisions for assistance under AAA are sharply limited by their constrained budgets and the competing demands for programs.

The extent of services under these several programs is still limited at present, although enthusiasm for in-home care is growing. The total sum of public dollars spent on home care remains only a fraction of that devoted to nursing homes.

OTHER SERVICES

A number of other modes of care can be tapped on behalf of elderly patients. Table 16-5 lists some of these services. However, despite their growing availability, they are still not widely used. Figure 16-9 shows the rates of use by age group. The most frequently used service in that set is the senior center, a service designed for the well elderly person.

Table 16-5   Examples of Community LTC Programs

Home care (home nursing and homemaking)	Caregiver support
Adult day care	Congregate housing
Adult foster care	Home repairs
Geriatric assessment	Meals (congregate and in-home)
Hospice / terminal care	Respite care
Telephone reassurance	Emergency alarms

Day care can fulfill a number of needs. Most day care programs provide some combination of recreational and restorative activity. In contrast to senior centers, which are usually sponsored by recreational departments and targeted at the well elderly, day care programs serve persons with limited functional ability. Some are for cognitively impaired persons. The programs provide supervised activ-

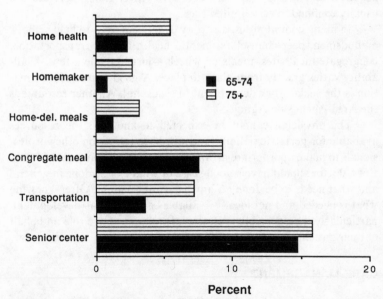

Figure 16-9   Proportion of persons aged 65 and older using community services, 1984. (*From Stone, 1986.*)

ities, which may improve basic ADL skills and social skills. At the very least, they provide an important respite for the primary care giver and thus may make the critical difference for allowing an impaired elderly person to remain at home. To increase efficiency, most programs serve any given client less than 5 days a week, usually 2 or 3 days.

Other forms of day care can include a larger medical component. Some areas have developed day hospitals for seniors, where virtually all the services of the hospital are available on an ambulatory basis. Emphasis is usually placed on rehabilitation, especially occupational and physical therapy. The adult day health center is an intermediate model, which combines day care with nursing, physical therapy, and perhaps social work. Such sites can also be used for periodic ambulatory care clinics.

A problem common to all day care programs is transportation. It is hard to arrange, expensive, and time-consuming. Special vans are usually needed, and, to avoid excessive travel times, services are usually confined to very limited areas.

In many communities, a variety of services exist to help seniors: ombudsmen, peer counselors, mental health clinics, transportation, congregate meal sites, meals on wheels—just to name a few. Availability varies greatly from place to place. A good source of information is the social work department in a hospital. Another resource is the Area Agency on Aging.

The physician cannot be expected to know all the resources available for geriatric patients and will have to rely on other professionals to make appropriate arrangements to take advantage of them. But a doctor should have a good sense of what can be done in general and what needs to be done for any particular patient. Often knowing what is needed and not locally available can lead to its development, particularly if responsible professionals take an active role on behalf of their patients.

CASE MANAGEMENT

The growing interest in the plethora of community long-term-care services has sparked some concerns about the need to control use. A frequent answer is case management. This term has been widely and variously used. The basic components of case management are assessment, prescription, authorization, coordination, and monitoring. These are issues very close to activities of primary care and hence may lead to some concern about role overlap between the case manager and the primary care physician. It is possible for physicians to serve as case managers, but most do not have the interest or the resources to perform this task. It is usually more efficient to look to other disciplines to perform this function but to recognize the important role of the physician in the overall care of the long-term-care patient. Where a full range of geriatric services is available, case management is usually included.

Regardless of discipline, the case manager faces some difficult tasks. There is often a discrepancy between responsibility and authority. It is very different to prescribe, authorize, or mandate. Case managers may or may not have the purchasing authority to pay for services they feel are necessary. Case managers may easily find themselves in the same bind as physicians. Specifically, they are expected to serve simultaneously as patient advocates and gatekeepers. The two roles are not compatible. For everyone's peace of mind, it is important to clarify at the outset who is the principal client. Because many decisions involve advocating on behalf of one group over another, this distinction is critical. It is very different to work on behalf of a client to obtain all the resources you believe they need and to work to distribute a fixed pool of resources to those who will best use them.

Another frequently heard concern about case management is the need to affix responsibility. On the one hand, the easiest way to do this is to give the case manager a budget and expect him or her to work within it to achieve the most possible. However, some have expressed anxieties that the person charged with authorizing services should be at arm's length from those providing them. Specific concerns are heard about hospital discharge planners' decisions as to when to refer patients to services owned or operated by the hospital. There is a real potential for client skimming. Similarly, if the case manager works for a care giving agency, there is the risk that that agency may get a disproportionate share of the choicest clients. On the other hand, even when case managers are separated from direct care, they are not immune to pressure from the purveyors, just as the physician is pursued by the drug companies.

REFERENCES

Feller BA: Americans needing home care, in *United States Vital and Health Statistics* Series 10, No. 153. DHHS Publ. No. (PHS) 86-1581, Public Health Service. Washington, DC, U.S. Government Printing Office, March 1986.

Hing E: Use of nursing homes by the elderly: Preliminary data from the 1985 National Nursing Home Survey, in *Advance Data from Vital and Health Statistics*, No. 135. DHHS Publ. No. (PHS) 87-1250. Hyattsville, MD, Public Health Service, May 1987.

Hing E, Sekscenski ES: Use of health care—nursing care, in Havlik RJ, Liu BM, Kovar MG (eds): *Health Statistics on Older Persons, United States, 1986, Vital and Health Statistics*, Series 25, No. 25. DHHS Publ. No. (PHS) 87-1409. Public Health Service, Washington, DC, U.S. Government Printing Office, June 1987.

Institute of Medicine Committee on Regulation of Nursing Homes: *Improving the Quality of Care in Nursing Homes*, Washington, DC, National Academy Press, 1986.

Kane RL, Jorgensen LA, Teteberg B, et al: Is good nursing-home care feasible? *JAMA* 235:516–519, 1976.

Kovar MG: Aging in the eighties, age 65 and over and living alone, contacts with family, friends, and neighbors. Preliminary data from the Supplement on Aging to the National Health Interview Survey: United States, January 1–June 1984, in *Advance Data from Vital and Health Statistics*, No. 116. DHHS Publ. No. 86-1250. Hyattsville, MD, Public Health Service, May 9, 1986.

Master RJ, Feltin M, Jainchill J, et al: A continuum of care for the inner city: Assessment of its benefits for Boston's elderly and high-risk populations. *N Engl J Med* 302:1434–1440, 1980.

Sekscenski ES: Discharges from nursing homes: Preliminary data from the 1985 National Nursing Home Survey, in *Advance Data from Vital and Health Statistics*, No. 142. DHHS Publ. No. (PHS) 87-1250, Hyattsville, MD, Public Health Service, 1987.

Sirrocco A: Nursing and related care homes as reported from the 1986 Inventory of Long-Term Care Places, in *Advance Data from Vital and Health Statistics*, No. 147. DHHS Publ. No. (PHS) 88-1250, Hyattsville, MD, Public Health Service, 1988.

Stone R: Aging in the eighties, age 65 years and over—use of community services. Preliminary data from the Supplement on Aging to the National Health Interview Survey: United States, January–June 1984, in *Advance Data from Vital and Health Statistics,* No. 124. DHHS Publ. No. 86-1250. Hyattsville, MD, Public Health Service, September 30, 1986.

U.S. Comptroller General: *The Well-Being of Older People in Cleveland, Ohio.* HRD 77–70. General Accounting Office, 1977.

U.S. Comptroller General: *Conditions of Older People: National Information System Needed.* HRD 79–95. General Accounting Office, 1979.

U.S. General Accounting Office: *Medicare Home Health Services: A Difficult Program to Control.* HRD 82–4. General Accounting Office, 1981.

Waldo DR, Lazenby HC: Demographic characteristics and health care use and expenditures by the aged in the United States: 1977–1984. *Health Care Fin Rev* 6(1):1–30, 1984.

Woolley FR, Warnick R, Kane RL, et al: *Problem-Oriented Nursing.* New York: Springer, 1974.

SUGGESTED READINGS

Callahan JJ, Jr, Diamond LD, Giele JZ, et al: Responsibility of families for their severely disabled elders. *Health Care Fin Rev* 1:29–73, Winter 1980.

Kane RA, Kane RL: *Long-term Care: Principles, Programs and Policies.* New York, Springer, 1987.

O'Brien CL: *Adult Day Care: A Practical Guide.* Monterey, CA, Wadsworth Health Sciences, 1982.

Silverstone B, Hyman HK: *You & Your Aging Parent.* New York, Pantheon, 1976.

Somers AR: Long-term care for the elderly and disabled: A new health priority. *N Engl J Med* 307:221–226, 1982.

Trager B: *Home Health Care and National Health Policy* (special issue of *Home Health Care Services Quarterly*). New York, Haworth Press, 1980.

Vladeck BG: *Unloving Care: The Nursing Home Tragedy.* New York, Basic Books, 1980.

Chapter 17

Nursing Home Care

Some of the basic demographic and economic aspects of nursing home care are discussed in Chapters 2 and 15. The focus of this chapter will be the clinical care of nursing home residents.

Numerous reports have documented that medical care in the nursing home is often inadequate (Moss and Halamandaris, 1977; Vladek, 1980; Rabin, 1981; Institute of Medicine, 1986). Physician visits are usually brief and superficial, documentation in medical records is scanty, treatable conditions are underdiagnosed or misdiagnosed, and psychotropic drugs are overused and misused in part because of the absence of mental health interventions by appropriately trained professionals (Ray et al., 1980; Borson et al., 1987).

Despite the logistical, economic, and attitudinal barriers that can foster inadequate medical care in the nursing home, many relatively straightforward principles and strategies can lead to improvements in the quality of medical care provided to nursing home residents. Fundamental to achieving these improvements is a clear

425

perspective on the goals of nursing home care, which are in many respects quite different from the goals of medical care in other settings and patient populations.

THE GOALS OF NURSING HOME CARE

The key goals of nursing home care are listed in Table 17-1. While the prevention, identification and treatment of chronic, subacute, and acute medical conditions are important, most of these goals focus on the functional independence, autonomy, quality of life, comfort, and dignity of the residents. Physicians who care for nursing home residents must keep these goals in perspective at the same time the more traditional goals of medical care are being addressed.

The heterogeneity of the nursing home population must also be recognized in order to focus and individualize the goals of care. Nursing home residents can be subgrouped into five basic types (see Figure 17-1). Over half of the admissions to nursing homes are "short stayers," remaining in the facility for less than 6 months. Short stayers can be further subdivided into residents who enter the nursing home very ill with a short life expectancy, and residents who enter the nursing home for short-term rehabilitation, such as after a hip fracture. The focus and goals of care for these two subgroups of nursing home residents are obviously very different. At any one time, most

Table 17-1   Goals of Nursing Home Care

Provide a safe and supportive environment for chronically ill and dependent people

Restore and maintain the highest possible level of functional independence

Preserve individual autonomy

Maximize quality of life, perceived well-being, and life satisfaction

Provide comfort and dignity for terminally ill patients and their loved ones

Stabilize and delay progression, whenever possible, of chronic medical conditions

Prevent acute medical and iatrogenic illnesses and identify and treat them rapidly when they do occur

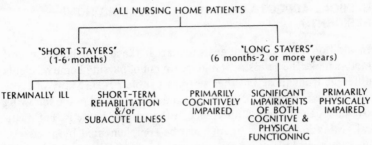

Figure 17-1 Basic types of nursing home patients. (*Reprinted with permission from Ouslander and Martin, 1987.*)

nursing home residents are "long stayers," individuals who will be in the facility longer than 6 months. As many as one-quarter of residents remain in the nursing home for 2 or more years. Long stayers can be further subdivided into residents with impairments of primarily cognitive functioning (e.g., the ambulatory, wandering resident with dementia), impairments of physical functioning (e.g., the resident with severe degenerative joint disease and osteoporosis, or end-stage heart failure), or residents with impairments of both cognitive and physical functioning (e.g., residents with stroke and significant residual deficits, residents with dementia and concomitant disabling medical conditions, or residents with end-stage dementia).

Many nursing homes attempt to geographically isolate these different types of residents. This strategy has several advantages, including the specialized training of staff caring for residents with specific types of problems, and the separation of residents with severe dementia and behavioral disturbances from cognitively intact residents. The latter often find interactions with severely demented residents very distressing.

While it is not always possible to geographically isolate these different types of residents, and residents often overlap or change between the types described, subgrouping nursing home residents in this manner will help the physician and interdisciplinary team to focus the care planning process on the most critical and realistic goals for individual residents.

CLINICAL ASPECTS OF CARE FOR NURSING HOME RESIDENTS

In addition to the different goals for care in the nursing home, several factors make the assessment and treatment of nursing home residents different from those in other settings (Table 17-2). Many of these factors relate to the process of care and are discussed in the following section. A fundamental difference in the nursing home is that medical evaluation and treatment must be complemented by an assessment and care planning process involving staff from multiple disciplines. Data on medical conditions and their treatment are integrated with assessments of the functional, mental, and behavioral status of the resident in order to develop a comprehensive data base and individualized plan of care.

Medical evaluation and clinical decision making for nursing home residents is complicated for several reasons. Unless the physician has cared for a resident before nursing home admission, it may be difficult to obtain a comprehensive medical data base. Residents may be unable to accurately relate their medical histories or describe their symptoms, and medical records are frequently unavailable or incomplete, especially for residents who have been transferred between nursing homes and acute hospitals. When acute changes in status occur, initial assessments are often performed by nursing home staff with limited skills and are transmitted to physicians by telephone. Even when the diagnoses are known or strongly suspected, many diagnostic and therapeutic procedures have an unacceptably high risk-to-benefit ratio among nursing home residents. For example, a barium enema may cause dehydration or severe fecal impaction, nitrates and other cardiovascular drugs may precipitate syncope or disabling falls in frail ambulatory residents with baseline postural hypotension, and adequate control of blood sugar may be extremely difficult to achieve without a high risk for hypoglycemia among diabetic residents with marginal or fluctuating nutritional intake who may not recognize or complain of hypoglycemic symptoms.

Further compounding these difficulties is the inability of many nursing home residents to effectively participate in important decisions regarding their medical care. Their prior expressed wishes are often not known, and an appropriate or legal surrogate decision

Table 17-2   Factors That Make Assessment and Treatment in the Nursing Home Different from Other Settings

1. The goals of care are often different (see Table 17-1)
2. Specific clinical disorders are prevalent among nursing home residents (see Table 17-3)
3. The approach to health maintenance and prevention differs (see Table 17-6)
4. Mental and functional status are just as, if not more important than, medical diagnoses
5. Assessment must be interdisciplinary, including:
   Nursing
   Psychosocial
   Rehabilitation
   Nutritional
   Other (e.g., dental, pharmacy, podiatry, audiology, ophthalmology)
6. Sources of information are variable:
   Patients often cannot give a precise history
   Family members and nurses' aides with limited assessment skills may provide the most important information
   Information is often obtained over the telephone
7. Administrative procedures for record keeping in both nursing homes and acute care hospitals can result in inadequate and disjointed information
8. Clinical decision making is complicated for several reasons:
   Many diagnostic and therapeutic procedures are expensive, unavailable, or difficult to obtain and involve higher risks of iatrogenic illness and discomfort than are warranted by the potential outcome
   The potential long-term benefits of "tight" control of certain chronic illnesses (e.g., diabetes mellitus, congestive heart failure, hypertension) may be outweighed by the risks of iatrogenic illness in many very old and functionally disabled residents
   Many residents are not capable (or questionably capable) of participating in medical decision making, and their personal preferences based on previous decisions are often unknown (see Table 17-7)
9. The appropriate site for and intensity of treatment are often difficult decisions that involve medical, emotional, ethical, economic, and legal considerations that may be in conflict with each other in the nursing home setting
10. Logistical considerations, resource constraints, and restrictive reimbursement policies may limit the ability of and incentives for physicians to carry out optimal medical care of nursing home residents

maker has often not been appointed. Several strategies described later in this chapter may help to overcome many of these difficulties.

Table 17-3 lists the most commonly encountered clinical disorders in the nursing home population. They represent a broad spectrum of chronic medical illnesses; neurological, psychiatric and behavioral disorders; and problems which are especially prevalent in the frail elderly (e.g., incontinence, falls, nutritional disorders, chronic pain syndromes). Although the incidence of iatrogenic ill-

Table 17-3   Common Clinical Disorders in the Nursing Home Population

Medical conditions
   Chronic medical illnesses
   Congestive heart failure
   Degenerative joint disease
   Diabetes mellitus
   Obstructive lung disease
   Renal failure
   Infections
      Lower respiratory tract
      Urinary tract
      Skin (pressure sores, vascular ulcers)
      Conjunctivitis
      Gastroenteritis
      Tuberculosis
   Gastrointestinal disorders
      Ulcers
      Reflux esophagitis
      Constipation
      Diarrhea
   Malignancies
Neuropsychiatric conditions
   Dementia
   Behavioral disorders associated with dementia
      Wandering
      Agitation
      Aggression
   Depression
   Neurological disorders other than dementia
      Stroke
      Parkinsonism
      Multiple sclerosis
      Brain or spinal cord injury

**Table 17-3 Common Clinical Disorders
in the Nursing Home Population (*Continued*)**

Functional disabilities requiring rehabilitation
  Stroke
  Hip fracture
  Joint replacement
  Amputation
Geriatric problems
  Delirium
  Incontinence
  Gait disturbances, instability, falls
  Malnutrition, feeding difficulties, dehydration
  Pressure sores
  Insomnia
  Chronic pain: musculoskeletal conditions, neuropathies,
    malignancy
  Iatrogenic disorders
    Adverse drug reactions
    Falls
    Nosocomial infections
    Induced disabilities
    Restraints and immobility, catheters, unnecessary
      help with basic ADLs
  Death and dying

nesses has not been systematically studied in nursing homes, it is likely to be as high as if not higher than that in acute hospitals (see Chapter 13). The management of many of the conditions listed in Table 17-3 is discussed in some detail in other chapters of this text (see Table of Contents and Index regarding specific conditions). Clinicians caring for nursing home residents should be especially well versed in the medical aspects of managing these conditions in the frail dependent elderly.

In addition to the numerous factors already mentioned that render the medical assessment and treatment of these conditions different, the process of care in nursing homes also differs substantially from that in acute hospitals, clinics, and home care settings.

PROCESS OF CARE IN THE NURSING HOME

The process of care in nursing homes is strongly influenced by numerous state and federal regulations, the highly interdisciplinary nature of nursing home residents' problems, and the training and skills of the staff that delivers most of the hands-on care.

Physician involvement in nursing home care and the nature of medical assessment and treatment offered to nursing home residents are often limited by logistical and economic factors. Few physicians have offices based either inside the nursing home or in close proximity to the facility. Many physicians who do visit nursing homes care for relatively small numbers of residents, often in several different facilities. Most nursing homes, therefore, have numerous physicians who make rounds once or twice per month and who are not generally present to evaluate acute changes in resident status, and attempt to assess these changes over the telephone. Many nursing homes do not have the ready availability of laboratory, radiological, and pharmacy services with the capability of rapid response, further compounding the logistics of evaluating and treating acute changes in medical status. Thus, nursing home residents are often sent to hospital emergency rooms where they are evaluated by personnel who are generally not familiar with their baseline status, and who frequently lack training and interest in the care of frail and dependent elderly patients.

Restrictive Medicare and Medicaid reimbursement policies may also dictate certain patterns of nursing home care. While physicians are required to visit nursing home residents only every 30 to 60 days, many residents require more frequent assessment and monitoring of treatment—especially with the shorter acute care hospital stays brought about by the prospective payment system [Diagnosis-Related Groups (DRGs)]. Yet, Medicare will generally reimburse a physician for only one routine visit per month, and perhaps one additional visit for an acute problem. Reimbursement for the routine visit is hardly adequate for the time that is required to provide good medical care in the nursing home, including travel to and from the facility, assessment and treatment planning for residents with multiple problems, communication with members of the interdisciplinary team and the resident's family, and proper documentation in the medical record. Activities which are often essential to good care in the nursing home, such as attendance at interdisciplinary conferences, family meetings, complex assessments of decision-making capacity, and counseling residents and surrogate decision makers on treatment plans in the event of terminal illness are generally not reimbursable at all. Medicare intermediaries often restrict reimbursement for rehabilitative services in what seems to be a variable and inequitable manner, thus limiting the treatment options for many residents (Smits et al., 1981). Although Medicaid programs vary considerably, most provide minimal coverage for ancillary services that are critical for optimum medical care, and many restrict reimbursement for several types of drugs which may be especially helpful for nursing home residents.

Amid these logistical and economic constraints, expectations for the care of nursing home residents are high. Table 17-4 outlines the various types of assessment generally recommended for the optimal care of nursing home residents. Physicians are responsible for completing an initial assessment within 48 h of admission and for monthly visits thereafter. Licensed nurses assess new residents as soon as they are admitted, on a daily basis, and generally summarize the status of each resident weekly. The extent of involvement of other disciplines in the assessment and care planning process varies depending on the residents' problems, the availability of various professionals, and state regulations. Most states require some type of involvement by the disciplines listed in Tables 17-2 and 17-4.

Representatives from nursing, social service, dietary, activities, and rehabilitation therapy (physical and/or occupational) participate in an interdisciplinary care planning meeting. Residents are generally discussed at this meeting within 2 weeks of admission and quarterly thereafter. The product of these meetings is an interdisciplinary care plan. The interdisciplinary care plan separately lists interdisciplinary problems (restricted mobility, incontinence, wandering, diminished food intake, poor social interaction, etc.), goals for the resident related to the problem, approaches to achieving these goals, target dates for achieving the goals, and assignment of responsibilities for working toward the goals among the various disciplines. These care plans are frequently the subject of careful scrutiny by state and federal auditors. The interdisciplinary care planning process serves as a cornerstone for resident management in many facilities but is a difficult and time-consuming process which requires leadership and tremendous interdisciplinary (and interpersonal) cooperation (Baldwin and Tsukuda, 1985). Staffing limitations in relation to the amount of time and effort required makes intensive interdisciplinary care planning

Table 17-4 Important Aspects of Various Types of Assessment in the Nursing Home

Type of assessment	Timing	Major objectives	Important aspects
Medical Initial	Within 48 h of admission	Verify medical diagnoses	A thorough review of medical records and physical examination are necessary
		Document baseline physical findings, mental and functional status, vital signs, and skin condition	Relevant medical diagnoses and baseline findings should be clearly and concisely documented in the patient's record
		Attempt to identify potentially remediable, previously unrecognized medical conditions	Medication lists should be carefully reviewed and only essential medications continued
		Get to know the resident and family (if this is a new resident)	Requests for specific types of assessment and inputs from other disciplines should be made
		Establish goals for the admission and a medical treatment plan	An initial medical problem list should be established (see example in Figure 17-2)
Periodic	Usually monthly	Monitor progress of active medical conditions	Progress notes should include clinical data relevant to active medical conditions and focus on changes in status
		Update medical orders	Unnecessary medications, orders for care, and laboratory tests should be discontinued
		Communicate with patient and nursing home staff	Mental, functional, and psychosocial status should be reviewed with nursing home staff and changes from baseline noted
			The medical problem list should be updated

434

As needed	When acute changes in status occur	Identify and treat causes of acute changes	On-site clinical assessment by the physician (or nurse practitioner or physician's assistant), as opposed to telephone consulation, will result in more accurate diagnoses, more appropriate treatment, and fewer unnecessary emergency room visits and hospitalization
			Vital signs, food and fluid intake, and mental status often provide essential information
			Infection, dehydration, and adverse drug effects should be at the top of the differential diagnosis for acute changes in status
Major reassessment	Annual	Identify and document any significant changes in status and new potentially remediable conditions	Targeted physical examination and assessment of mental, functional, and psychosocial status and selected laboratory tests should be done (see Table 17-6)
Nursing	Within hours of admission, and then routinely with monitoring of daily and weekly progress	Identify biopsychosocial and functional status strengths and weaknesses	Particular attention should be given to emotional state, personal preferences, and sensory function
		Develop an individualized care plan	Careful observation during the first few days of admission is important to detect effects of relocation
		Document baseline data for ongoing assessments	Potential problems related to other disciplines should be recorded and communicated to appropriate members of the interdisciplinary care team

Table 17-4   Important Aspects of Various Types of Assessment in the Nursing Home (*Continued*)

Type of assessment	Timing	Major objectives	Important aspects
Psychosocial	Within 1–2 weeks of admission and as needed thereafter	Identify any potentially serious psychological signs or symptoms and refer to mental health professional, if appropriate Determine past social history, family relationships, and social resources Become familiar with personal preferences regarding living arrangement	Getting to know the family and their preferences and concerns are critical to good nursing home care Relevant psychosocial data should be communicated to the interdisciplinary team
Rehabilitation (physical and occupational therapy)	Within days of admission and daily or weekly thereafter (depending on the rehabilitation program)	Determine functional status as it relates to basic activities of daily living Identify specific goals and time frame for improving specific areas of function Monitor progress toward goals Assess progress in relation to potential for discharge	Small gains in functional status can improve chances for discharge as well as quality of life Not all residents have areas in which they can reasonably be expected to improve; strategies to maintain function should be developed for these residents Assessment of and recommendations for modifying the environment can be critically important for improving function and discharge planning

Nutritional	Within days of admission and then periodically thereafter	Determine nutritional status and needs Identify dietary preferences Plan an appropriate diet	Restrictive diets may not be medically necessary and can be unappetizing Weight loss should be identified and reported to nursing and medical staff
Interdisciplinary care plan	Within 1–2 weeks of admission and every 3–4 months thereafter	Identify interdisciplinary problems Establish goals and treatment plans Determine when maximum progress toward goals has been reached	Each discipline should prepare specific plans for communication to other team members based on their own assessment
Capacity for medical decision making*	Within days of admission and then whenever changes in status occur	Determine which types of medical decision the resident is capable of participating in A resident who is still capable of making decisions independently should be encouraged to identify a surrogate decision maker in the event the resident later loses this decision-making capability If the resident lacks capacity for many or all decisions, appropriate surrogate decision makers should be identified (if not already done)	Residents with varying degrees of dementia may still be capable of participating in many decisions regarding their medical care Attention should be given to potentially reversible factors that can interfere with decision-making capacity (e.g., depression, fear, delirium, metabolic and drug effects) Family and health professional concerns should be considered, but the resident's desires should be paramount The resident's capacity may fluctuate over time because of physical and emotional conditions

Table 17-4 Important Aspects of Various Types of Assessment in the Nursing Home (Continued)

Type of assessment	Timing	Major objectives	Important aspects
Preferences regarding treatment intensity* and nursing home routines	Within days of admission and periodically thereafter	Determine residents' wishes as to the intensity of treatment they would want in the event of acute or chronic progressive illness	Specificity is important (e.g., "No heroic measures" is ambiguous) Attempt to identify specific procedures the resident would or would not want This assessment is often made by ascertaining the resident's prior expressed wishes (if known), or through surrogate decision makers (legal guardian, durable power of attorney for health care, family)

*See Table 17-7; these issues are also discussed in more detail in Chapter 18.

and teamwork unrealistic in many nursing homes. Although physicians are seldom directly involved in the care planning meetings in most facilities, they are generally required to review and sign the care plan and may find the team's perspective very valuable in planning subsequent medical care.

STRATEGIES TO IMPROVE MEDICAL CARE IN NURSING HOMES

Several strategies might improve the process of medical care delivered to nursing home residents. Three such strategies will be briefly described: the use of a comprehensive face sheet and documentation standards; the use of nurse practitioners or physicians' assistants; and a systematic approach to screening, health maintenance, and preventive practices for the elderly dependent nursing home population. In addition to these strategies, strong leadership of a medical director who is appropriately trained and dedicated to improving the facilities' quality of medical care is essential in order to develop, implement, and monitor policies and procedures for medical services. The role of the medical director in nursing homes is discussed in detail elsewhere (Levenson, 1988). The medical director should set standards for medical care and serve as an example to the medical staff by caring for some of the residents in the facility. The medical director should also be involved in various committees (pharmacy, infection control, quality assurance) and should involve interested medical staff in these committees as well as educational efforts through formal in-service presentations, teaching rounds, and appropriate documentation procedures.

One of the fundamental problems with the medical care delivered to nursing home residents is, in fact, documentation. As already mentioned, nursing home residents often have multiple coexisting medical problems and long previous medical histories. Residents often cannot relate their medical histories, and their previous medical records are frequently unavailable or incomplete. Thus, it is difficult, and sometimes impossible, to obtain a comprehensive medical data base. The effort should, however, be invested, and not wasted. Critical aspects of the medical data base should be recorded on one page or face sheet of the medical record. An example of a format for a face sheet is shown in Figure 17-2. The face sheet should also contain some information on the resident's neuropsychiatric and usual mental status, social information such as individuals to contact at critical times, and information about the resident's treatment status in the event of acute illness. These are data essential to the care of the resident and should be readily available in one place in the record so that when emergencies arise, medical consultants see the resident, or members of the interdisciplinary team need an overall perspective, it is easy to locate. The face sheet should be copied and sent to the hospital or other health care facilities to which the resident might be transferred. Time and effort will be required in order to keep the face sheet updated. For facilities with access to computers and/or word processing, incorporating the face sheet into a data base should be relatively easy and facilitate its rapid completion and periodic updating.

Medical documentation in progress notes for routine visits and assessments of acute changes is frequently scanty and/or illegible. "Stable," or "No change" are too frequently the only documentation for routine visits. While time constraints may preclude extensive notes, certain standard information should be documented. The "SOAP" (*s*ubjective, *o*bjective, *a*ssessment, *p*lan) format for charting routine notes is especially appropriate for nursing home residents (Table 17-5). In facilities in which microcomputers are available, simple data bases with word-processing capabilities can be used to enable physicians to efficiently produce legible, concise, yet comprehensive progress notes.

Another area in which medical documentation is often inadequate relates to the residents' decision-making capacity and treatment preferences. These issues are discussed briefly at the end of this chapter as well as in Chapter 18. In addition to placing critical information on the face sheet and other areas (e.g., identifying residents on "No CPR status" on the front and/or spine of the medical record), it is essential that physicians thoroughly and legibly document all discussions they have had with the resident, family, legal guardians, and/or durable power of attorney for health care about these issues. Failure to do so may result not only in poor communication and inappropriate treatment but also in substantial legal liability. Notes about

IDENTIFYING DATA

Name_____ Age_____

Record No. _____

Date of original admission to facility_____/___/_____ Most recent readmission ____/___/___

Primary physician _____ *(if applicable)*

ACTIVE MEDICAL PROBLEMS

1._____
2._____
3._____
4._____
5._____
6._____
7._____
8._____

NEUROPSYCHIATRIC STATUS

A. Dementia
____Absent ____Present
If present:
____Alzheimer's type
____Multi—infarct
____Mixed
____Other (_____)
____Uncertain

B. Psychiatric/behavioral disorders
1._____
2._____

C. Usual Mental Status
_____Alert, oriented, follows direction
_____Alert, disoriented, but follows directions
_____Alert, disoriented, cannot follow
_____Not alert (lethargic, comatose)

TREATMENT STATUS   (See note dated____/___/___)

____Full code   ____DNR, do not hospitalize, treat infections, etc. in facility
____DNR, but hospitalize   ____Supportive care
                                      ____ including enteral feeding
                                      ____ no enteral feeding

PAST HISTORY

A. Acute hospitalizations (since original admission to facility)

Diagnoses	Date (mos/yr)
1._____	_____
2._____	_____
3._____	_____

B. Major Surgical Procedures

Procedure	Date (yr)
1._____	_____
2._____	_____
3._____	_____

C. Allergies
1._____
2._____

SOCIAL INFORMATION

Name	Phone No.

Closest relative (relationship)
_____ _____

Other relative or friend
_____

Legal guardian
_____

Durable Power for Health Care
_____

Religious Preference:_____

Signature _____ Date:____/___/___

Figure 17-2   Example of a face sheet for a nursing home medical record.

Table 17-5   SOAP Format for Medical Progress Notes on Nursing Home Residents

Subjective	New complaints
	Symptoms related to active medical conditions
	Reports from nursing staff
	Progress in rehabilitative therapy
	Reports of other interdisciplinary team members
Objective	General appearance
	Weight
	Vital signs
	Physical findings relevant to new complaints and active medical conditions
	Laboratory data
	Consultant reports
Assessment	Presumptive diagnosis(es) for new complaints or changes in status
	Stability of active medical conditions
Plans	Changes in medications or diet
	Nursing interventions (e.g., monitoring of vital signs, skin care)
	Assessments by other disciplines
	Consultants
	Laboratory studies
	Discharge planning (if relevant)

these issues should not be thinned from the medical record and are probably best kept on a separate page behind the face sheet.

A second approach to improving medical care in nursing homes is the development and implementation of selected screening, health maintenance, and preventive practices. Table 17-6 lists examples of such practices. With few exceptions, the efficacy of these practices has not been well-studied in the nursing home setting. In addition, not all the practices listed in Table 17-6 are relevant for every nursing home resident. For example, some of the annual screening examinations are not appropriate for short stayers, or for many long-staying residents with end-stage dementia (Figure 17-1). Thus, the practices outlined in Table 17-6 must be tailored to the specific nursing home population as well as the individual resident and must be creatively incorporated into routine care procedures as much as possible in order to be time-efficient, cost-effective, and reimbursable by Medicare.

Table 17-6 Screening, Health Maintenance, and Preventive Practices in the Nursing Home

Practice	Minimum recommended frequency*	Comments
	Screening	
History and physical examination	Yearly	Generally required, but yield of routine annual history and physical is debated Focused exam probably beneficial, including rectal, breast, and, in some women, pelvic exam
Weight	Monthly	Generally required Persistent weight loss should prompt a search for treatable medical, psychiatric, and functional conditions
Functional status assessment, including gait and mental status testing, and screening for depression†	Yearly	Functional status usually assessed periodically by nursing staff Systematic global functional assessment should be done at least yearly in order to detect potentially treatable conditions (or prevent complications) such as early dementia, depression, gait disturbances, urinary incontinence
Visual screening	Yearly	Assess acuity, intraocular pressure, identify correctable problems
Auditory	Yearly	Identify correctable problems
Dental	Yearly	Assess status of any remaining teeth, fit of dentures, and identify any pathology
Podiatry	Yearly	More frequently in diabetics and residents with peripheral vascular disease Identify correctable problems and ensure appropriateness of shoes

Table 17-6   Screening, Health Maintenance, and Preventive Practices in the Nursing Home (Continued)

Practice	Minimum recommended frequency*	Comments
Screening (continued)		
Tuberculosis	On admission and yearly	All residents and staff should be tested Control skin tests and booster testing is generally recommended for nursing home residents (see text)

Laboratory tests
  Stool for occult blood
  Complete blood count
  Fasting glucose
  Electrolytes
  Renal function tests
  Albumin, calcium, phosphorous
  Thyroid function tests (including TSH level)
	Yearly	These tests appear to have reasonable yield in the nursing home population (see references)

Monitoring in selected residents		
All residents Vital signs, including weight	Monthly	More often if unstable or subacutely ill
Diabetics: Fasting and postprandial glucose, glycosylated hemoglobin		Fingerstick tests may also be useful if staff can perform reliably
Residents on diuretics or with renal insufficiency (creatinine >2, or BUN >35): Electrolytes, BUN, creatinine	Every 2–3 months	Nursing home residents are more prone to dehydration, azotemia, hyponatremia, and hypokalemia
Anemic residents who are on iron replacement or who have hemoglobin <10: Hemoglobin/hematocrit	Monthly until stable, then every 2–3 months	Iron replacement should be discontinued once hemoglobin value stabilizes

Blood level of drug for residents on specific drugs, e.g.:
  Digoxin
  Dilantin
  Quinidine
  Procainamide
  Theophylline
  Nortriptyline
	Every 3–6 months	More frequently if drug treatment has just been initiated

Table 17-6   Screening, Health Maintenance, and Preventive Practices in the Nursing Home (*Continued*)

Practice	Minimum recommended frequency*	Comments
	Prevention	
Influenza		
Vaccine	Yearly	All residents and staff with close resident contact should be vaccinated
Amantadine	Within 24–48 h of outbreak of suspected influenza A	Dose should be reduced to 100 mg per day in elderly; further reduction if renal failure present
		Unvaccinated residents and staff should be treated throughout outbreak; vaccinated can be treated until their symptoms resolve
Pneumococcal/pneumonia bacteremia Pneumococcal vaccine	Once	Efficacy in nursing home residents is debated
Tetanus booster	Every 10 years, or every 5 years with tetanus-prone wounds	Many elderly people have not received primary vaccinations; they require tetanus toxoid, 250–500 units of tetanus immune globulin, and completion of the immunization series with toxoid injection 4–6 weeks later and then 6–12 months after the second injection
Tuberculosis Isoniazid 300 mg per day for 1 year	Skin test conversion in selected residents	Residents with abnormal chest film (more than granuloma), diabetes, end-stage renal disease, hematological malignancies, steroid or immunosuppressive therapy, or malnutrition should be treated
Antimicrobial prophylaxis for residents at risk‡	Generally recommended for dental procedures, genitourinary procedures, and most operative procedures	Chronically catheterized residents should not be treated with continuous prophylaxis (see Chapter 6)

Table 17-6   Screening, Health Maintenance, and Preventive Practices in the Nursing Home (*Continued*)

Practice	Minimum recommended frequency*	Comments
Prevention (*continued*)		
Body positioning and range of motion for immobile residents	Ongoing	Frequent turning of very immobile residents is necessary to prevent pressure sores
		Semi-upright position is necessary for residents with swallowing disorders or enteral feeding to help prevent aspiration
		Range of motion to immobile limbs and joints is necessary to prevent contractures
Infection control procedures and surveillance	Ongoing	Policies and protocols should be in effect in all nursing homes
		Surveillance of all infections should be continuoûs to identify outbreaks and resistance patterns
Environmental safety	Ongoing	Appropriate lighting, colors, and the removal of hazards for falling are essential in order to prevent accidents
		Routine monitoring of potential safety hazards and accidents may lead to alterations which may prevent further accidents

*Frequency may vary depending on resident's condition.
†See Chapters 3 and 4 and Appendix for examples of assessments.
‡See Yoshikowa and Norman (1987) for detailed recommendations.

All long-staying residents should have some type of comprehensive, multidisciplinary reevaluation yearly. The efficacy of a routine standard annual history and physical examination and large panels of laboratory tests has been questioned (Gambert et al., 1982; Irvine et al., 1984; Domoto et al., 1985; Wolf-Klein et al., 1985; Levenstein et al., 1987). A targeted physical examination and functional assessment and selected laboratory tests are probably beneficial (Levenstein et al., 1987). Because reactivated tuberculosis is relatively common among the chronically ill elderly, all nursing home residents should have a skin test (with controls) on admission and yearly (unless they have a known prior positive test) (Stead et al., 1985). Recently, testing for the "booster phenomenon" has been recommended 10 to 14 days after an initial negative test because there is some incidence (probably in the range 5 to 15 percent) of conversion to a positive response during this time period which could be falsely interpreted as conversion on subsequent annual testing. Many nursing home residents are anergic, which can create difficulty in detecting active cases. Details about recommendations for tuberculosis screening in nursing homes can be found elsewhere (Cooper, 1986; Stead et al., 1987; Stead and To, 1987).

Because most nursing home residents have chronic medical conditions which are being actively treated, monitoring and treatment of these conditions becomes an important aspect of medical care. Several examples are presented in Table 17-6. Vital signs and weight are extremely important for accurate assessment on a routine basis, so that when acute or subacute changes occur, they can be compared to the resident's baseline.

Despite the old age and prevalence of chronic medical conditions and functional disabilities among the nursing home population, several preventive health practices may be effective. Most of these are related to infectious diseases (Table 17-6). One important exception relates to body positioning and range of motion for immobile residents, with the hope of preventing pressure sores, contractures, and aspiration pneumonia. In addition to preventive practices for nursing home residents, prevention is also relevant for nursing home staff as well as the facility as a whole. All nursing home staff who have close contact with residents should be vaccinated against influenza annually (Patriarca et al., 1987). The nursing home staff must also be intensively educated about infection control procedures such as hand washing, wound care (Garibaldi et al., 1981; Crossley et al., 1985), and catheter care (see Chapter 6).

The facility should have sound policies and procedures for infection control and should monitor patterns of infection and antimicrobial susceptibility. Because of the prevalent and often inappropriate use of antimicrobials, resistant organisms and *Clostridium difficile* diarrhea have become important problems in nursing homes (Zimmer et al., 1986). Another example of facilitywide prevention relates to environmental safety. Recommendations for assessing and altering the home environment in order to prevent falls are also relevant to nursing homes. Facilities should monitor falls and other accidents and make routine "environmental rounds" in order to identify potential hazards.

The third strategy that may help to improve medical care in nursing homes is the use of nurse practitioners and physician assistants. Although the cost-effectiveness of this approach has not been well documented, these health professionals may be especially helpful in carrying out specific functions in the nursing home setting. Recent legislation has enabled physician assistants to bill for services under Medicare. Nurse practitioners cannot bill Medicare directly; however, several states will reimburse their care and individual facilities and/or physician groups will hire them on a salaried basis. Although there is substantial overlap in training and skills, nurse practitioners may have an especially helpful perspective in interacting with nursing staff about the nonmedical aspects of nursing home resident care. On the other hand, physicians' assistants may be especially helpful in facilities where there is a high concentration of subacutely ill patients who require frequent medical assessment and intervention. Both can be very helpful in implementing some of the screening, monitoring, and preventive practices outlined in Table 17-6, and in communicating with interdisciplinary staff, families, and residents at times when the physician is not in the facility. One of the most appropriate roles for nurse practitioners and physicians' assistants is in the initial assessment of acute or subacute changes in resident status. They can perform a focused history and physical examination and order appropriate diagnostic studies. Several algorithms have been developed for this purpose (Martin et al., 1988), one of which is shown in Figure 17-3. This strategy enables the on-site assessment of acute change, the detection and treatment of new problems early in their course, more appropriate utilization of acute care hospital emergency rooms, and the rapid identification of residents who need to be hospitalized.

ACUTE ABDOMINAL PAIN

Symptoms: Sudden onset of diffuse or localized pain with or without nausea, vomiting, diarrhea

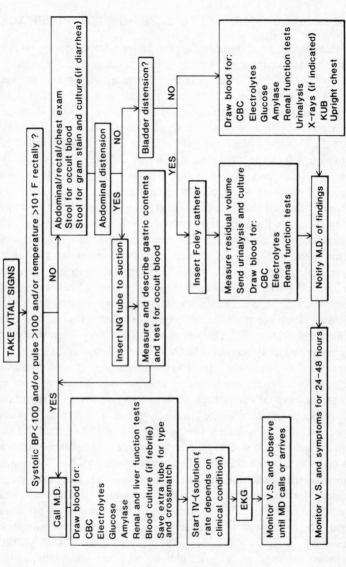

Figure 17-3 Example of an algorithm protocol for the management of acute abdominal pain in the nursing home by a nurse practitioner or physician's assistant.

THE NURSING HOME–ACUTE CARE HOSPITAL INTERFACE

Nursing home residents are frequently transferred back and forth between the nursing home and one or more acute care hospitals. The major reasons for transfer include infection and the need for parenteral antimicrobials and hydration, as well as acute cardiovascular conditions and hip fractures. Transfer to an acute care hospital is often a very disruptive process for a chronically ill nursing home resident. In addition to the effects of the acute illness, nursing home residents are subject to acute mental status changes and a myriad of potential iatrogenic problems (see Chapter 13). Probably the most prevalent of these iatrogenic problems are related to immobility, including deconditioning and difficulty regaining ambulation and/or transfer capabilities, and the development of pressure sores.

Because of the risks of acute care hospitalization, the decision to hospitalize a nursing home resident must carefully weigh a number of factors. A variety of medical, administrative, logistical, economic, and ethical issues can influence decisions to hospitalize nursing home residents. It is beyond the scope of this chapter to discuss these issues in detail; they are reviewed at length elsewhere (Rubenstein et al., 1988; Ouslander, 1988; Zimmer et al., 1988). Very often when nursing home residents become acutely ill, they simply need a few days of close observation with intravenous antimicrobials and hydration, such as for a lower respiratory or urinary tract infection. Decisions regarding hospitalization in these situations boil down to the capabilities of the physician and the nursing home staff to provide these services in the nursing home, the preferences of the resident and the family, and the logistical and administrative arrangements for acute hospital care. If, for example, the nursing home staff has been trained and has the personnel to institute intravenous therapy without detracting from the care of the other residents, and there is a nurse practitioner or physician's assistant to perform follow-up assessments, the resident with an acute infection who is otherwise medically stable may best be managed in the nursing home. Many facilities have limited nurse staffing, do not run continuous intravenous infusions, and do not have nurse practitioners or physicians' assistants and will, therefore, not be capable of managing these situations adequately.

One of the greatest difficulties arising from the frequent transfer of nursing home residents to acute care hospitals is the disruption in the continuity of medical records at a time when major changes in the residents' status are occurring. Hospitals often receive inadequate information from the nursing home records on transfer and vice versa when the resident is transferred back to the nursing home. Most nursing homes begin an entirely new medical record after a resident has been readmitted from an acute care hospital stay of longer than 7 to 14 days, which further compounds the difficulty in obtaining an adequate medical data base. Utilizing a face sheet similar to the one depicted in Figure 17-2 will help to provide hospital personnel and physicians (who may be covering the primary physician) with critical data and to update these data when the face sheet is completed at the nursing home when the resident is readmitted. Physician's hospital discharge summaries are rarely available within 24 to 48 h of the resident's nursing home admission, and standard intrafacility transfer forms often contain incomplete or ambiguous information. The development of a standard discharge summary form with data tailored to the nursing home's needs will greatly improve information transfer and the assessment process. An example of such a discharge summary form is included in the Appendix.

ETHICAL ISSUES IN NURSING HOME CARE

Ethical issues arise as much, if not more often, in the day-to-day care of nursing home residents than in the care of patients in any other setting. Several of the most common ethical dilemmas that occur in the nursing home are outlined in Table 17-7. Nursing homes care for an extraordinarily high concentration of individuals who are unable or questionably capable of participating in decisions concerning their current and future health care. It is among these same individuals that severe functional disabilities and terminal illnesses are very prevalent. Thus, questions regarding individual autonomy, decision-making capacity, surrogate decision makers, and the intensity of treatment that should be given at the end of life arise on a daily basis. These questions are both troublesome and complex but must be dealt with in a straightforward and systematic manner in order to provide optimal medical care to nursing home residents within the context of

Table 17-7   Common Ethical Issues in the Nursing Home

Ethical issue	Examples
Preservation of autonomy	Choices in many areas are limited in most nursing homes (e.g., mealtimes, sleeping hours)
	Families, physicians, and nursing home staff tend to become paternalistic
Decision-making capacity	Many nursing home residents are incapable or questionably capable of participating in decisions about their care
	There are no standard methods of assessing decision-making capacity in this population
Surrogate decision making	Many nursing home residents have not clearly stated their preferences or appointed a surrogate before becoming unable to decide for themselves
	Family members may be in conflict, have hidden agendas, or be incapable of or unwilling to make decisions
Quality of life	This concept is often entered into decision making, but it is difficult to measure, especially among those with dementia
	Ageist biases can influence perceptions of nursing home residents' quality of life
Intensity of treatment	A range of options must be considered, including cardiopulmonary resuscitation and mechanical ventilation, hospitalization, treatment of specific conditions (e.g., infection) in the nursing home without hospitalization, enteral feeding, comfort or supportive care only

*Approaches to these ethical issues are listed further in Table 17-4 and discussed in Chapter 18.

ethical principles and state and federal laws. Some practical methods of approaching these complex issues are discussed in Chapter 18. In addition, several helpful references are provided in the Suggested Readings sections of the bibliography at the end of this chapter as well as in Chapter 18.

REFERENCES

Baldwin D, Tsukuda R: Interdisciplinary teams, in Cassel C, Walsh J (eds): *Geriatric Medicine,* vol 2. New York, Springer-Verlag, 1985.

453

Borson S, Liptzin B, Nininger J, et al: Psychiatry in the nursing home. *Am J Psychiatr* 144:1412–1418, 1987.

Cooper JK: Decision analysis for tuberculosis prevention treatment in nursing homes. *J Am Geriatr Soc* 34:814–817, 1986.

Crossley KB, Irvine P, Kaszar DJ, et al: Infection control practices in Minnesota nursing homes. *JAMA* 254:2918–2921, 1985.

Domoto K, Ben R, Wei JY, et al: Yield of routine annual laboratory screening in the institutionalized elderly. *Am J Public Health* 75:243–245, 1985.

Gambert SR, Duthie EH, Wiltzius F: The value of the yearly medical evaluation in a nursing home. *J Chronic Dis* 35:65–68, 1982.

Garibaldi RA, Brodine RN, Matsumiya S: Infections among patients in nursing homes. *N Engl J Med* 305:731–735, 1981.

Institute of Medicine: *Improving the Quality of Care in Nursing Homes.* Washington, DC, National Academy Press, 1986.

Irvine PW, Carlson K, Adcock M, et al: The value of annual medical examinations in the nursing home. *J Am Geriatr Soc* 32:540–545, 1984.

Levenson S (ed): *Medical Direction in Long Term Care.* Owings Mills, MD, National Health Publishing, 1988.

Levenstein MR, Ouslander JG, Rubenstein LZ, et al: Yield of routine annual laboratory tests in a skilled nursing home population. *JAMA* 258:1909–1941, 1987.

Martin SE, Turner CL, Mendelsohn S, et al: Assessment and initial management of acute medical problems in a nursing home, in Basku G (ed): *Principals and Practice of Acute Geriatric Medicine.* St Louis, Mosby, 1988.

Moss FE, Halamandaris VJ: *Too Old, Too Sick, Too Bad: Nursing Homes in America.* Germantown, PA, Aspen Systems, 1977.

Ouslander JG: Reducing the hospitalization of nursing home residents. *J Am Geriatr Soc* 36:171–173, 1988.

Ouslander JG, Martin SE: Assessment in the nursing home. *Clin Geriatr Med* 3:155–174, 1987.

Patriarca PA, Arden NH, Koplan JP, Goodman RA: Prevention and control of type A influenza infections in nursing homes. *Ann Int Med* 107:732–740, 1987.

Rabin DL: Physician care in nursing homes. *Ann Intern Med* 94:126–128, 1981.

Ray WA, Federspeil CF, Schaffner W: A study of antipsychotic drug use in nursing homes: Epidemiologic evidence suggesting misuse. *Am J Public Health* 70:485–491, 1980.

Rubenstein LZ, Ouslander JG, Wieland D: Dynamics and clinical implications of the nursing home–hospital interface. *Clin Geriatr Med* 4:471–492, 1988.

Smits HL, Feder J, Scanlon W: Medicare's nursing-home benefit: Variations in interpretation. *N Engl J Med* 307:353–356, 1981.

Stead WW, To T: The significance of the tuberculin skin test in elderly persons. *Ann Intern Med* 107:837–842, 1987.

Stead WW, Lofgren JP, Warren E, et al: Tuberculosis as an endemic and nosocomial infection among the elderly in nursing homes. *N Engl J Med* 312:1483–1487, 1985.

Stead WW, To T, Harrison RW, et al: Benefit-risk considerations in preventive treatment for tuberculosis in elderly persons. *Ann Intern Med* 107:843–845, 1987.

Vladek B: *Unloving Care: The Nursing Home Tragedy*. New York, Basic Books, 1980.

Wolf-Klein GP, Holt T, Silverstone FA, et al: Efficacy of routine annual studies in the care of elderly patients. *J Am Geriatr Soc* 33:325–329, 1985.

Yoshikowa TT, Norman DC: *Aging and Clinical Practice: Infectious Diseases*. New York, Igaku-Shoin, 1987.

Zimmer JG, Bentley DW, Valenti WM, et al: Systemic antibiotic use in nursing homes: A quality assessment. *J Am Geriatr Soc* 34:703–710, 1986.

Zimmer JG, Eggert GM, Treat A, et al: Nursing homes as acute care providers: A pilot study of incentives to reduce hospitalizations. *J Am Geriatr Soc* 36:124–129, 1988.

SUGGESTED READINGS

Nursing Home Care (General)

Aiken LH, Mezey MD, Lynaugh JE, et al: Teaching nursing homes: Prospects for improving long-term care. *J Am Geriatr Soc* 33:196–201, 1985.

Avorn J, Langer E: Induced disability in nursing home patients: A controlled trial. *J Am Geriatr Soc* 30:397–400, 1982.

Ciocon JO, Silverston FA, Graver M, et al: Tube feedings in elderly patients: Indications, benefits, and complications. *Arch Intern Med* 148:429–433, 1988.

Cohen-Mansfield J, Billig N: Agitated behaviors in the elderly: I. A conceptual review. *J Am Geriatr Soc* 34:711–721, 1986.

Fries BE, Cooney LM: Resource utilization groups: A patient classification system for long-term care. *Med Care* 23:110–122, 1985.

Lewis MA, Kane RL, Cretin S, et al: The immediate and subsequent outcomes of nursing home care. *Am J Public Health* 75:758–762, 1985.

Lewis MA, Cretin S, Kane RL: The natural history of nursing home patients. *Gerontologist* 25:382–388, 1985.

Sloane PD, Pickard CG: Custodial nursing home care: Setting realistic goals. *J Am Geriatr Soc* 33:864–868, 1985.

Somers AR: Long-term care for the elderly and disabled: A new health priority. *N Engl J Med* 307:221–226, 1982.

Wieland GD, Rubenstein LZ, Ouslander JG, et al: Organizing an academic nursing home: impacts of institutionalized elderly. *JAMA* 255:2622–2627, 1986.

Williams C: Teaching nursing homes: Their impact on public policy, patient care and medical education. *J Am Geriatr Soc* 33:189–195, 1985.

Zimmer JG, Watson N, Treat A: Behavioral problems among patients in skilled nursing facilities. *Am J Public Health* 74:1118–1121, 1984.

Zweibel NR, Cassel CK (eds): Clinical and policy issues in care of the nursing home patient. *Clin Geriatr Med* Vol 4, No. 3, 1988.

Ethical Issues in Nursing Homes

Besdine RW: Decisions to withhold treatment from nursing home residents. *J Am Geriatr Soc* 30:602–606, 1983.

Brown NK, Thompson DJ: Nontreatment of fever in extended-care facilities. *N Engl J Med* 300:1246–1250, 1979.

Glasser G, Zweibel NR, Cassel CK: The ethics committee in the nursing home: Results of a national survey. *J Am Geriatr Soc* 36:150–156, 1988.

Haycox JA: Late care of the demented patient: The question of nursing-home placement. *N Engl J Med* 303:165–166, 1980.

Hilfiker D: Allowing the debilitated to die. *N Engl J Med* 308:716–719, 1983.

Lo B, Dornbrand L: Guiding the hand that feeds: Caring for the demented elderly. *N Engl J Med* 311:402–404, 1984.

Lo B, Dornbrand L: The case of Claire Conroy: Will administrative review safeguard incompetent patients? *Ann Intern Med* 104:869–873, 1986.

Lynn J: Dying and dementia. *JAMA* 256:2244–2245, 1986.

Mott PD, Barker WH: Hospital and medical care use by nursing home patients: The effect of patient care plans. *J Am Geriatr Soc* 36:47–53, 1988.

Nevins MA: Analysis of the Supreme Court of New Jersey's decision in the Claire Conroy case. *J Am Geriatr Soc* 34:140–143, 1986.

Steinbrook R, Lo B: Artificial feeding—solid ground, not a slipping slope. *N Engl J Med* 318:286–290, 1988.

Uhlman RF, Clark H, Pearlman RA, et al: Medical management decisions in nursing home patients: Principles and policy recommendations. *Ann Intern Med* 106:879–885, 1987.

Volicer L, Rheaume Y, Brown J, et al: Hospice approach to the treatment of patients with advanced dementia of the Alzheimer's type. *JAMA* 256:2210–2213, 1986.

Chapter 18

Ethical Issues in the Care of the Elderly

Ethics is a fundamental part of geriatrics. While it is central to the practice of medicine itself, the dependent nature of the geriatric patient makes it a special concern. The issues that tend to attract the greatest attention are those affecting life-and-death decisions: Should one withhold or withdraw treatment? Do you resuscitate? What about tube feeding? These are each important and taxing questions posed in the context of real people. However, they arise much less often than do the less heralded ethical dilemmas that confront us each day as we decide about discharge from hospital, arrange placement in a nursing home, or recommend therapies. Consideration of the ethics of geriatric care must address the full spectrum of these issues.

AUTONOMY AND BENEFICENCE

Table 18-1 provides a framework for discussing ethical issues. Two principal components to ethical discussions are the concepts of auton-

Table 18-1   Major Ethical Principles

Beneficence
  The obligation to do good
Nonmaleficence
  The obligation to avoid harm
Autonomy
  Duty to respect persons and their right to independent self-determination
    regarding the course of their lives and issues concerning the integrity of their
    bodies and minds
Justice
  Nondiscrimination: duty to treat individuals fairly; not to discriminate on the
    basis of irrelevant characteristics
  Distribution: duty to distribute resources fairly, nonarbitrarily, noncapriciously
Fidelity
  Duty to keep promises

---

omy and beneficence. *Autonomy* refers to one's right to control one's destiny, to exert one's will. Obviously there are limits to how freely such control can be expressed, but for geriatric purposes the principal issue revolves around whether the patient is able to assess the situation and make a rational decision independently. This raises the second concept. *Beneficence* refers to the duty to do good for others, to help them directly and in avoiding harm. This idea comes very close to paternalism, where one becomes the agent of another to make decisions as a father might do for a child. Such action directly conflicts with the principle of autonomy.

Physicians face a difficult set of choices in practice when they seek to walk these often fine lines. As Meier and Cassel (1986) note:

Although the medical community has frequently been attacked for its paternalistic attitude toward patients, it is usually conceded that paternalism can be justified if certain criteria are met: if the dangers averted or benefits gained for the person outweigh the loss of autonomy resulting from the intervention; if the person is too ill to choose freely; and if other persons in similar circumstances would likely choose the same intervention.

The challenge then comes down to several fundamental issues:

1   Is the patient capable of understanding the dilemma?
2   Is the patient able to express a preference?

3 Has the patient received accurate information about the benefits and risks?

4 Are there clear options? Have they been made clear?

5 What happens when the patient's preferences are contrary to the physician's or the patient's family's?

USING INFORMATION—COMPETENCE AND INFORMED CONSENT

In the case of the elderly, much of the concern is directed toward the issue of understanding and expressing opinions. The two most extreme cases are the comatose patient, who clearly cannot communicate, and the aphasic patient, who may not be able to communicate effectively. In the former case, we must look for other ways to preserve autonomy. In the latter, we must be very careful to assess and separate areas of communication from reasoning.

There is an important difference between the concepts of competence and decision-making capability. The former is a legal term. One not competent to act on one's own behalf requires an agent to act for oneself. In the case of dementia, persons may or may not be capable of understanding and interpreting complex situations and making a rational decision. We know that intellectual deficits are spotty. A person may get lost easily or forget things but still can make decisions. Just think of the classic absent-minded professor. The presence of a formal diagnosis of dementia, even by type, may not be a sufficient indicator of the individual's ability to comprehend and express a meaningful preference. Just as it is wrong to infantilize such patients by directing questions to others more quick to respond, so, too, might it be inappropriate to prejudge their ability to participate in decisions about their own care.

Determining cognitive ability and decision-making capacity is not easy. One must distinguish memory from understanding. The literature is not very helpful. Taub (1986) found that younger age and more education were predictors of understanding informed consents but that simplifying the form did not consistently improve understanding. Tymchuk et al. (1986) found too that varying the mode of presentation of information was not very helpful. However, major deficits in short-term memory or verbal knowledge were associated with reduced understanding. Neither study attempted any form of assistance such as reminders or prompts. Patients with memory deficits may need special help in recalling the components of the issue, but once reminded can often express a clear, sensible opinion.

One criterion for decision making, often presented with regard to informed consent, is the confirmation of the decision after a period of time for the patient to consider the issues at hand. Clearly, memory is an important ingredient in such an approach. Its feasibility will vary greatly with circumstances. The pressures of contemporary funding sadly prohibit such a reasonable approach to many crucial decisions. Contrast the situation for deciding about posthospital placement with that about discontinuing treatment or pursuing a high-risk treatment. The former decision is typically made under great duress with utilization review looming. Choices are frequently poorly described and the consequences of the alternatives, when such are even presented, not well defined.

The other side of the coin is the question of how information is presented. In order to make a rational decision, we all need a clear sense of the alternatives, including their benefits and risks. The physician is a major source of this information. More often than not the range of alternatives is foreshortened to emphasize those deemed most appropriate. Rarely are patients given the full description of the benefits and risks. In some instances this is appropriate, since the entire list of all possible risks may be excessive, and a discussion of very serious yet very rare conditions may inappropriately frighten a patient. When decisions about nursing home entry are made, they are not given the same level of serious attention accorded those about surgery. In many cases the physician may not know all the risks and benefits, but we never will until we are forced to address them.

When patients face decisions about entering a nursing home, for example, they need to understand the options at several levels. First, is a nursing home the best answer? What are the trade-offs between safety, privacy, and loss of autonomy? What other service configurations might work? At what cost, financial and otherwise? Next, they need to choose among nursing homes. Which one offers the social environment that suits their life-styles as well as having available resources to meet their physical needs? In too many cases, patients get to choose in neither category. Decisions, especially decisions made in hospitals, are made under great time pressure. Availability often takes precedence. A physician was heard to remark that a good discharge plan was one where patients knew where they were going. Surely something better than that should be expected.

ADVANCE DIRECTIVES

What happens when the patient cannot express a preference? One way of trying to deal with this situation is to encourage the development of advance directives, in which persons indicate what they want done under such circumstances (High, 1987). The two most common forms of these are living wills and durable power of attorney. The former indicates in as much detail as possible what actions should or should not be taken under specific circumstances. These living wills have been criticized as being too vague or too specific, and some research shows that a person's intentions and preferences change with circumstances. People usually are more anxious to avoid a bad condition than to get rid of it once it occurs. Similarly, it is difficult to know for certain how you would feel if faced with a certain life-threatening choice.

Living wills most often address the issue of extraordinary actions to sustain life, generally the question of resuscitation. They provide a means to indicate whether the patient prefers that heroic measures not be undertaken. In one sense, the more specific are such orders the better. Under what conditions? What constitutes an heroic measure? Another class of extraordinary measures is the use of artificial life supports. Again there is a need for specificity. Is a feeding tube the equivalent of a respirator? Some would argue that it is (Steinbrook and Lo, 1987).

Forgoing heroic measures need not mean abrogating all interest in surviving. One terrible anecdote is told about a nursing home staff that allowed a patient to choke to death on aspirated food because he had signed a "do not resuscitate" (DNR) request. Does not wanting cardiopulmonary resuscitation mean that the patient does not want pneumonia treated? DNR is not synonymous with "do not care."

Although there is a desire for specificity, both ethical and practical considerations enter into the picture. Few persons are prepared to sit down with a list of circumstances and actions to indicate in a calm, rational way if this occurs, this is what I want done or not done. At best, one may get a sense of a person's priorities and feelings about active efforts. Some advocate, for example, including provisions for advance directives on admission to a nursing home, while others suggest that it is unrealistic to expect that persons can make clear, thoughtful determinations at such a time of high stress. The danger of not building the decision into the admission routine, or at least the admission data collection process, is that it goes unattended. If the decision is best postponed until a calmer time after a period of adjustment, it should not be forgotten.

There are standard forms available to guide you in making choices and indicating preferences, but filling out such a list may be disconcerting. More than two-thirds of the states have some form of living will legislation, but the precise nature of those laws varies greatly in terms of what must be specified and under what conditions the delineated preferences can be followed.

An alternative to the living will approach of prespecification is the designation of a proxy, who is authorized to act on the patient's behalf if that person is unable to communicate. This designation can be done by using a durable power of attorney, previously used to transfer control of property. States must specifically extend their durable power of attorney statutes to cover medical decisions. Under this approach one can specify both the person one wishes to act as agent and the conditions under which such a proxy should be exercised. The components of a Durable Power of Attorney for Health Care are shown in Table 18-2.

With both the living will and the durable power of attorney there is some potential for misuse. Decisions once made can be difficult to revoke. What is the test of mental competence that allows one to change one's mind about a decision to not use life support systems? Stories are told about families who followed the patient's instructions even when the patient appeared to have a change of mind.

In the absence of any specification of actions or agents, someone must be identified to act for one who is unable to act on one's own behalf. There are legal procedures to accomplish this, which vary from state to state. In general, the two major classes of legally empowered agents are conservators and guardians. The latter usually have greater powers. A formal legal decision is needed to establish such a condition.

Table 18-2   Components of Durable Power of Attorney for Health Care

Creation of durable power of attorney for health care
  Statement that gives intention and refers to statute(s) authorizing such
Designation of health care agent
  Statement naming and facilitating access to (address, telephone number)
    agent; state laws will vary as to who may serve as agent—some states
    preclude providers of health care or employees of institutions where care is
    given; person designated as agent should have agreed to assume this role
General statement of authority granted
  Statement about circumstances under which the agent is granted power and
    indications of the power the agent will have in that event (usually a general
    statement about right to consent or refuse or withdraw consent for care,
    treatment, service or procedure, or release of information subject to any
    specific provisions and limitations indicated)
Statement of desires, special provisions, and limitations
  Opportunity to indicate general preferences (e.g., wish not to have life
    prolonged if burdens outweigh benefits; wish for life sustaining treatment
    unless in coma which physicians believe to be irreversible, then no such
    efforts; wish for all possible efforts regardless of prognosis); opportunity for
    specific types of things wanted done or not done and indications for such
    actions
Signatures
  Individual dated signature
  Witnesses (better notarized): witnesses cannot be those named as agents,
    providers of health care, or employees of facilities giving such care
Conditions
  Form should have place where person signing indicates awareness of rights,
    including the right to revoke the document and the conditions under which the
    document comes into force; some states require a mandatory maximum period
    such a document can be valid without renewal

Note: A copy of a basic form of a durable power of attorney for health care can be obtained from the California Medical Association (44 Gough Street, San Francisco CA 94103).

A critical question is, who is the person best qualified to assume that responsibility? Common wisdom suggests that it is the next of kin, but the ethical community argues that it should be the person most familiar with the patient's preferences, the person who can most closely estimate what the patient would have wanted. A rarely seen relative might know much less about the patient's wishes or life-style than might a close friend, clergyman, or even the attending physician. The choice should rest on the level of knowledge possessed. Where there are multiple contenders for the role, the courts may have to decide who is best positioned to know the patient's preferences. In cases where there is no one appropriate, the court may appoint a public guardian.

Agents, whether designated by durable power of attorney or chosen as the best available person, are vulnerable to pursuing their own interests rather than the patient's. At best, they must make inferences about the patient's wishes from their knowledge of the patient or the choice indicated in the durable power document. Surrogates' decisions may not be congruent with the wishes of the individuals they represent. They can be sincerely torn between acting in what they perceive to be the individual's wishes and best interests, two different perspectives on the issue.

Recent court decisions suggest that families and physicians may not have the last word in decisions about the care of incompetent persons. In the case of a demented woman with a legal guardian, the court ordered that a state ombudsman had to become involved in the decision to prevent premature discontinuation of tube feeding (Lo and Dornbrand, 1986).

THE PHYSICIAN'S ROLE

The physician may feel under great pressure. At times the physician's preferences will differ from those of the patient or the patient's agent. Nor are there only two poles to work between. Especially in the care of dependent older persons, family may exert strong influences to pursue what they perceive as the best interests of the patient or for other reasons. The physician must keep in mind who is the client.

One important issue is how actively should physician preferences be voiced. Physicians have an obligation to provide patients with a full set of information: the alternatives and the risks and benefits associated with each option, and to be sure that the patient appreciates that information. It is difficult to be fully objective in many instances. Values may unconsciously distort the way options are portrayed; risks may be minimized or even overlooked. Some physicians prefer to think of themselves as simply conduits of information, but others believe strongly that their opinions should be counted. They argue that the physician is often the most knowledgeable person involved and has a duty to guide and at least suggest a course of therapy. In some cases, patients may specifically ask for advice, or even indicate that they want the doctor to make the decision. Despite efforts to maintain a shared decision-making relationship, physicians will often find themselves unequal partners because of their authoritarian position. This deference is especially true with the current group of geriatric patients who were raised with a much more respectful set of beliefs about physicians than is currently the case among younger generations. The contemporary geriatrician must struggle hard to encourage the maximum autonomy from patients.

In an era of litigation, many physicians are understandably wary of taking charge. Fearful of being held responsible, they may wash their hands of the decision. Physicians find themselves smack in the middle of the pulls between autonomy and beneficence. Physicians who want to do what is best for their patients will offer their opinions and give their reasons. But in the end, they cannot override the patient. If they find themselves in strong disagreement, they can assist patients to find new sources of care, but they cannot abandon a patient because of a difference of opinion. Physicians and hospitals facing patients who want to act in a way different from their convictions have often worked very hard to transfer the locus of care, but until that transfer is accomplished, they are stuck with dealing with patients on their terms or going to court. A recent court decision affirmed that "competent patients have the right to decline life-prolonging treatment, even if physicians disagree because of conscience or ethics." Moreover, the hospitals and physicians involved would not be criminally or civilly liable if they carried out the patient's wishes in these matters (Lo, 1986).

A difficult problem for most physicians is when to introduce the topic of the patient's need to consider some form of advance directive. Speaking about such topics may seem like conceding defeat, but it represents a significant service to the patient, who needs to plan for the future appropriately. A legal vehicle designating who has legal responsibility can save much heartache later, even when it may not be legally binding.

SPECIAL PROBLEMS WITH NURSING HOME RESIDENTS

Nursing home patients present some special problems. They are usually admitted to nursing homes because of reduced capacity to cope. Many suffer from some degree of cognitive impairment. In one sense they are subject to a cruel paradox: because the quality of their daily lives may be so miserable, their lives are seen to have less value. It is easier to justify inattention or withholding extensive care (Brown and Thompson, 1979).

Table 18-3 lists four areas where clinical decisions in treating long-term-care patients may pose the greatest ethical dilemmas. As noted in Chapter 17, beyond the usually considered question of resuscitation, the physician faces difficult decisions in determining when it is appropriate to transfer a patient from the nursing home to hospital or when to intervene aggressively to treat changes in physiological status from fluid imbalance or infection. Perhaps one of the most perplexing areas is when to pursue heroic measures to maintain nutritional supports. Especially with the tremendous growth in technology for establishing effective, but expensive nutritional regimens in persons incapable of eating on their own for sustained periods, this issue is faced with increasing frequency. Artificial feeding decisions seem to arouse more controversy than other life-sustaining treatment issues. The growing consensus seems to favor the view that tube and intravenous feeding are more akin to a medical intervention than to routine nursing care or comfort (Steinbrook and Lo, 1988).

Physicians must be diligent in working to preserve the patient's personhood. Essentially nursing home residents should not lose any of their rights as people just because they enter a nursing home. They should be eligible to participate in a full range of activities and to make choices about their lives and their health care. They should be the first ones consulted about changes in their condition or therapy. Visits to a nursing home should be more like home calls or office visits than hospital visits.

In practice, this freedom is often not allowed. One set of arguments for constraining nursing home resident choice is the limitations

Table 18-3 Major Topics for Clinical Ethical Decisions

Resuscitation
Transfer to more intensive level of care
Treatment of infections and other intercurrent physiological derangements
Nutrition and hydration

Source: After Lynn, 1986.

imposed by any institution. Just as college students must eat at certain times and choose from a menu, so, too, must nursing home residents. But the similarity breaks down when one appreciates the limited options available to the residents. They cannot easily order in a pizza or go out for a beer. Again part of the restriction is imposed by their medical status. Pizza and beer may be prohibited from their diet. Often this medicalization represents its own set of ethical dilemmas. When is dietary control a greater good than culinary pleasure? But too often medical orders become excuses for not individualizing regimens. Few conditions are aggravated by different hours of going to bed. In fact, sleeping medications might be less often prescribed if there were more flexibility in bedtimes. Similarly, participation in activities or the right to privacy become major issues in a world shrunk to nursing home proportions. How much say should a resident have in the choice of a roommate? Some would argue that single rooms should be the norm. The same people who would not deign to share a hotel room with a stranger for a single night seem to have no problem committing nursing home residents to roommates for years. An often repressed subject is the nursing home resident's rights to sexual privacy. Neither age nor dependency means a need to abrogate all rights to a sexual life. Sexual intimacy requires privacy. Too often nursing home staffs are insensitive and intolerant to these needs (McCartney et al., 1987).

There is a danger that the physician will treat the staff's needs rather than the patient's. Care should be exercised to avoid prescribing prn restraints or sedatives to offer easy ways for staff to deal with behaviors they find disruptive. Too available recourse to such orders strips the patient of personhood and makes the patient simply an object to be controlled.

Because nursing home residents are vulnerable, special care is needed to protect their rights. Uhlmann and his colleagues (1987) have developed an excellent set of principles and practices for this purpose. The general goal is to maximize the resident's autonomy in making decisions about treatment. Several ombudsman groups have created a parallel set of concerns in the form of a resident's bill of rights, which outlines the choices that should be available and the protections that can be sought. The recent Institute of Medicine study (1986) of nursing home quality took special pains to emphasize the need to integrate quality of life considerations with quality of care. The former is an essential component of the latter. As such, it is the responsibility of the physician to see that these elements are addressed as part of basic care.

One useful approach to buffer the relations between the nursing home, outside investigators and practitioners, and the residents is to establish an ethics committee composed of persons within and without the home. Traditionally such committees began with the major charge of overseeing research activities, but they have increasingly begun to take responsibility for reviewing and facilitating standards for other aspects of the institution's activities and to serve as resources to establish guidelines for managing decision making around ethically difficult areas. Such committees are especially useful when they operate in a proactive manner, exploring issues in advance rather than assessing actions already taken. In many instances, they offer a disinterested forum where these very sensitive matters can be discussed with maximum dispassion and all sides of an issue aired.

SPECIAL CASE OF DEMENTIA

Because dementia implies a loss of humanness, there are special questions to be raised about how much treatment is appropriate (Rango, 1985). As already noted, the severe loss of cognitive function makes patient participation in decision making very difficult. Those left to act as agents for the demented patient must struggle with the difficult issue of when the loss of self-awareness and ability to maintain relationships constitutes substantial suffering. The loss of intellect is perhaps the most serious loss experienced by people. In one effort to explore the value of alternative outcomes among nursing home residents, if the resident was described as having loss of cognitive ability, all outcomes were substantially lower rated by a variety of persons, including care providers, family, policymakers, and the general public (Kane, 1986).

The management of demented patients poses additional problems. Demented persons are frequently intrusive. They threaten the privacy of those cognitively intact residents who must live with them. It does not seem right to diminish the quality of life for the latter in the name of efficiency or in some hope that they will stimulate the demented. Separate programs or units seem much more humane and sensible. Some have expressed concern about the burden on staff, but this anxiety does not seem to be borne out by experience. The separation allows more appropriate programming and facility design. In fact, the basic plans for facilities for the physically impaired and the cognitively impaired are also diametrically opposed. The former need ready access to nursing stations and short distances to walk, whereas the latter are best left to wander unimpeded in an eventually enclosed area with as much space as possible. In the continuum of special care facilities for the demented, we are now seeing the extension of the principles of hospice care to this group and their families (Volicer et al., 1986).

POLICY ISSUES

Age has become a major issue in policy. Growing concern about the high cost of health care, especially at the end of life, has prompted discussion as to whether age should be a criterion for rationing services (Scitovsky and Capron, 1986). The concern expressed over the reports of withholding services like renal dialysis in the United Kingdom's National Health Service (Aaron and Schwartz, 1984) suggests that our country is uncomfortable with such an approach, but it is being proposed (Callahan, 1987). At a more subtle level, measures of program effectiveness tend to use something equivalent to the quality-adjusted life-year (QALY). This term implies that valuable life is that lived free of dependency. Gerontologic researchers have called it *active life expectancy* (Katz, 1983). Such proxies for program effectiveness incorporate ethical components subtly. We have not established the base on which to put a value on life lived at some level of dependency. To assume that it has no value, as is implied by active life years, appears to contradict the very purpose for geriatrics. As advocates for the elderly, geriatricians must be extremely vigilant to how such terms are used both in everyday speech and in analyses. It is important to bear in mind that any measure that uses life expectancy will tend to be biased against the elderly (Avorn, 1984). At a time when there is an effort to pit one generation against another, care must be taken to avoid setting the terms of the debate such that the outcome is inevitable.

SUMMARY

In summary, elderly patients should not lose their rights to full consideration of options and participation in decisions. The principles of autonomy and beneficence, which form a central part of the ethics of medicine in general, are strained with the dependent elderly because the temptation toward paternalism is greater in the presence of the tendency to infantilize elderly patients, especially when they cannot readily communicate. Concerns about how to make decisions for persons unable to express their own preferences are often couched in terms of fear of litigation, but the growing body of experience suggests that carefully pursued efforts to establish agency and act accordingly will not put physicians or institutions at great risk of lawsuits. Finally, it is important to recognize that the life of dependent elderly persons, especially those in nursing homes, is composed of many little incidents. The daily loss of dignity, privacy, and self-respect may be too readily ignored. To be truly the patient's advocate, the physician must be vigilant to these small but critical ethical insults. It would be the greatest irony if the elderly patient were daily abused while living, only to become the subject of profound ethical analysis about dying. This is precisely the kind of behavior geriatrics is in business to prevent.

REFERENCES

Aaron, HJ, Schwartz WB: *The Painful Prescription: Rationing Hospital Care*. Washington, DC, Brookings Institution, 1984.

Avorn J: Benefit and cost analysis in geriatric care: Turning age discrimination into health policy. *N Engl J Med* 310:1294–1301, 1984.

Brown NK, Thompson DJ: Nontreatment of fevers in extended-care facilities. *N Engl J Med* 300:1248–1250, 1979.

Callahan D: *Setting Limits*. New York: Basic Books, 1987.

High DM: Planning for decisional incapacity: A neglected area in ethics and aging. *J Am Geriatr Soc* 35:814–820, 1987.

Institute of Medicine: *Improving the Quality of Care in Nursing Homes*. Washington, DC, National Academy Press, 1986.

Kane RL, Bell RM, Riegler SZ: Value preferences for nursing home outcomes. *Gerontologist* 26:303–308, 1986.

Katz S, Branch LG, Branson MH, et al: Active life expectancy. *N Engl J Med* 309:1218–1224, 1983.

Lo B: The Bartling case: Protecting patients from harm while respecting their wishes. *J Am Geriatr Soc* 34:44–48, 1986.

Lo B, Dornbrand L: The case of Claire Conroy: Will administrative review safeguard incompetent patients? *Ann Intern Med* 104:869–873, 1986.

Lynn J: Dying and dementia. *JAMA* 256:2244–2245, 1986.

McCartney JR, Izeman H, Rogers D, et al: Sexuality and the institutionalized elderly. *J Am Geriatr Soc* 35:331–333, 1987.

Meier DE, Cassel CK: Nursing home placement and the demented patient: A case presentation and ethical analysis. *Ann Intern Med* 104:98–105, 1986.

Rango N: The nursing home resident with dementia: Clinical care, ethics and policy implications. *Ann Intern Med* 102:835–841, 1985.

Scitovsky AA, Capron AM: Medical care at the end of life; The interaction of economics and ethics. *Ann Rev Publ Health* 7:59–75, 1986.

Steinbrook R, Lo B: Artificial feeding—solid ground, not a slippery slope. *N Engl J Med* 318:286–290, 1988.

Taub HA, Baker MT, Sturr JF: Informed consent for research: Effects of readability, patient age and education. *J Am Geriatr Soc* 34:601–606, 1986.

Tymchuk AJ, Ouslander JG, Rader N: Informing the elderly: A comparison of four methods. *J Am Geriatr Soc* 34:818–822, 1986.

Uhlmann RF, Clark H, Pearlman RA, et al: Medical management decisions in nursing home patients. *Ann Intern Med* 106:879–885, 1987.

Volicer L, Rheaume Y, Brown J, et al: Hospice approach to the treatment of patients with advanced dementia of the Alzheimer's type. *JAMA* 256:2210–2213, 1986.

SUGGESTED READINGS

Beauchamp TL, Childress JF: *Principles of Biomedical Ethics*. New York, Oxford University Press, 1979.

Cassel CK, Meier DE, Traines ML: Selected bibliography of recent articles in ethics and geriatrics. *J Am Geriatr Soc* 34:399–409, 1986.

Ciocon JG, Silverstone FA, Graver LM, et al: Tube feedings in elderly patients: Indications, benefits and complications. *Arch Intern Med* 148:429–433, 1988.

Elford RJ: *Medical Ethics and Elderly People*. Edinburgh, Churchill Livingstone, 1987.

Emanuel EJ: A review of the ethical and legal aspects of terminating medical care. *Am J Med* 84:291–301, 1988.

Jonsen AR, Siegler M, Winslade WJ: *Clinical Ethics*. New York, Macmillan, 1982.

Lynn J: *By No Extraordinary Means: The Choice to Forgo Life-sustaining Food and Water*. Bloomington, IN, Indiana University Press, 1986.

Suggested Geriatric Medical Forms

BASIC MEDICAL HISTORY AND PHYSICAL ASSESSMENT

A. Medical History

1. Patient's major complaint(s) (in patient's own or care giver's language)

   _____
   _____
   _____
   _____
   _____

2. Prior surgery

   Date   Surgical procedure
   _____ / _____ / _____   _____
   _____ / _____ / _____   _____
   _____ / _____ / _____   _____
   _____ / _____ / _____   _____

3. Other hospitalizations

   Date   Hospital   Diagnoses
   _____ / _____ / _____   _____   _____
   _____ / _____ / _____   _____   _____
   _____ / _____ / _____   _____   _____
   _____ / _____ / _____   _____   _____

4. Other medical history

   a. TB test status _____

   b. Immunization status

      1. Pneumococcal _____
      2. Tetanus _____
      3. Influenza _____

   c. Last dental visit _____

   d. Last Papanicolaou (Pap) test _____

5. Allergies: _____

6. Habits

	No	Yes
a. Smoking	_____	_____
b. Alcohol consumption	_____	_____

   If yes, specify amount and duration _____

   c. Diet _____

   d. Exercise _____

475

7. Current medications

Prescribed drugs   Dosage and frequency

_____   _____

_____   _____

_____   _____

_____   _____

_____   _____

_____   _____

Over-the-counter drugs   Dosage and frequency

_____   _____

_____   _____

_____   _____

_____   _____

8. Symptom review

a. Patient's overall rating of own health:

_____ Excellent   _____ Very good   _____ Good
_____ Fair   _____ Poor

b. Selected symptom review (enter C for chronic, N for new). If positive, describe briefly.

_____ Anorexia
_____ Fatigue
_____ Weight loss
_____ Insomnia
_____ Headache
_____ Visual impairment
_____ Hearing impairment
_____ Dental / denture discomfort
_____ Cough or wheezing
_____ Dyspnea
_____ Exertional chest discomfort
_____ Orthopnea
_____ Edema
_____ Claudication
_____ Dizziness / unsteadiness
_____ Falls*
_____ Syncope
_____ Dysphagia
_____ Abdominal pain
_____ Change in bowel habit or constipation
_____ Blood in stool
_____ Urinary frequency and / or urgency
_____ Nocturia
_____ Hesitancy, straining, or intermittent stream
_____ Incontinence*
_____ Foot problems
_____ Focal weakness or sensory loss

_____ Transient visual disturbance
_____ Forgetfulness*
_____ Depression
_____ Disruptive behavior / wandering

*See other assessment forms

9. Depression screen

For each of the following questions, which description comes closest to the way you have been feeling *during the past month*?

	All the time	Most of the time	Some of the time	A little of the time	None of the time
a. How much of the time, *during the past month,* has your health limited your social activities (like visiting relatives)?	_____	_____	_____	_____	_____
b. How much of the time, *during the past month,* have you been a very nervous person?	_____	_____	_____	_____	_____
c. *During the past month,* how much of the time have you felt calm and peaceful?	_____	_____	_____	_____	_____
d. How much of the time, *during the past month,* have you felt downhearted and blue?	_____	_____	_____	_____	_____
e. *During the past month,* how much of the time have you been a happy person?	_____	_____	_____	_____	_____
f. How often, *during the past month,* have you felt so down in the dumps that nothing could cheer you up?	_____	_____	_____	_____	_____
g. *During the past month,* how often has feeling depressed interfered with what you usually do?	_____	_____	_____	_____	_____
h. *During the past month,* how often did you feel that you had nothing to look forward to?	_____	_____	_____	_____	_____
i. How often have you felt like crying *during the past month*?	_____	_____	_____	_____	_____
j. *During the past month,* how often did you feel like life isn't worth living anymore?	_____	_____	_____	_____	_____

Answers of "all the time" or "most of the time" should raise suspicion of depression (except to questions c and e).

477

10. Functional status

   a. Basic and instrumental activities of daily living

	Fully independent*	Needs some human assistance (including supervision)	Totally dependent
Bathing	————	————	————
Ambulation	————	————	————
Transfer	————	————	————
Dressing	————	————	————
Personal grooming	————	————	————
Toileting	————	————	————
Eating	————	————	————
Preparing meals	————	————	————
Managing money	————	————	————
Managing medications	————	————	————
Using telephone	————	————	————

Is the patient incontinent?

Bladder Yes _____ No _____   Bowel Yes _____ No _____

*Indicate whether mechanical aid used and what type(s)

   b. Functional limitations

For how long (if at all) has your health limited you in each of the following activities? (Check the category which is the best description.)

	Limited for more than 3 months	Limited for 3 months or less	Not limited at all
The kinds or amounts of *vigorous* activities you can do, like lifting heavy objects, running, or participating in strenuous sports	————	————	————
The kinds or amounts of *moderate* activities you can do, like moving a table or carrying groceries	————	————	————
The kinds of work or housework you can do around your home	————	————	————
Working at a job	————	————	————
Walking uphill or climbing stairs	————	————	————
Bending, lifting, or stooping	————	————	————

Walking one block _____ _____ _____

Eating, dressing, bathing, or
using the toilet _____ _____ _____

B. Physical Examination

1. Vital signs

	Supine	Sitting	Standing
Blood pressure	/	/	/
Pulse (per minute)	_____	_____	_____
Respiratory rate (per minute)	_____	_____	_____

Weight (lb)_____ Height_____
Weight last examination (lb)_____(date of last examination___ / ___ / ___)

2. Skin

_____Excessive dryness
_____Rash (Describe: _____)
_____Lesions—suspected malignant (Location:_____)
_____Pressure sores

Location	Size (cm)	Stage (I-IV)
_____	_____	_____
_____	_____	_____
_____	_____	_____

3. Hearing

_____Hears normal voice   _____Wears hearing aid
_____Impaired   _____Cerumen impacted in ear canals
_____Hears 1024-Hz tuning fork

Frequency threshold at 40 dB_____

4. Vision:

Able to read newsprint

_____With corrective lenses   _____Without corrective lenses

Visual acuity

	Reading	Distance
Right	_____ / _____	_____ / _____
Left	_____ / _____	_____ / _____

Cataract present: _____Right   _____Left

Funduscopic findings

	Normal	Abnormal (describe)	Unable to visualize
Right	_____	_____	_____
Left	_____	_____	_____

5. Mouth

_____Poor oral hygiene

Dentures
_____None _____Good fit _____Poor fit
_____Sores under dentures _____Other lesion (describe)

6. Neck

	Normal	Abnormal
Range of motion	_____	_____
Thyroid	_____	_____

_____Thyroid scar
_____Mass (describe]

7. Lymph nodes

_____No lymphadenopathy
_____Enlarged nodes (Describe: _____)

8. Breasts

Mass present? _____Yes _____No
If yes: _____Right _____Left (Describe: _____)

Other abnormality _____

9. Lungs

	No	Yes		No	Yes
Rales	_____	_____	Bronchospasm	_____	_____
Rhonchi	_____	_____	Other (specify)	_____	_____

If yes, describe: _____

10. Cardiovascular

a. Heart

	No	Yes
Irregular rhythm	_____	_____
Murmur	_____	_____
S_3	_____	_____
S_4	_____	_____
Other (specify)	_____	_____

If yes, describe: _____

b. Bruits

_____None
Carotid _____Right _____Left
Femoral _____Right _____Left

c. Distal pulses

	Present	Absent
Right dorsalis pedis	_____	_____
Right posterior tibial	_____	_____
Left dorsalis pedis	_____	_____
Left posterior tibial	_____	_____

d. Edema

	None	1+	2+	3+	4+
Pedal	_____	_____	_____	_____	_____
Tibial	_____	_____	_____	_____	_____
Sacral	_____	_____	_____	_____	_____

11. Abdomen

Liver size_____cm
Abdominal masses _____None _____Pulsatile _____Other
Bruits _____Yes _____No
Tenderness _____Yes _____No

Describe positive findings: _____
_____

12. Rectal

_____Diminished/absent sphincter tone
_____Enlarged prostate (Describe:_____)
_____Prostate mass
_____Rectal mass
_____Fecal impaction

Occult blood _____Negative _____Positive

13. Genital/pelvic

a. Men
_____Normal
_____Abnormal (Describe: _____)

b. Women
_____Normal
_____Abnormal (Describe: _____)
_____Vaginal atrophy _____Mass
_____Atrophic vaginitis _____Tenderness
_____Pelvic prolapse _____Other

Pap test done _____Yes _____No

14. Musculoskeletal

	None	Spine	Shoulders	Elbows	Hands	Hips	Knees	Feet
Deformity	___	___	___	___	___	___	___	___
Limited range of motion	___	___	___	___	___	___	___	___
Tenderness	___	___	___	___	___	___	___	___
Prominent swelling or inflammation	___	___	___	___	___	___	___	___

Description of deformity or limited range of motion: _____
_____
_____

15. Neurological

    a. Mental status

	Intact	Impaired
Orientation		
Person	_____	_____
Place	_____	_____
Time	_____	_____
Situation	_____	_____
Memory	_____	_____
Remote	_____	_____
Recent	_____	_____
Object recall after 5 minutes	_____	_____
Immediate (repetition)	_____	_____

Short Portable Mental Status Questionnaire
(Many other standardized tests are also available.)

Right	Wrong	
_____	_____	What is the date today (month/day/year)?
_____	_____	What day of the week is it?
_____	_____	What is the name of this place?
_____	_____	What is your telephone number? (If no telephone, what is your street address?)
_____	_____	How old are you?
_____	_____	When were you born (month/day/year)?
_____	_____	Who is the current president of the United States?
_____	_____	Who was the president just before him?
_____	_____	What was your mother's maiden name?
_____	_____	Subtract 3 from 20 and keep subtracting 3 from each number you get, all the way down.

Number of errors:_____

0-2 errors = intact
3-4 errors = mild intellectual impairment
5-7 errors = moderate intellectual impairment
8-10 errors = severe intellectual impairment

(If dementia is suspected, further assessment should be undertaken. See Dementia Assessment.)

    b. Mood/affect:

_____Appropriate _____Labile _____Depressed _____Agitated
_____Anxious

c. General

	Normal	Abnormal (describe)
Cranial nerves	_____	_____
Motor		
Strength	_____	_____
Tone	_____	_____
Sensation		
Pin	_____	_____
Touch	_____	_____
Vibration	_____	_____
Reflexes	_____	_____
Cerebellar	_____	_____
Finger to nose	_____	_____
Heel to shin	_____	_____
Romberg	_____	_____
Gait	_____	_____ (see Falls Assessment Form)

Description of abnormal findings: _____
_____
_____

d. Other signs

	Absent	Present (describe)
Resting tremor	_____	_____
Cogwheel rigidity	_____	_____
Bradykinesia	_____	_____
Intention tremor	_____	_____
Involuntary movements	_____	_____
Pathological reflexes	_____	_____

Description of findings present: _____
_____
_____

C. Laboratory Data

Test/procedure	Date	Normal	Abnormal (describe)
_____	____/____/____	_____	_____
_____	____/____/____	_____	_____
_____	____/____/____	_____	_____
_____	____/____/____	_____	_____
_____	____/____/____	_____	_____

D. Problem List

Problem/diagnosis	Date identified	Comments
_____	____/____/____	_____
_____	____/____/____	_____
_____	____/____/____	_____
_____	____/____/____	_____
_____	____/____/____	_____
_____	____/____/____	_____
_____	____/____/____	_____
_____	____/____/____	_____
_____	____/____/____	_____
_____	____/____/____	_____
_____	____/____/____	_____
_____	____/____/____	_____
_____	____/____/____	_____
_____	____/____/____	_____

SOCIAL ASSESSMENT

1. Has any of the following happened in the last year (describe if yes)?

_____Death of spouse
_____Death of other close family member
_____Change in health of family member
_____Change in living situation
_____Divorce or separation
_____Marriage or "pairing up"
_____Change in financial state

2. Living situation

a. _____House
   _____Apartment
   _____Other

b. _____Alone
   _____With another person or others

   If so, who lives with patient?

   Name   Relationship
   1. _____
   2. _____
   3. _____

c. Telephone
   _____None
   _____Yes [phone number (_____)_____-_____]

d. Stairs
   _____No
   _____Yes
   If yes, how many?_____
   Is elevator available? _____No _____Yes

3. a. Does patient require help in any of the following? If so, who provides it?

	Help needed	Provided by
Meal preparation	_____	_____
Shopping	_____	_____
Light housecleaning	_____	_____
Laundry	_____	_____
Getting out of bed	_____	_____
Getting into bed	_____	_____
Dressing	_____	_____
Bathing	_____	_____

b. Describe what the patient ate yesterday:

Breakfast	Lunch	Dinner
_____	_____	_____
_____	_____	_____

4. How often in past week did patient leave the house (other than this visit)?
At least daily_____ Several times_____ Once_____ Never_____

5. How often do visitors come to patient's house?
Daily_____ Weekly_____ Less often_____ Never_____

6. Whom would patient call in an emergency (nonprofessional)?
_____

7. Does patient have a legal guardian or durable power of attorney for health care?
_____No _____Yes (If yes, list name, address and telephone number.)
_____
_____
_____

8. Is patient's care covered by
Medicaid
Supplemental private insurance (beyond Medicare)   _____

9. Does the patient receive
Social Security   _____
Supplemental Security Income (SSI)   _____
Private pension   _____
Other income   _____

10. Does income permit purchase of needed
Food   _____
Clothing   _____
Housing   _____
Heating   _____
Transportation   _____
Drugs   _____
Is money a problem for the patient   _____No _____Yes

11. Does patient receive services from any social agency?
Yes_____ No_____
Name and phone number of agency _____

ENVIRONMENTAL ASSESSMENT

1. How many rooms are available to patient? _____
   Own bedroom _____ If shared, with whom? _____
   Bathroom _____
   Kitchen _____
   Living/sitting room_____

2. Must patient climb stairs to enter or leave house?
   Yes_____ No_____
   If yes, are they well lit and in good repair?
   Yes_____ No_____

3. Is neighborhood dangerous?
   Yes_____ No_____

4. Is house clean?
   Yes_____ No_____

5. Does house seem adequately insulated and ventilated?
   Yes_____ No_____

6. Are there signs of neglect?
   Old food in refrigerator _____
   Unwashed dishes _____
   Accumulated dirty clothing _____
   Other (describe): _____

7. Is there a sufficient supply of food for at least several days?
   Yes_____ No_____

8. Safety checklist

	Yes	No
a. Can the patient		
Lock and unlock the door	_____	_____
Reach light switches	_____	_____
Call for help (telephone and numbers accessible)	_____	_____
Safely transfer from bed, chair, toilet, tub	_____	_____
b. Are there obvious dangers:		
Overloaded electrical outlets	_____	_____
Frayed electrical wires	_____	_____
Poor lighting	_____	_____
Cluttered furniture	_____	_____
Unsafe furniture	_____	_____
Frayed carpets or broken floors	_____	_____
Missing or broken smoke alarm	_____	_____

9. Fall Hazard Checklist (after *Clinical Report on Aging,* Volume 1, Number 5, 1987)

a. Throughout the household, check that the following is in order:

_____ 1. Flooring and carpeting are in good condition without protruding obstacles that may cause tripping and falling.

_____ 2. Lighting is bright and without glare.

_____ 3. Nightlights are strategically placed throughout the house, especially on stairways and along routes between bedroom and bathroom. Illuminated light switches are used when possible in similar high-risk locations.

_____ 4. Telephones are positioned so that persons do not have to hurry to answer a ringing telephone.

_____ 5. Electric cords are not located in walkways. When possible, they are shortened and tacked down to baseboards.

_____ 6. Clutter does not obstruct walkways.

b. Bathroom

_____ 7. Railings are installed in the bathtub and toilet areas and are easily accessible for use.

_____ 8. A nonslip surface is on the floor of the tub and shower. If a bath mat is used, it is of substantial quality.

_____ 9. If a throw rug is used, it has a nonskid rubber backing.

_____10. Water drainage is appropriate to prevent the development of slippery floors after bathing.

c. Bedroom

_____11. Throw rugs do not represent a slip or trip hazard, particularly those en route to the bathroom.

_____12. Bedside table is present for placement of glasses and other items rather than cluttering the floor beside the bed.

d. Kitchen

_____13. The floor is made of a nonslip material.

_____14. Spills are cleaned up quickly to prevent slipping.

_____15. Cleaning and cooking supplies are stored in locations that are not too high (for shorter persons who would otherwise climb) or too low (for persons who develop lightheadedness after stooping).

_____16. A high chair is available for doing dishes.

_____17. A sturdy step stool is available for reaching high places.

e. Living room

_____18. Throw rugs are not present over a carpet or otherwise scattered about.

_____19. Furniture is placed in positions that allow for wide walkways.

_____20. Chairs and sofas are of a height sufficient to permit easy sitting and standing for elderly persons.

f. Stairways

_____21. Sturdy railings are provided along both sides of stairways, including the stairway to the basement.
_____22. Step surfaces are nonskid.
_____23. Materials are not stored on stair landings or thresholds.
_____24. When possible, bright nonskid tape is placed on the top and bottom steps to indicate where the steps begin and end.

g. Outside the house

_____25. Front and back steps are in good condition. During the winter, sand and/or salt are available for slippery surfaces to ensure safety.
_____26. Walkways are shoveled free of ice and snow in the winter to prevent slips and falls.
_____27. Stairways and railings are sturdy.

DEMENTIA ASSESSMENT

A. History

1. Active medical conditions

   _____
   _____
   _____

2. Medications

   _____
   _____
   _____

3. History of (describe):

   _____Hypertension
   _____Stroke
   _____Transient ischemic attack
   _____Depression
   _____Other psychiatric disorder

4. Current symptoms (complaints of patient or family)

   _____Memory loss
   _____Forgets recent events
   _____Forgets things just said
   _____Forgets names of people
   _____Forgets words
   _____Gets lost
   _____Asks questions or tells stories repeatedly
   _____Confused about date or place
   _____Can't do simple calculations
   _____Can't understand what is read or said
   _____Impairment of other cognitive functions
   _____Anxiety / agitation
   _____Paranoia
   _____Delusions / hallucination
   _____Wandering
   _____Disruptive behavior
   _____Incontinence

5. Onset of symptoms

   _____Recent (days to few weeks)
   _____Longer duration (months)
   _____Uncertain

6. Progression of symptoms

   _____Rapid
   _____Gradual
   _____Stepwise (irregular, stuttering deteriorations)
   _____Uncertain

7. Activities of daily living (ADL)

Does the impairment of cognitive function interfere with instrumental ADL?
_____Yes _____No
If yes, which ones? _____
Basic ADL? _____Yes _____No
If yes, which ones? _____

B. Physical Examination

1. General appearance

   _____Normal
   _____Abnormal (Describe: _____)

2. Blood pressure

   Right arm _____/_____
   Left arm _____/_____

3. Hearing

	Normal	Abnormal
Normal voice		
1024-Hz tuning fork		

4. Orientation

	No	Yes
Person		
Place		
Time		
Situation		

5. Memory function

	Normal	Impaired
Remote		
Recent (object recall after 5 minutes)		
Immediate (digit repetition)		

6. Short Portable Status Questionnaire
   (Many other standardized tests are also available)

Right	Wrong	
_____	_____	What is the date today (month/day/year)?
_____	_____	What day of the week is it?
_____	_____	What is the name of this place?
_____	_____	What is your telephone number? (If no telephone, what is your street address?)
_____	_____	How old are you?
_____	_____	When were you born (month/day/year)?
_____	_____	Who is the current president of the United States?
_____	_____	Who was the president just before him?
_____	_____	What was your mother's maiden name?
_____	_____	Subtract 3 from 20 and keep subtracting 3 from each new number you get, all the way down.

Number of errors_____

0-2 errors = intact
3-4 errors = mild intellectual impairment
5-7 errors = moderate intellectual impairment
8-10 errors = severe intellectual impairment

7. Other cognitive functions

	Normal	Impaired
General fund of knowledge	_____	_____
Simple calculations	_____	_____
Ability to write name	_____	_____
Ability to copy diagrams	_____	_____
Interpretations of proverbs	_____	_____
Naming common objects	_____	_____
Insight	_____	_____
Judgment	_____	_____
Ability to follow simple written commands (e.g., "Close your eyes")	_____	_____
Ability to follow simple verbal commands (e.g., "Touch your left ear with your right hand")	_____	_____

8. Thought content

_____Normal
_____Delusions
_____Paranoid ideation
_____Other (Describe: _____)

9. Mood/affect

_____Appropriate _____Depressed _____Labile _____Agitated
_____Other (Describe: _____)

10. Behavior during examinations

	Yes	No
Good attention and concentration	_____	_____
Good effort to answer questions and perform tasks	_____	_____
Many "don't know" answers	_____	_____

11. Remainder of neurological examination
_____Focal neurological signs (Describe:_____
_____)
_____Signs of parkinsonism (Describe: _____
_____)

Pathological reflexes:
_____Babinski
_____Hoffman
_____Grasp
_____Palmomental

493

Gait:
_____Normal
_____Abnormal (Describe: _____)
_____Other abnormality (Describe: _____)

Sensory examination:
_____Normal
_____Abnormal (Describe: _____)

12. Hachinski ischemia score

Characteristic	Point score
Abrupt onset	2
Stepwise deterioration	1
Somatic complaints	1
Emotional incontinence	1
History or presence of hypertension	1
History of strokes	2
Focal neurological symptoms	2
Focal neurological signs	2

Total score: _____

(Score of 4 or more suggests multi-infarct dementia.)

C. Diagnostic Studies

	Normal	Abnormal
Blood:		
CBC	_____	_____
Sedimentation rate	_____	_____
Glucose	_____	_____
BUN	_____	_____
Electrolytes	_____	_____
Calcium	_____	_____
Liver function tests	_____	_____
Free thyroxine index	_____	_____
TSH	_____	_____
VDRL	_____	_____
Vitamin B_{12}	_____	_____
Folate	_____	_____
Radiographic:		
Chest film	_____	_____
CT scan	_____	_____
Other:		
Urinalysis	_____	_____
EKG	_____	_____
EEG	_____	_____
Lumbar puncture	_____	_____
Audiology	_____	_____

D. Diagnosis

_____Probable primary degenerative dementia (Alzheimer's type)
_____Multi-infarct dementia
_____Mixed
_____Other (describe)
_____Depression
_____Other potentially reversible cause of dementia (describe)

INCONTINENCE ASSESSMENT

I. Assessment of acute incontinence

If incontinence is of recent onset (within a few days) and / or associated with an acute illness, check for any of the following:

_____Acute urinary tract infection
_____Fecal impaction
_____Acute confusion (delirium)*
_____Immobility*
_____Drug effects (e.g., excessive sedation, polyuria caused by diuretics, urinary retention, other autonomic effects)
_____Metabolic abnormality with polyuria (e.g., hyperglycemia, hypercalcemia)

*Such that ability to get to a toilet (or toilet substitute) is impaired.

If incontinence persists despite management of any of these conditions and / or resolution of an acute illness, further assessment (as shown in Part II) should be pursued.

II. Assessment of persistent incontinence

A. History

1. Do you ever leak urine when you don't want to?

   _____No, never   _____Yes

2. Do you ever have trouble getting to the toilet on time or have accidents getting your clothes or bed wet?

   _____No, never   _____Yes

3. How long have you had a problem with urinary leakage?

   _____Less than 1 week
   _____1 to 4 weeks
   _____1 to 3 months
   _____4 to 12 months
   _____1 to 5 years
   _____Longer than 5 years

4. How often do you leak urine?

   _____Less than once per week
   _____More than once per week, but less than once per day
   _____About once per day
   _____More than once per day
   _____Continual leakage
   _____Variable

5. Does the leakage occur

   _____Mainly during the day
   _____Mainly at night
   _____Both night and day

6. When you leak urine, how much leaks?

_____Just a few drops
_____More than a few drops, but less than a cupful
_____More than a cupful (enough to wet clothes and/or bed linens)
_____Variable
_____Unknown

7. Do any of the following cause you to leak urine?

_____Coughing
_____Laughing
_____Exercise or other forms of straining
_____Inability to get to the toilet in time

8. How often do you normally urinate?

_____Every 6 to 8 hours or less often
_____About every 3 to 5 hours
_____About every 1 or 2 hours
_____At least every hour or more often
_____Frequency varies
_____Unknown

9. Do you wake up at night to urinate?

_____Never or rarely
_____Yes, usually between one and three times
_____Yes, four or more times per night
_____Yes, but frequency varies

10. Once your bladder feels full, how long can you hold your urine?

_____As long as you want (several minutes at least)
_____Just a few minutes
_____Less than a minute or two
_____Not at all
_____Cannot tell when bladder is full

11. Do you have any of the following when you urinate?

_____Difficulty in getting the urine started
_____Very slow stream or dribbling
_____Straining to finish
_____Discomfort or pain
_____Burning
_____Blood in the urine

12. Are you using any of the following to help with the urinary leakage?

_____Bed or furniture pads
_____Sanitary napkins
_____Other types of pads in your underwear
_____Special undergarments
_____Medication
_____Bedside commode
_____Urinal
_____Other (Describe: _____)

498

13. Is the urinary leakage enough of a problem that you would like further evaluation and treatment?

_____Yes _____No

14. Do you ever have uncontrolled loss of stool?

_____No, never _____Yes

15. Relevant medical history

_____Stroke
_____Dementia
_____Parkinson's disease
_____Prior CNS trauma / surgery
_____Other neurological disorder
_____Diabetes
_____Congestive heart failure
_____Other (Specify: _____)

16. Prior genitourinary history

_____Multiple vaginal deliveries
_____Cesarean section(s)
_____Abdominal hysterectomy
_____Vaginal hysterectomy
_____Bladder suspension
_____TURP (transurethral prostate resection)
_____Suprapubic prostatectomy
_____Urethral stricture / dilatation
_____Bladder tumor
_____Pelvic irradiation
_____Recurrent urinary tract infections

17. Medications

Diuretic   _____

_____

Antihypertensive   _____

_____

Other drugs that _____
affect the autonomic _____
nervous system _____

B. Physical Examination

1. Mental status

_____Normal
_____Mild / moderate cognitive impairment
_____Severe cognitive impairment (unaware of toileting needs)

2. Mobility

_____Ambulates independently, with adequate speed
_____Ambulates independently, but slowly (so that ability to get to a toilet is impaired)
_____Not independently ambulatory, but able to use urinal, bed pan, or bedside commode independently
_____Chair- or bed-bound, but able to use urinal or bed pan independently
_____Dependent on others for toileting

3. Abdominal examination

_____Bladder enlarged and palpable
_____Bladder not palpable

4. Neurological examination of lower extremities

_____Normal
_____Evidence of upper motor neuron lesion
_____Evidence of lower motor neuron lesion
_____Peripheral neuropathy

5. Rectal examination

_____Decreased rectal sphincter tone
_____Decreased perianal sensation
_____Absent bulbocavernosus reflex
_____Prostate enlarged
_____Prostate cancer suspected

6. External genitalia

_____Skin irritation
_____Diminished sensation
_____Abnormal (Describe: _____)

7. Vaginal examination

_____Atrophic vaginitis
_____Mild prolapse
_____Moderate / severe prolapse
_____Rectocele
_____Adenexal or uterine mass

C. Diagnostic Studies

1. Pad test with full bladder

_____No leakage
_____Leakage, small amount
_____Leakage, large amount
_____Delayed leakage

2. Voided volume

_____Unable   _____ml

3. Post void residual

_____ml (or volume in bladder _____ml)

4. Bladder filling (if done)
Capacity: _____ml

_____Stable
_____Involuntary contraction (at _____ml)
Amount lost: _____ml

5. Stress maneuvers
Volume in bladder: _____ml

Supine	Standing	
_____	_____	No leakage
_____	_____	Leak small amount
_____	_____	Leak large amount
_____	_____	Delayed leakage

6. Voided volume
_____ml

7. Calculated residual
_____ml

8. Urinalysis

_____Normal
_____Hematuria (>2 RBC per high-power field)
_____Pyuria (>5 WBC per high-power field)
_____Bacteriuria (>1+)

9. Urine culture

_____Sterile
_____Insignificant growth ($<10^5$ colonies/ml)
_____Significant growth ($>10^5$ colonies/ml)
    Organism(s) _____
    Sensitive to _____
    _____

D. Disposition

_____Treat reversible factors (describe)
_____Treat for urge incontinence
_____Treat for stress incontinence
_____Treat for mixed incontinence
_____Manage supportively
_____Refer for further evaluation
    Reason: _____
List specific treatment program
_____
_____

ASSESSMENT FOR PATIENTS WHO FALL

1. Current medical problems

   _____
   _____
   _____
   _____

2. Medications

   _____
   _____
   _____

3. Is there a previous history of falls?
   _____Yes _____No
   If yes:
   Number of previous falls_____
   Is there a pattern?
   _____Yes _____No
   Frequency

   _____

   Time of day

   _____

   Position

   _____

   Activity

   _____

   Circumstances

   _____
   _____

4. Circumstances surrounding current fall

   Time of day

   _____

   Location

   _____

   Relationship to specific activities (e.g., toileting, climbing or descending
   stairs, exercise, turning head)

   _____
   _____

   Witness(es)

   _____

   Environmental hazards (e.g., poor lighting, loose rug, uneven floor, other
   obstacles)

   _____
   _____
   _____

5. Patient's description of and reasons for the fall (in patient's words)

_____

_____

_____

_____

6. Questions to the patient (and / or witness)

a. Did you know you were going to fall?
_____Yes _____No

b. After you fell, did you know what happened?
_____Yes _____No

c. Did you lose consciousness (pass out?)
_____Yes _____No
If yes, how long were you unconscious? _____minutes.
Were you aware of what happened after you awoke?
_____Yes _____No
Had you lost control of your bowel or bladder?
_____Yes _____No

d. Were you able to get up right away?
_____Yes _____No

e. Did you have any pain or injury after the fall?
_____Yes _____No

f. Did you do any of the following just before the fall?

_____Trip
_____Slip
_____Stand up quickly
_____Turn your head suddenly
_____Cough
_____Urinate
_____Have a bowel movement
_____Eat a large meal

g. Did you have any of the following symptoms just before you fell?

_____Lightheadedness
_____Vertigo (spinning around the room or vice versa)
_____Palpitations
_____Shortness of breath
_____Weakness or numbness on one side of the body
_____Sudden weakness of both legs
_____Slurred speech
_____Difficulty saying what you wanted to say
_____Strange smells
_____Flashing lights (scotomata)

7. Physical assessment

   a. Postural vital signs

	Supine	Sitting	Standing
Blood pressure	_____/_____	_____/_____	_____/_____
Pulse	_____	_____	_____
Blood pressure other arm			_____/_____

   b. Skin

   _____Bruises
   _____Diminished turgor

   c. Vision

   _____Adequate for independent ambulation
   _____Limits mobility, but still independent
   _____Inadequate for independent ambulation

   d. Neck

   _____Supple
   _____Full range of motion
   _____Symptoms with rotation

   e. Cardiovascular

   _____Arrhythmia
   _____Murmur suggestive of aortic stenosis
   _____Signs of heart failure (Describe: _____)
   _____Carotid bruit(s)

   f. Musculoskeletal

   _____Trauma and / or suspected fracture
   _____Deformity
   _____Limited range of motion
   _____Joint inflammation

   g. Podiatric
   Are any of the following impairing ambulation?

   _____Callouses
   _____Bunions
   _____Nail deformity
   _____Ulceration
   _____Poorly fitted or otherwise inadequate shoes

   h. Neurological

   _____Abnormal mental status
   _____Focal neurological sign(s)
   _____Muscular weakness
   _____Muscular rigidity / spasticity
   _____Bradykinesia
   _____Resting tremor

_____Peripheral neuropathy
_____Ataxia, finger to nose
_____Ataxia, heel to shin

Describe positive findings: _____
_____

i. Mobility

_____Ambulates independently
_____Uses aid
        _____Cane
        _____Quad-cane
        _____Walker
_____Wheelchair, able to transfer independently
_____Wheelchair, needs help to transfer

j. Stability and gait (see also Chapter 7)

	Normal	Abnormal
Sitting balance	_____	_____
Rising from sitting to standing	_____	_____
Standing balance with eyes open	_____	_____
Standing balance with eyes closed (Romberg test)	_____	_____
Initiation of walking	_____	_____
Length of stride	_____	_____
Distance feet apart	_____	_____
Turning	_____	_____
Sitting down	_____	_____

Describe positive findings: _____
_____
_____

8. Diagnostic studies

Test / procedure	Result
_____	_____
_____	_____
_____	_____
_____	_____
_____	_____
_____	_____
_____	_____
_____	_____
_____	_____

Index

Page numbers in *italic* indicate tables and figures